Coccidioidomycosis

A Text

CURRENT TOPICS IN INFECTIOUS DISEASE

Series Editors:

William B. Greenough III
Chief, Infectious Disease Division
The Johns Hopkins University
School of Medicine
Baltimore, Maryland

Thomas C. Merigan
Head, Division of Infectious Disease
Stanford University Medical Center
Stanford, California

The Atypical Mycobacteria and Human Mycobacteriosis
   John S. Chapman

Infections of the Gastrointestinal Tract: Microbiology,
   Pathophysiology, and Clinical Features
   Herbert L. DuPont and Larry K. Pickering

Coccidioidomycosis: A Text
   Edited by David A. Stevens

A Continuation Order Plan is available for this series. A continuation order will bring delivery of each new volume immediately upon publication. Volumes are billed only upon actual shipment. For further information please contact the publisher.

Coccidioidomycosis

A Text

Edited by

David A. Stevens, M.D.

Chief, Division of Infectious Diseases
Santa Clara Valley Medical Center
San Jose, California
and
Associate Professor, Dept. of Medicine
Stanford University, Medical School
Stanford, California
and
Principal Investigator
Infectious Disease Research Laboratory
Institute for Medical Research of Santa Clara County
San Jose, California

Springer Science+Business Media, LLC

Library of Congress Cataloging in Publication Data

Main entry under title:

Coccidioidomycosis.

    (Current topics in infectious disease)
    Bibliography: p
    Includes index.
    1. Coccidioidomycosis. I. Stevens, David A. II. Series. [DNLM: 1. Coccid-
ioidomycosis. WC460 C6577]
RC136.3.C6   616.2'4   80-15855
ISBN 978-1-4757-1714-3   ISBN 978-1-4757-1712-9 (eBook)
DOI 10.1007/978-1-4757-1712-9

© 1980 Springer Science+Business Media New York
Originally published by Plenum Publishing Corporation, New York in 1980
Softcover reprint of the hardcover 1st edition 1980

Contributors

Antonino Catanzaro, M.D., Assistant Professor of Medicine, Department of Medicine, Pulmonary Division, University of California Medical School, San Diego, California

Stanley C. Deresinski, M.D., Clinical Assistant Professor of Medicine, Stanford University School of Medicine, Stanford, California; and Palo Alto Veterans Administration Hospital, Palo Alto, California

David J. Drutz, M.D., Chief, Infectious Diseases Section, Audie L. Murphy Memorial Veterans' Hospital; and Chief, Division of Infectious Diseases, Professor of Medicine and Microbiology, University of Texas Health Science Center, San Antonio, Texas

John N. Galgiani, M.D., Assistant Professor of Medicine, University of Arizona College of Medicine; and Chief, Section of Infectious Diseases, Veterans Administration Medical Center, Tucson, Arizona

Robert P. Harvey, M.D., Clinical Instructor, Allergy and Immunology, University of Colorado Health Sciences Center, Denver, Colorado

Robert W. Huntington, M.D., Consulting Pathologist; and Director of Medical Services, Emeritus, Kern Medical Center, Bakersfield, California; and Clinical Professor of Pathology, Emeritus, University of Southern California School of Medicine, Los Angeles, California

Milton Huppert, Ph.D., Chief, Mycology Research Laboratory, Audie L. Murphy Memorial Veterans' Hospital; and Professor, Department of Microbiology, University of Texas Health Science Center, San Antonio, Texas

Paul H. Jacobs, M.D., Director, Dermatology Clinic; Director, Superficial Mycoses Laboratory; and Professor, Clinical Dermatology, Stanford University Medical Center, Stanford, California

Peter C. Kelly, M.D., Chief, Infectious Diseases; and Associate Chairman, Department of Medicine, Maricopa County General Hospital, Phoenix, Arizona

Allan Lavetter, M.D., Staff Pediatrician and Infectious Disease Consultant, Santa Clara Kaiser Medical Center, Santa Clara, California; and Clinical Associate Professor, Departments of Medicine and Pediatrics, Stanford University School of Medicine, Stanford, California

Demosthenes Pappagianis, M.D., Ph.D., Professor and Chairman, Department of Medical Microbiology, University of California School of Medicine, Davis, California

Eskild Antoni Petersen, M.D., Assistant Professor, Department of Internal Medicine, University of Arizona, Tucson, Arizona; and Visiting Scientist, Laboratory of Clinical Investigation, National Institute of Allergy and Infectious Diseases, National Institutes of Health, Bethesda, Maryland

David Salkin, M.D., Director of Medical Research, La Viña Hospital, Altadena, California; and Clinical Professor of Medicine, University of Southern California, Los Angeles, California; and Clinical Professor of Medicine, Loma Linda University, Loma Linda, California

David A. Stevens, M.D., Chief, Division of Infectious Diseases, Santa Clara Valley Medical Center, San Jose, California; and Associate Professor, Department of Medicine, Stanford University, School of Medicine, Stanford, California

Sung H. Sun, Ph.D., Associate Chief, Mycology Research Laboratory, Audie L. Murphy Memorial Veterans' Hospital, San Antonio, Texas

Preface

The idea for compiling a book on coccidioidomycosis first began to take shape in my mind in 1976 at an annual meeting of the Coccidioidomycosis Study Group (see Chapter 23) in Palo Alto. In my discussions with the chairman, Demosthenes Pappagianis, we agreed that considerable data had accumulated in the almost 20 years since the publication of Marshall Fiese's landmark book, *Coccidioidomycosis* (Charles C Thomas, Springfield, Ill., 1958). Pappagianis encouraged me to consider writing a new book.

Also about this time, my Stanford colleague Tom Merigan was collaborating in assembling a series of texts on infectious diseases, and he added his encouragement to that of Pappagianis. I planned to enlist the collaboration of my colleagues for the multiauthored work I had conceived to encompass the various facets of coccidioidomycosis. The more I worked, the more I appreciated the effort that had gone into the Fiese book.

I hope the final product is a useful, readable, and comprehensive text and reference source for this disease and a worthy successor to the Fiese book. This volume places greater emphasis on the basic science background of present clinical experience and attempts to examine critically the data base and how it fits with recommendations made in the clinical literature. In some of the contributed chapters, I made virtually no changes; in others, I battered them to fit my preconceptions. I only hope my colleagues involved in the latter will eventually forgive my bullying them. In any case, I take the blame for any faults in all these chapters—in the ones unchanged, by sins of omission, and in the others, by sins of commission.

The volume proceeds from basic and general aspects to the sequence of events in the human disease, i.e., primary infection and then specific clinical syndromes, and concludes with discussions of prophylaxis and therapy. The bibliography chapter is offered to provide additional sources in searching for a point, as is the bibliography in each chapter (particularly review articles).

I thank my colleagues at the Santa Clara Valley Medical Center for providing an environment of high-level medical practice that made possible care of our own coccidioidomycosis patients, whose multisystem involvement requires many specialists and generalists. This book would not have been possible without the contribution of my wife Julie and my children, Joseph and Emily. They forebore holiday and weekend days that I worked on the book, periodic ill humor, and tripping over stacks of books, files, reprints, chapters, and correspondence on the den floor.

David A. Stevens

San Jose and Stanford, California

Contents

Chapter 3

MYCOLOGICAL DIAGNOSIS OF COCCIDIOIDOMYCOSIS 47
M. Huppert and S. H. Sun

Chapter 4

EPIDEMIOLOGY OF COCCIDIOIDOMYCOSIS 63
Demosthenes Pappagianis

Chapter 5

IMMUNOLOGY OF COCCIDIOIDOMYCOSIS 87

David A. Stevens

Chapter 6

SEROLOGY AND SERODIAGNOSIS OF
COCCIDIOIDOMYCOSIS 97

Demosthenes Pappagianis

Chapter 7

PATHOLOGY OF COCCIDIOIDOMYCOSIS 113

Robert W. Huntington

Chapter 8

CLASSIFICATION OF COCCIDIOIDOMYCOSIS 133

David Salkin

Chapter 9
PRIMARY COCCIDIOIDOMYCOSIS 139
Antonino Catanzaro and David J. Drutz

Chapter 10
PULMONARY COCCIDIOIDOMYCOSIS 147
Antonino Catanzaro and David J. Drutz

Chapter 11

COCCIDIOIDAL MENINGITIS 163

Peter C. Kelly

Chapter 12

COCCIDIOIDOMYCOSIS OF BONE AND JOINTS 195

Stanley C. Deresinski

Chapter 21
IMMUNOTHERAPY-TRANSFER FACTOR IN
COCCIDIOIDOMYCOSIS 261
David A. Stevens

Chapter 22
VACCINATION-IMMUNOPROPHYLAXIS IN
COCCIDIOIDOMYCOSIS 269
David A. Stevens

Chapter 23
BIBLIOGRAPHY OF COCCIDIOIDOMYCOSIS 273
David A. Stevens

1

History of Coccidioidomycosis: "Dust to Dust"

Stanley C. Deresinski

1. PROLOGUE

In the tumult following Pearl Harbor, tens of thousands of persons of Japanese ancestry in the United States were placed in camps throughout the country as part of the infamous World War II policy of "internment." Among the locations used was one on the Gila River in the desert of southern Arizona. Since this area was known to be endemic for coccidioidomycosis, there was little surprise when many cases of the disease appeared among the unwilling residents of the camp.

Meanwhile, a similar outbreak of coccidioidomycosis occurred at a nearby prisoner-of-war camp in Florence, southeast of Phoenix. Not only did Florence serve as the prisoner-of-war headquarters for Arizona, but the Florence Station Hospital, because of its climate, was the referral center for all prisoners with tuberculosis. Investigation at Florence by Charles Smith uncovered at least two deaths from coccidioidomycosis as well as ten infections in tuberculous prisoners who had been confined to the hospital wards. One of these, a U-boat officer, had entered with a unilateral tuberculous pleural effusion and promptly developed a coccidioidal effusion on the contralateral side. The camp hospital was finally closed after the government of Germany invoked the Geneva Convention.

Meanwhile, in the San Joaquin Valley of California, prisoner-of-war work camps were established near Minter and Lemoore Fields—also in known endemic areas. As a consequence, in 2 months and 10 days in the summer of 1945, 22 American personnel and 150 German prisoners (one-tenth of the local POW population) were hospitalized with coccidioidomycosis at Minter Field, where the German prisoners had been assigned to harvest potatoes and sugar beets.[1]

2. IN THE BEGINNING

In January 1888, Domingo Escurra, then a 32-year-old cavalryman, left for the Chaco frontier of Northern Argentina. It was at least a year later when, after awakening from his siesta, he noticed what he thought was a spider bite on his right cheek. Despite treatment with tobacco, the lesion progressed, becoming somewhat verrucous. Inguinal adenopathy and multiple additional skin lesions (one of which he incised with a penknife) appeared before he presented himself at the Military Hospital, where a diagnosis of lupus vulgaris was made and he was treated with nitric acid. Because his disease continued to progress he was sent to Buenos Aires, where he was admitted to the Rawson Hospital under the care of Dr. M. Bengolea, who made a diagnosis of mycosis fungoides. After administration, without response, of a mixture of protiodide of mercury and potassium iodide for 20 days, as well as mercurial liniments, he referred the patient to Alejandro Posadas, Intern of the University Hospital Clinics, for further study.

The 21-year-old Posadas obtained tissue from Escurra and examined it in the laboratory assigned to Drs. Robert Wernicke and Guillermo Udaondo which was adjacent to wards five and nine of the Hospital Clinics. Examining the lesions with a microscope, he noted multinucleate giant cells and "psorospermiae." The "sporangia" were spherical, of variable size, with a doubly refractile outer membrane and granular contents, and were apparently nonmotile. The constancy with which these strange organisms were found within the lesions led Posadas to state: "I have therefore found a new *Psorospermia,* very probably causing mycotic tumors" (mycosis fungoides).*[2]

---

*Posadas was to die in Paris just 10 years later, on November 21, 1902, of "consumptive" lung disease at the age of 31. In his brief life he was able to develop several innovative surgical techniques in addition to describing the new "psorospermiae." He was described as being a strange and reserved man with enormous discipline, the latter possibly as a result of his Jesuit secondary education at the College of El Salvador. Despite this, he did have detractors who thought of him as a poseur because of his large collars and ties, the tails he wore to the hospital in the morning, and his enormous moustache. Indeed in the last years of his life, undoubtedly because of the knowledge that the time left to him was short, he abandoned his earlier ascetic life style for a more epicurean one [J. Arce, Alejandro Posadas, in: *The Complete Works of Alejandro Posadas* (trans. by F. Botero), Institute of Surgical Clinics, Buenos Aires (1928)]

Joas Furtado-Silveira had left his home in Fayal, in the Azores, and emigrated to California in 1886, where he became a farm laborer in the San Joaquin Valley. During that time he developed a persistent sore on his neck. Five years later this lesion was still present and another had appeared on his forehead. Although he felt quite well he was shunned by his fellow workmen and was therefore compelled to seek medical aid and so came under the care of Dr. A. W. Rickey of Porto Costa, California. Furtado-Silveira's condition gradually deteriorated, and in July 1893 he was admitted to the service of Dr. C. N. Ellingwood at the San Francisco City and County Hospital. His disease continued to generally progress, but its capricious nature was noted: "At intervals, without any assignable cause, the disease would make rapid progress, while again it would apparently remain stationary for weeks at a time" (Fig. 1). Also noted was the apparent resistance to involvement of the conjuctiva and mucous membranes. Furtado-Silveira's physicians, confused by the clinical picture, performed a biopsy of a neck lesion. The tissue, examined by Dr. Emmett Rixford of the Cooper Medical College (subsequently Stanford Medical School) and Dr. T. C. Gilchrist at Johns Hopkins, revealed organisms which resembled those illustrated in the report of the case of Domingo Escurra by Wernicke.*[3] (Rixford had originally sent some tissue to Welch at Johns Hopkins, "who expressed doubt as to the organisms being protozoa,"[4] before referring the materials to Gilchrist). Rixford and Gilchrist, however, while accepting the protozoan nature of the organisms (a mistake Darling was to repeat 10 years hence in his description of *Histoplasma capsulatum*), rejected the diagnosis of mycosis fungoides. They also considered and rejected diagnoses of syphilis, tuberculoid leprosy, and tuberculosis verrucosa cutis.

Unfortunately for the patient, his physicians next embarked on a series of therapeutic adventures, some benign, some hideous. Secondarily infected surfaces were treated with antiseptic solution with good effect. Next came topical applications and then intralesional injection of methyl violet, which had no effect other than to stain the lesions. Iodine had no effect. Bromine topically produced "superficial necrosis, which was, if anything, more pronounced in the neighboring healthy skin than upon the diseased parts." Despite this, the same solution was administered by intralesional injection "with considerable apparent improve-

---

* In 1932 a case report described an aviator in whom coccidioidomycosis had once again been misdiagnosed as mycosis fungoides [E. P. Zeisler, 1932, Chronic coccidioidal dermatitis, *Arch. Dermatol. Syphilol.* 25: 53–71 (1932)]. The story came full circle in 1955 when Garb and Miller described a patient with mycosis fungoides who developed disseminated coccidioidomycosis [J. Garb and D. B. Miller, Mycosis fungoides, tumor stage, co-existent with disseminated coccidioidomycosis, *Arch. Dermatol.* 71:59–65 (1955)].

ment, but the injections were attended with so much suffering, not withstanding the previous use of cocaine, that the attempt to continue them was abandoned.'' Oil of turpentine with olive oil, 10% carbolic acid, potassium permanganate topically, and bichloride solution intralesionally were successively used without significant effect. One lesion was excised *in toto* with subsequent healing. Several others were curetted and then "thoroughly sealed with the actual cautery" with encouraging results. As a consequence, on March 17, 1894, under chloroform narcosis, "all the infected areas, save the one about the mouth, were most thoroughly scraped with a sharp spoon. The raw surfaces were then vigorously scrubbed with a bristle brush and an abundance of bichloride solution . . . was applied.'' The results, some 3 months later, can be seen in Fig. 2 (compare to Fig. 1). The disease progressed, and Joas Furtado-Silveira, having lost both his eyes, his nose, and part of an ear, lost what was left of his life on January 31, 1895, 3 years before Escurra was to succumb to the same disease.*[5]

Five months before Furtado-Silveira's death, 33-year-old José Teix-

---

* Escurra's head, preserved in formalin, was discovered in 1948 in the anatomical museum at the University of Buenos Aires School of Medicine and became Exhibit No. 1 in the Institute of Parasitology.

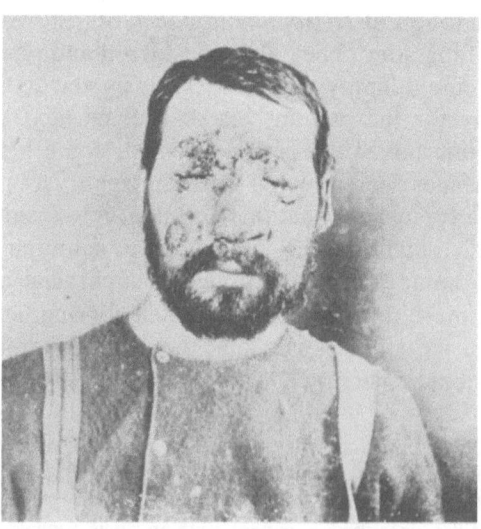

Figure 1. Photograph of Silveira taken November 1893, 4 months after his admission to the San Francisco City and County Hospital.[5]

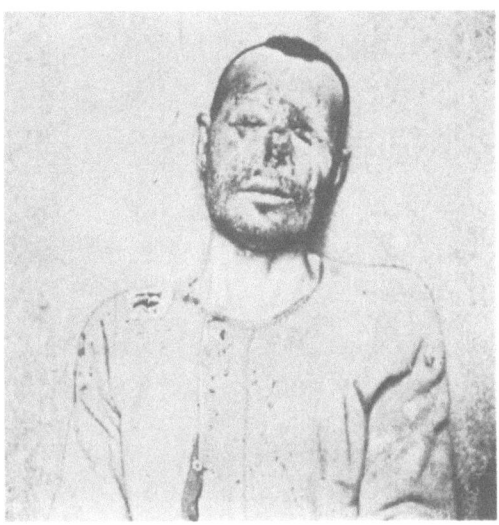

Figure 2. Silveira on June 26, 1894, 7 months before his death. Rixford and Gilchrist wrote that this photograph "shows what extensive ravages this frightful disease produced . . ."[5]

ara Pereira was admitted to St. Mary's Hospital in San Francisco by Drs. W. S. Thorne and L. Robinson. Pereira had migrated, also from the Azores, to the San Joaquin Valley at age 19, working first as a farm laborer and then as a bartender. Two months prior to admission the patient had noted two small "pimples on his forehead." Lesions rapidly appeared at other sites, and he became febrile, developed night sweats, and lost 35 lb. After admission, Pereira, whose biopsy led to the same diagnosis as in the previous two cases, had a rapid downhill course and died on September 21, 1894, less than 3 months after the onset of his illness and just a few days after his case had been read before the California Academy of Medicine by Thorne and by Rixford.[5-7]

Rixford and Gilchrist, from their study of both Furtado-Silveira and Pereira, concluded that the skin was the portal of entry of the infection despite their repeated failure to produce new skin lesions in Furtado-Silveira by autoinoculation experiments. They also concluded that the disease was only minimally contagious. While their animal inoculation experiments were, by their own account, "not very satisfactory," they did manage to produce localized skin lesions by inoculation in one dog and one rabbit.

Rixford and Gilchrist provided extensive illustrations of the organism they observed (see Figs. 3 and 4) and were convinced that it was a protozoan of the class Sporozoa. Because of its resemblance to the

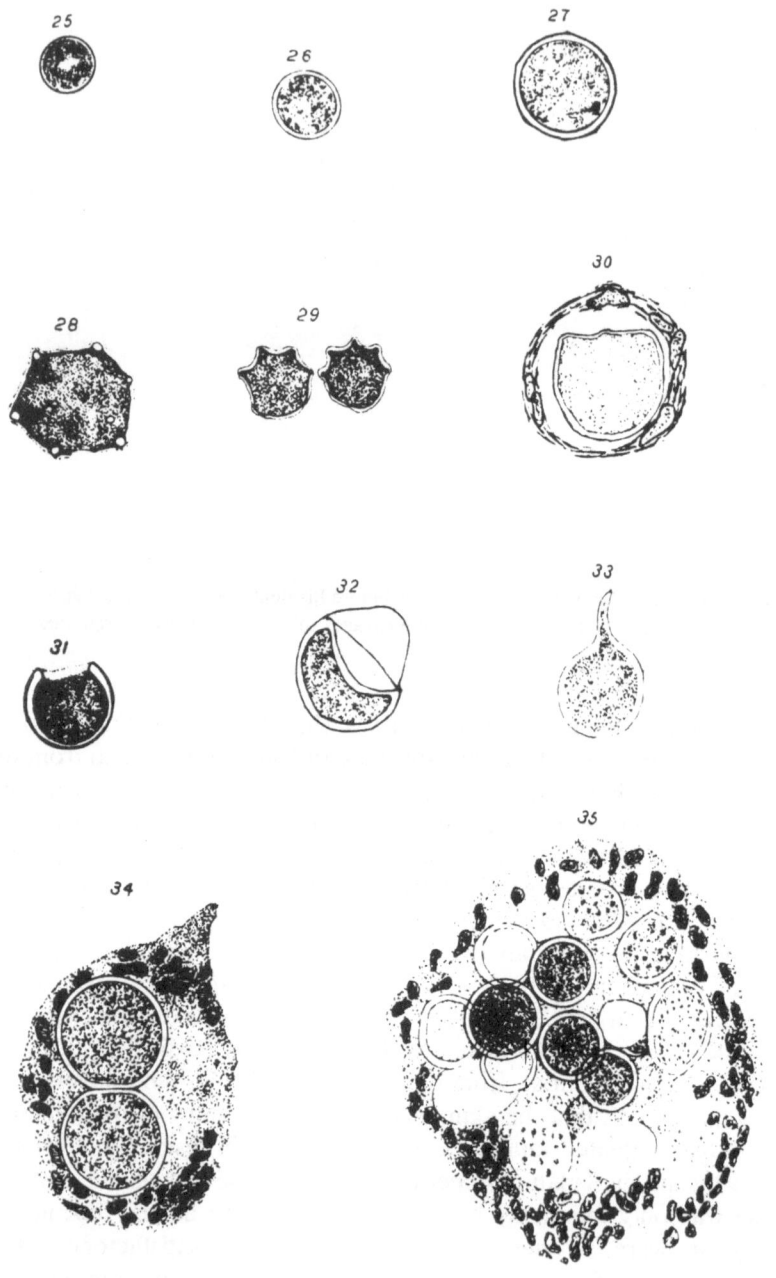

Figure 3. Photograph of Plate XXX from Rixford and Gilchrist[5] containing some of their illustrations of the "protozoan."

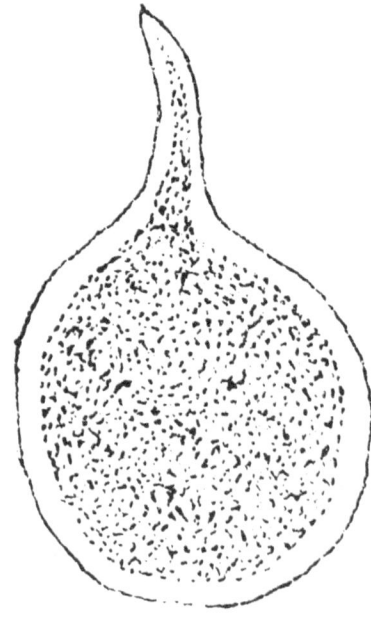

Figure 4. Enlarged view of Figure 33 from Plate XXX from Rixford and Gilchrist.[5] The authors interpreted this as possibly being a motile amoeboid from. It appears that this may have been a spherule in the very early stage of conversion to the mycelial phase.

coccidia they named it *Coccidioides*. They were, however, clearly "splitters" and not "lumpers": while they gave the additional appellation *"immitis"* to Silveira's organism, Pereira's was entitled *"pyogenes"* because of the differences in the clinical course and cellular responses seen. The source of these appellations was Stiles, an authority on protozoa, whose consultation had been requested by Gilchrist.[4] Furthermore, their conviction that the organism was a protozoan led them to regard the "mould" which overgrew culture plates obtained from the clinical material by Montgomery as a contaminant.

William Ophüls was at first similarly skeptical when Herbert Moffitt and May Ash showed him the "white mouldy growth" they had recovered in culture after 2 days from the pleura and spleen of a 19-year-old farm laborer (another emigrant from the Azores) who had died of an acute disseminated infection on February 6, 1900. However, Ophüls, then Professor of Pathology and Bacteriology at the Cooper Medical College, and Moffitt were able to present a paper to the Thirteenth Annual Meeting of the California State Medical Society on April 17, 1900, just 70 days later (the paper was published in another 74 days!), in which they confirmed the fungal nature of the organism, described its life cycle, and satisfied Koch's postulates by guinea-pig inoculation.[8]

While Ophül's first paper came to print rapidly, his next publication

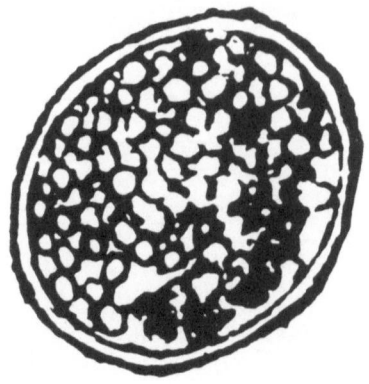

Figure 5. Enlargement of Figure 27 from Ophüls.[9]

on this disease was written in 1901 but not published until 1905.[9] In this comprehensive treatise (Fig. 5–8 are photographs of some of the illustrations), Ophüls stated his belief that the disease was a zoonosis, with man as an accidental host. He believed that, in his cases at least, "the infection had evidently started in the lungs and thence spread to other organs." He discounted Rixford and Gilchrist's division of *Coccidioides* into two species. In one important experiment he observed the transition from mould to the "protozoan" form of the organism in a subcutaneous abscess induced in a rabbit, and in another, noted the spherical forms to sprout hyphae in a coverslip preparation, thus providing direct evidence for the final link in the life cycle he had earlier postulated. From his

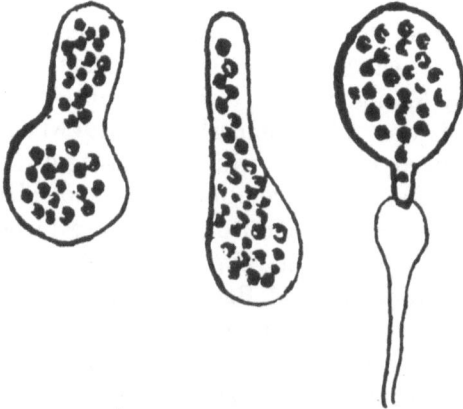

Figure 6. Enlargement of Figure 26 from Ophüls showing intermediate forms.[9]

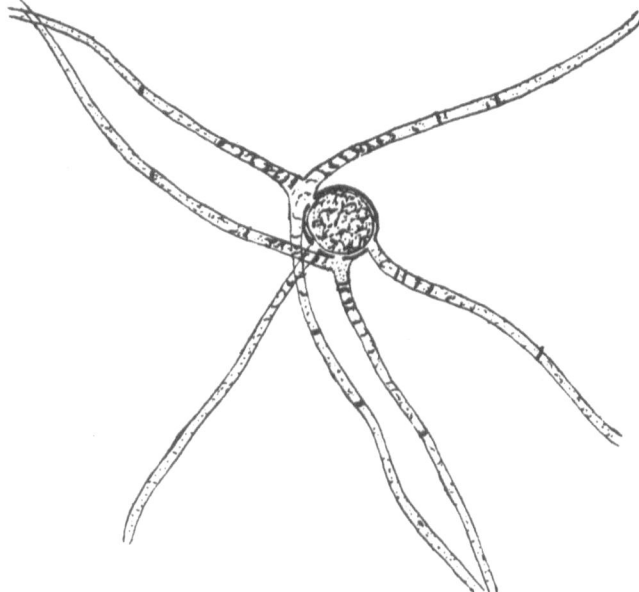

Figure 7. Enlargement of Figure 33 from Ophüls showing spherule converting to mycelial phase.[9]

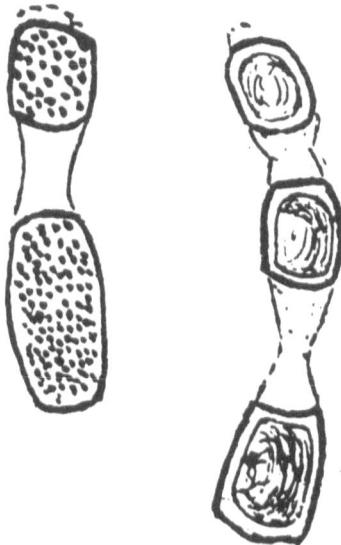

Figure 8. Enlargement of Figure 25 from Ophüls.[9]

microscopic observations he concluded "that the sporulating forms contain a substance which has a strong positive chemotactic influence upon the polymorphonuclear leukocytes." He proposed the term "coccidioidal granuloma" because some of the cases seen resembled glanders.

In that same year, in a separate publication (the opening sentence of which stated, "We have in California a peculiar form of oidiomycosis . . ."), Ophüls reviewed his 6 cases and summarized 7 others from the literature.[10] Adequate information was available in 12 cases, and of these, 1 appeared to have been cured by amputation of an infected foot, 1 still had active infection, 1 had been lost to follow-up, and 9 had died! In a comment on this paper, Dr. H. A. L. Ryfkogel of San Francisco conjectured that while it seemed the disease was rare (and fatal), "It may be demonstrated later that in California and in certain other parts of the universe the disease is fairly prevalent."

3. DECIPHERING THE EPIDEMIOLOGIC PUZZLE

Determination of the true prevalence of this disease, however, awaited a series of almost serendipitous observations. On August 28, 1929, a 26-year-old Stanford University medical student carelessly opened a petri dish containing a several months' old culture of *C. immitis*. He became ill 9 days later, and on October 8, 1929, the *San Francisco Examiner* reported, under the heading "Modern Hero," that Harold C. Chope, a "youthful scientific research man, faces death in a local hospital because of a mysterious mould breathed in while making an important experiment." However, the *Examiner* on December 2, 1929, was able to state that Chope (who was not to die until April 25, 1976, at the age of 72), "stricken with a rare and little known disease while seeking its cure, is on the road to recovery. And the experience gained from his case may be a step forward in the treatment of the malady." In a separate newspaper report, Dr. W. J. Cummins of the Southern Pacific Hospital was quoted as saying that while Chope's disease "exists principally in the San Joaquin Valley, it is not to be considered a San Joaquin Valley disease."

Chope's illness proved to be a self-limited one consisting principally of pneumonia and erythema nodosum.[11] Within the next 5 months, Ernest Dickson, in whose laboratory Chope's accident had occurred, observed similar self-limited illness in two patients from whom he was also able to recover *C. immitis*. In 1937 he reported these as well as two other similar cases; of the five patients, from all of whom the fungus was isolated, four had developed erythema nodosum. The title of Dickson's paper was " 'Valley Fever' of the San Joaquin Valley and Fungus Coccidioides," and in it he concluded that the cases he reported "prove conclusively that Fungus *Coccidioides* is sometimes the cause of a symptom complex of acute illness (which is) identical with what has been known locally in the San Joaquin Valley as Valley Fever."[12]

·In a somewhat pompous comment on Dickson's paper Dr. Roland Tupper of Fresno stated: "The coccidioidal granuloma that we see here is found in persons who are in close contact with the soil, whereas the erythema nodosum is usually found among those of a better class." (Stewart and Meyer[13] had reported, 5 years earlier, the isolation of *C. immitis* from the soil under a Delano bunkhouse where four Filipino farm workers had contracted serious coccidioidal infection.) Dr. Karl Meyer speculated that the apparent immunity of long-term residents of the San Joaquin Valley to coccidioidal disease is "conditioned by a previous, in all likelihood subclinical immunizing infection by the saprophyte." He then went on to suggest large-scale use of coccidioidin skin testing in order to examine this hypothesis.[12]

Dr. Dickson had arranged a meeting in January 1936 with the physicians of the Kern County Health Department to ask their cooperation in the study of *Coccidioides* infection in order to follow up on the observation that a pneumonia preceded coccidioidal granuloma. Dr. Myrnie Gifford, who had been searching for *Ascaris lumbricoides* in patients with Valley Fever since joining the staff 17 months before, in examining case histories in preparation for Dickson's visit discovered that 3 of 15 cases of "*Coccidioides* Fungus Infection" had had erythema nodosum early in their course. According to Smith,[11] this triggered Dickson's memory of Chope's clinical course leading to the 1937 paper described above.

This Bakersfield meeting led to immediate studies in Kern County as well in Dickson's laboratory. In fact, the Kern County Health Department preempted Dickson by getting their finding in print first. As Dickson stated in an addendum to his publication, shortly after presenting this paper to the California Medical Association in May 1937,[12] his attention was called to the 1935–1936 annual report of the Kern County Health Department. In it was described the isolation of *C. immitis* from six cases diagnosed as San Joaquin fever or erythema nodosum, as well as strongly positive reactions in the patients when skin tested with Kessel's coccidioidin preparation.[14]

In their annual report of the subsequent year, the Kern County Health Department more fully described their findings. They reported a coccidioidin skin test survey on 60 migrant workers, described the seasonal variation in incidence of the disease, and pointed out the apparent greater virulence of infection in various nonwhite races.[15]

3.1. The Flying Chlamydospore and "The Mystery of the Deadly Dust"

Ophüls "begat" Dickson, who "begat" Smith. In 1931 Dickson acquired a Rockefeller Fellowship for study at the Harvard School of Public Health for the newly graduated Chope. Chope recruited his classmate (Chope having dropped back a class due to his illness) and medical fraternity brother, Charles E. Smith, to substitute for him in his work for Dickson until his return. Chope, however, did not return and Dickson obtained for Smith another Rockefeller Fellowship but provided two conditions: (1) that Smith obtain his D.P.H. at Dickson's alma mater in Toronto, and (2) that upon completion of his studies he return to Stanford for at least 2 years to work on "fungus Coccidioides." Smith agreed, and it was during this period (1934–1936) of work on the fungus at Stanford that he acquired his personal coccidioidal infection.[11]

Smith was back in Toronto during the exciting times of the Gifford and Dickson reports. Dickson, meanwhile, had obtained funding from the Rosenberg Foundation, which, quite appropriately, was endowed by the Rosenberg Brothers Dried Fruit Company, whose fortune had derived primarily from prunes and raisins grown in the San Joaquin Valley. Smith returned to Stanford in the autumn of 1937 after a 1-year absence only to discover that he had become the wandering epidemiologist of Kern and Tulare Counties. Each Sunday evening Smith would leave his home to tour one of the two counties in the "Flying Chlamydospore," a Ford purchased by Stanford, and would return either late Wednesday night or on Thursday morning. During a period of 18 months ending in May 1939, Smith saw over 400 patients with either erythema nodosum or multiforme, finding that all who were skin tested with coccidioidin had positive reactions. He also established the incubation period and confirmed the seasonal incidence of the disease.

It was also during this time that Smith's disdain for cleaning glassware led to another extremely important advance. Smith and Dickson had agreed that mycelial phase antigens would be useless for serological testing, so their development of such tests was delayed while attempts were made to produce spherules *in vitro* in quantity. In the meanwhile, Smith became engaged in experiments in which he unsuccessfully attempted to "inactivate" (presumably referring to antigenicity) coccidioidin (a mycelial phase preparation) with serum from both sensitive and desensitized guinea pigs. Having procrastinated in cleaning out the Wasserman tubes (disposable glassware not being available) for 1 week, Smith, upon finally bringing himself to this unpleasant task, discovered discrete buttons, indicating precipitin reactions, in the bottoms of the tubes containing coccidioidin and serum from infected guinea pigs. The tubes containing control serum possessed no such buttons. The coccidioidin was quickly tested as a complement-fixing antigen and proved successful in this test as well. The standardization of these tests, which had first been demonstrated by Cooke in 1914[16] and Davis in 1924,[17] respectively, led to the mammoth studies published a decade later.[18-20]

When World War II began and it appeared necessary to establish airfields in the southwestern United States, Smith became consultant to the Secretary of War. Seizing the opportunity, Smith began a wide-scale epidemiological program in July 1941 by skin testing all the personnel at Gardner and Minter Army Air Fields. While the headquarters of Minter was at Bakersfield Junior College, the men lived in tents at the Kern County Airport. At Gardner Field (in Taft, California) "dust was ankle deep and swirled in clouds over the fields."[1] Obviously such conditions led to enormous numbers of cases of coccidioidomycosis and also allowed the evaluation of simple preventive measures such as dust control. Smith managed to make an outstanding contribution to the military effort while, at the same time, gathering mountains of data which led to his definitive publications on skin and serological testing and on the manifestations of the disease. These studies demonstrated the broad clinical spectrum of the disease, the time course of the serological response to infection, the correlation of the height of the complement-fixing antibody titer with the extent of disease, and the prognostic importance of the development of delayed dermal hypersensitivity to coccidioidin. These studies were complemented by those of Negroni as well as those of Maddy,[21] who delineated the extent of endemicity in Arizona and suggested that it was coextensive with the Lower Sonoran Life Zone which had been outlined in the previous century by Merriam.[22] Smith's accomplishments had even led to the appearance of his photograph in the *Saturday Evening Post* as part of an article entitled "The Mystery of the Deadly Dust."[23] Unhappily, the caption concluded, "Thus far, no drug or vaccine has proved effective in prevention or cure."

4. THE ERA OF IMMUNOLOGY AND CHEMOTHERAPY

4.1. Immunoprophylaxis

During the World War II studies, Smith was able to demonstrate that self-limited, naturally acquired infection appeared to protect individuals from subsequent infection with *C. immitis*. Rixford and Gilchrist,[5] as well as Negroni *et at.*,[24] had previously attempted immunization of animals with live organisms with only limited success. In 1951 Smith reported that mice infected with a strain of low virulence survived an otherwise lethal intraperitoneal challenge with a virulent strain[25] and in 1956 reported, along with Lorraine Friedman, protective immunization of mice with killed arthrospores.[26] Demosthenes Pappagianis *et al.*, however, later showed that mice immunized in that fashion, while protected from intraperitoneal challenge, were poorly. protected from intranasal challenge.[27] Pappagianis, a disciple of Smith, demonstrated the ability to protect mice against intranasal challenge by subcutaneous vaccination with a viable, avirulent mutant arthrospore preparation.[27] Converse *et al.* at Fort Detrick, was able to reproduce these results using other strains of the fungus.[28]

However, in both laboratories it was found that the vaccinating organism persisted in the host. Furthermore, avirulence proved to be an unstable phenomenon, leading to the abandonment of live vaccines.

Hillel Benjamin Levine, another disciple of Smith, reasoned that since the spherule–endospore phase was the parasitic form of the fungus, perhaps immunization with spherules or endospores might prove superior to mycelial phase vaccination. Smith was skeptical. Had not Vogel *et al.*[29] failed to produce significant immunity to nasal challenge in guinea pigs by vaccination with heat-killed spherules harvested from embryonated eggs? However, in 1960, Levine, along with Smith and James Cobb (whose technical assistance was to prove as invaluable to Levine as Margaret Saito's had to Smith and then to Pappagianis), demonstrated the superior immunogenicity of a killed spherule–endospore vaccine.[30] Studies performed in the subsequent years demonstrated protective efficacy against intranasal challenge in monkeys,[31] as well as marked efficacy in mice.[32]

However, little notice was taken of these studies, and Levine had consequently become discouraged. Then, in 1963, the venerable Myrnie Gifford paid a visit to Levine. She had read his work and was excited by its potential. Levine, thus encouraged, proceeded with the studies leading to the first administration of the vaccine to humans. (H. B. Levine, personal communication).

The first to receive the vaccine were Levine and Smith, who must have approached this task with at least some trepidation, since both had long since developed dermal hypersensitivity to coccidioidin. Smith, who had become Professor of Public Health at Stanford (where, according to Broughton,[33] he was known to his students as "Snuffy") on Dickson's death in 1942, had more recently become Dean of the School of Public Health at the University of California in Berkeley.

While dean, he managed to continue his work on coccidioidomycosis without interfering with his administrative duties by performing his research between 5:00 and 8:00 each morning! The two met at 6:00 a.m. in Smith's office, and the first task was for Smith to teach Levine how to administer epinephrine, in case one of them should develop anaphylaxis. Immediately prior to injection of the vaccine Smith called to Margaret Saito, who was in the next room, that "if you hear a 'kerplunk' don't worry. If you hear two 'kerplunks' come running!" No "kerplunks" were heard (H. B. Levine, personal communication), and the safety of the vaccine was subsequently demonstrated, in collaboration with Pappagianis, by administration to a large group of volunteers.[34]

Further details concerning the vaccine can be found in Chapter 22.

4.2. Spherulin—A New Diagnostic and Epidemiologic Reagent

If a killed spherule vaccine was superior to a mycelial preparation as an immunogen, should not a spherulin-derived antigen be superior to coccidioidin as a reagent in the detection of dermal hypersensitivity? Although a previous study had been complicated by an early toxic reaction to the spherule-derived antigen, Levine set out to answer this question. Levine, again using Converse's method for maintenance of the organism in the spherule phase,[35] produced a reagent he called "spherulin." Subsequent studies have demonstrated spherulin to be superior to coccidioidin in the detection of dermal hypersensitivity to *C. immitis* in animals and in man, in both the epidemiological and the clinical setting.[36-38]

4.3. A Special Immortality

The first symposium on coccidioidomycosis, in honor of Myrnie Gifford, was held in 1957, just 1 year before Fiese's remarkable monograph[39] on the disease was published. The second symposium, held in Phoenix in December 1965, was convened in honor of Charles Smith. Seventeen months later, on April 18, 1967, Smith died, 6 months before he was to have become president of the American Public Health Association, and prior to publication of the symposium. Among the condolences received by his wife, Elizabeth, was a letter from his students which said: "His is the special kind of immortality reserved for those who devote their lives to the teaching of others."[33]

4.4. The Clinicians—Amphotericin B

Exactly 8 months after the loss of Smith, William A. Winn died. Winn, medical director of Springville Hospital in Tulare County, had complemented Smith's public health and basic science approach with his clinical descriptions of coccidioidomycosis, particularly those of cavitary disease and meningitis. His pioneering reports of the use of amphotericin B in meningeal[40] and nonmeningeal[41] coccidioidomycosis represented the first successful nonsurgical treatment of this infection.* Fortunately, other clinicians in the endemic area, such as David Salkin, Hans Einstein and Tom Larwood, followed in Winn's path. They were, of course, supplemented in their knowledge of the disease by the pathological studies of such as Forbus and Bestebreurtje[42] and Robert Huntington (see chapter 7), as well as the refinements in serological techniques produced by Milton Huppert. All clinicians leaned heavily on the serological services offered by Smith and then by Pappagianis and by Huppert.

4.5. Immunotherapy—Transfer Factor

In 1960, 5 years after his description of dialyzable transfer factor, Lawrence collaborated with Pappagianis and Smith in demonstrating transfer of delayed hypersensitivity to coccidioidin by administering leukocyte extracts obtained from coccidioidin-sensitive donors to coccidioidin-negative lifelong residents of New York.[43] Smith had previously demonstrated that while humoral antibody is not protective in this disease, the development and maintenance of delayed hypersensitivity is critical to the outcome.[18-20] Later studies were able to correlate *in vitro* defects of cellular immunity with defective delayed hypersensitivity.[44]

In the early 1970s the first reports of attempts of the use of transfer factor as a therapeutic agent in disseminated coccidioidomycosis appeared.[45-48] In January 1974 a meeting, bringing together various investigative groups from throughout the southwestern United States, was held at San Francisco Children's Hospital. Information on the use of transfer factor in more than 40 patients was exchanged. In response to the recognition of the need for a controlled trial, the Coccidioidomycosis Cooperative Treatment Group was formed. This group began collating their data on delayed hypersensitivity and cellular immunity in coccidioidomycosis.[49] At the Third International Coccidioidomycosis Sympos-

---

* The role of coccidioidomycosis in precipitating the first clinical trial of penicillin in the United States has been delightfully reported by Morris Tager [M. Tager, John F. Fulton, coccidioidomycosis, and penicillin, *Yale J. Biol. Med.* **49**:391–398 (1976)].

ium in Tucson, held in honor of David Salkin, in November 1976, more than one-fifth of the papers presented dealt with cellular immunology, and of these, half were reports on transfer factor.

4.6. Newer Chemotherapies

The introduction of amphotericin B had led to a revolution in the management of patients with coccidioidomycosis. However, it was soon recognized that, because of its toxicity and occasional therapeutic failure, it was not the ideal antifungal agent. While the search for such a chemotherapeutic agent was slow in the beginning, by the middle of the 1970s a number of candidates were under study. Of these only a few reached clinical trial by 1980. Amphotericin B methyl ester, while showing initial promise, had been administered to only a very small number of patients, and appeared to have new toxicities. Clotrimazole, the first of a number of imidazoles, has been generally abandoned. Miconazole, a phenethyl imidazole, appears promising in its initial clinical trials[50]. A variety of other drugs have been shown to have efficacy in animal models of coccidioidomycosis and await study in man. Of these, ambruticin appears to have potential,[51] as does ketoconazole, which is undergoing clinical trials at present, with promising results.[52]

5. THE FUTURE

We have covered vast distances in our understanding of coccidioidomycosis in the nearly nine decades since Domingo Escurra came to Buenos Aires for medical care. Our knowledge of clinical and epidemiologic aspects of the disease is quite good. Our knowledge of the cellular immune response to the fungus is burgeoning. Chemotherapeutic advances are being made. Transfer factor may prove to be a useful therapeutic modality. With Levine's vaccine, we have in our hands the potential ultimate means of control of the disease—preventing its occurrence.

6. EPILOGUE—A REPRISE

In the wake of the 1975 Viet Cong—North Vietnamese victory, tens of thousands of Vietnamese refugees were brought to the United States and placed in camps throughout the country. Camp Pendleton, despite its being in an area of Southern California long known to be endemic for coccidioidomycosis, was used as a major holding area, at one time accommodating 18,000 Vietnamese. These refugees were housed in tents which were frequently pitched on bare ground. Their children played in the dust and dirt outside. Soon, the first cases of coccidioidomycosis began appearing in this immunologically virgin population. And, in keeping with the known information concerning the course of the illness in other Oriental groups, cases of disseminated coccidioidomycosis began appearing in the Vietnamese, who by then had been dispersed throughout the country.

Meanwhile, the German Luftwaffe began sending selected pilots to the United States for advanced flight training by the U.S. Air Force. Since much of the training took place in the southwestern states, many of the pilots had their training interrupted or terminated by episodes of acute coccidioidomycosis.

ACKNOWLEDGMENTS.   The author wishes to acknowledge the assistance of Rosemarie Vila and Ada Bowen in the preparation of this chapter. Milton Huppert and Sue Sun directed my attention to reference 4 and to its helpful information.

REFERENCES

1. C. E. Smith, Coccidioidomycosis, in: *Preventive Medicine in World War II*, Vol. IV, *Communicable Diseases Transmitted Chiefly Through the Respiratory and Alimentary Tracts* (E. C. Hoff, ed.), Department of the Army, Washington, D.C., U.S. Government Printing Office (1958), pp. 285–316.
2. A. Posadas, Un nuevo caso de micosis fungoidea con psorospermias, *An. Circ. Med. Argent.* **15**:585–597 (1892).
3. R. Wernicke, Ueber einen protozoenbefund bei Mycosis fungoides *Zentrabl. Bakteriol.* **12**:859–861 (1892).
4. E. Rixford, Early history of coccidioidal granuloma in California, in: *Coccidioidal Granuloma, Calif. State Dep. Public Health Spec. Bull.* No. 57 (1931), pp. 5–8.
5. E. Rixford and T. C. Gilchrist, Two cases of protozoan (coccidioidal) infection of the skin and other organs, *Johns Hopkins Hosp. Rep.* **1**:209–268 (1896).
6. W. S. Thorne, A case of protozoic skin disease, *Occident. Med. Times* **8**:703–704 (1894).
7. E. Rixford, A case of protozoic dermatitis, *Occident. Med. Times* **8**:704–707 (1894).
8. W. Ophüls and H. C. Moffitt, A new pathogenic mould (formerly described as a protozoan: *Coccidioides immitis* pyogenes). Preliminary Report, *Philadel. Med. J.* **5**:1471–1472 (1900).
9. W. Ophüls, Further observations on a pathogenic mould formerly described as a protozoan *(Coccidioides immitis, Coccidioides pyogenes)*, *J. Exp. Med.* **6**:443–486 (1905).
10. W. Ophüls, Coccidioidal granuloma, *J. Am. Med. Assoc.* **45**:1201–1296 (1905).
11. C. E. Smith, Reminiscences of the flying chlamydospore and its allies, in: *Coccidioidomycosis* (L. Ajello, ed.), University of Arizona Press, Tucson (1967) pp. xiii–xxii.

12. E. C. Dickson, "Valley Fever" of the San Joaquin Valley and fungus *Coccidioides, Calif. West. Med.* **47**:151–155 (1937).
13. R. A. Stewart and K. F. Meyer, Isolation of *Coccidioides immitis* from soil, *Proc. Soc. Exp. Biol. Med.* **29**:937–938, 1932.
14. M. A. Gifford, San Joaquin fever, in: *Kern County Health Department Annual Report* (1935–1936), pp. 22–23.
15. M. A. Gifford, W. C. Buss, and R. J. Dowds, Data on *Coccidioides* fungus infection, Kern County, 1901–1936, in: *Kern County Health Department Annual Report* (1936–1937), pp. 39–54.
16. J. V. Cooke, Immunity tests in coccidioidal granuloma, *Proc. Soc. Exp. Biol. Med.* **12**:35 (1914).
17. D. J. Davis, Coccidioidal granuloma with certain serologic and experimental observations, *Arch. Dermatol. Syphilol.* **9**:577–588 (1924).
18. C. E. Smith, R. R. Beard, E. G. Whiting, and H. G. Rosenberger, Varieties of coccidioidal infection in relation to the epidemiology and control of the disease, *Am. J. Public Health* **36**:1394–1402 (1946).
19. C. E. Smith, E. G. Whiting, E. E. Baker, H. G. Rosenberger, R. R. Beard, and M. T. Saito, The use of coccidioidin, *Am. Rev. Tuberc.* **57**:330–360 (1948).
20. C. E. Smith, M. T. Saito, and S. A. Simmons, Pattern of 39,500 serologic tests in coccidioidomycosis, *J. Am. Med. Assoc.* **160**:546–552 (1956).
21. K. T. Maddy, The geographic distribution of *Coccidioides immitis* and possible ecologic implications, *Ariz. Med.* **15**:178–188 (1958).
22. C. H. Merriam, Results of a biological survey of the San Francisco mountain region and desert of the little Colorado in Arizona, in: *North American Fauna,* No. 3, U.S. Department of Agriculture (1890), pp. 1–34.
23. M. Silverman, The mystery of the deadly dust, *Saturday Evening Post,* December 17, 1949.
24. P. Negroni, D. Vivoli, and H. Bonfliglioli, Estudios sobre el *Coccidioides immitis* Rixford y Gilchrist. VII. Reacciones immunoalergicas en la infección experimental del cobayo, *Rev. Inst. Bacteriol. Dep. Nac. Hig. (Argent.)* **14**:273–286 (1949).
25. C. E. Smith, Annual Progress Report, Commission on Acute Respiratory Diseases, Armed Forces Epidemiological Board, Washington, D.C. (1951).
26. L. Friedman and C. E. Smith, Vaccination of mice against *Coccidioides immitis, Am. Rev. Tuberc.* **74**:245–248 (1956).
27. D. Pappagianis, H. B. Levine, C. E. Smith, R. J. Berman, and G. S. Kobayashi, Immunization of mice with viable *Coccidioides immitis, J. Immunol.* **86**:28–34 (1961).
28. J. L. Converse, M. W. Castleberry, A. R. Besemer, and E. M. Synder, Immunization of mice against coccidioidomycosis, *J. Bacteriol.* **84**:46–52 (1962).
29. R. A. Vogel, B. F. Fetter, N. F. Conant, and E. P. Lowe, Preliminary studies on artificial active immunization of guinea pigs against respiratory challenge of *Coccidioides immitis, Am. Rev. Tuberc.* **70**:498–503 (1954).
30. H. B. Levine, J. M. Cobb, and C. E. Smith, Immunity to coccidioidomycosis induced in mice by purified spherule, arthrospore and mycelial vaccines, *Trans. N.Y. Acad. Sci. II* **22**:436–449 (1960).
31. H. B. Levine, R. L. Miller, and C. E. Smith, Influence of vaccination on respiratory coccidioidal disease in cynomolgous monkeys, *J. Immunol.* **89**:242–251 (1962).
32. H. B. Levine, J. M. Cobb, and C. E. Smith, Immunogenicity of spherule-endospore vaccines of *Coccidioides immitis* for mice, *J. Immunol.* **87**:218–219 (1961).
33. P. Broughton, A special kind of immortality, *Am. J. Public Health* **57**:1087–1090 (1967).
34. D. Pappagianis and H. B. Levine, The present status of vaccination against coccidioidomycosis in man, *Am. J. Epidemiol.* **102**:30–41 (1975).

35. J. L. Converse, Growth of spherules of *Coccidioides immitis* in a chemically defined liquid medium, *Proc. Soc. Exp. Biol. Med.* **90:**709–711 (1955).
36. H. B. Levine, J. M. Cobb, and G. M. Scalarone, Spherule coccidioidin in delayed dermal sensitivity reactions of experimental animals, *Sabouraudia* 7:20–32 (1969).
37. D. A. Stevens, H. B. Levine, and D. R. Ten Eyck, Dermal sensitivity to different doses of spherulin and coccidioidin, *Chest* **65:**530–533 (1974).
38. D. A. Stevens, H. B. Levine, S. C. Deresinski, and L. J. Blaine, Spherulin in clinical coccidioidomycosis-comparison with coccidioidin, *Chest* **68:**697–702 (1975).
39. M. J. Fiese, *Coccidioidomycosis,* Charles C. Thomas, Springfield, Ill. (1958).
40. W. A. Winn, The treatment of coccidioidal meningitis—the use of amphotericin B in a group of 25 patients, *Calif. Med.* **10:**78–89 (1964).
41. W. A. Winn, Coccidioidomycosis and amphotericin B, *Med. Clin. North Am.* **47:**1131–1148 (1963).
42. W. D. Forbus and A. M. Bestebreurtje, Coccidioidomycosis: a study of 95 cases of the disseminated type with special reference to the pathogenesis of the disease, *Mil. Surg.* **99:**653–719 (1946).
43. F. T. Rappaport, H. S. Lawrence, J. W. Miller, D. Pappagianis, and C. E. Smith, Transfer of delayed hypersensitivity to coccidioidin in man, *J. Immunol.* **84:**358–367 (1960).
44. A. Catanzaro. L. E. Spitler, and K. M. Moser, Cellular immune response in coccidioidomycosis *Cell. Immunol.* **15:**360–371 (1975).
45. J. R. Graybill, J. Silva, Jr., R. H. Alford, D. E. Thor, Immunologic and clinical improvement of progressive coccidioidomycosis following administration of transfer factor, *Cell. Immunol.* **8:**120–135 (1973).
46. P. Cloninger, L. D. Thrupp, G. A. Granger, and H. S. Novey, Immunotherapy with transfer factor in disseminated coccidioidal osteomyelitis and arthritis, *West. J. Med.* **120:**322–325 (1974).
47. D. A. Stevens, D. Pappagianis, V. A. Marinkovich, and T. F. Waddell, Immunotherapy in recurrent coccidioidomycosis, *Cell. Immunol.* **12:**37–48 (1974).
48. A. Catanzaro, L. Spitler, K. M. Moser, Immunotherapy of coccidioidomycosis, *J. Clin. Invest.* **54:**690–701 (1974).
49. J. R. Graybill (for the Coccidioidomycosis Cooperative Treatment Group), The clinical course of coccidioidomycosis following transfer factor therapy, in: *Coccidioidomycosis: Current Clinical and Diagnostic Status* (L. Ajello, ed.), Symposia Specialists, Miami (1977), pp. 335–345.
50. D. A. Stevens, Miconazole in the treatment of systemic fungal infections, *Am. Rev. Resp. Dis.* **116:**801–806 (1977).
51. H. B. Levine, S. M. Ringel, and J. M. Cobb, Therapeutic properties of oral ambruticin (W7783) in experimental pulmonary coccidioidomycosis of mice, *Chest* 73:202–206 (1978).
52. D. Borelli, J. L. Bran, J. Fuentes, R. Legendre, E. Leiderman, H. B. Levine, A. Restrepo-M., and D. A. Stevens, Ketoconazole, an oral antifungal: laboratory and clinical assessment of imidazole drugs, *Postgrad. Med. J.* **55:**657–661 (1979).

2

Overview of Mycology, and the Mycology of *Coccidioides immitis*

M. Huppert and S. H. Sun

1. INTRODUCTION

Fungi are ubiquitous microorganisms found in terrestrial, freshwater, and marine habitats. Since they do not possess substances active in photosynthesis, they are limited to saprophytic, or symbiotic, or parasitic life cycles. The majority of fungus species are saprophytic and play an active role in the economy of nature by decomposing complex organic substances. The fungi as a group are extremely versatile and have served humans well in addition to plaguing them terribly. They have been used as a nutritional source for centuries and have been utilized effectively in fermentation, dairy, and chemical industries. On the other hand, the fungi also have caused widespread destruction of crops, contaminated food, fuels, and industrial products, and infected man and animals.

An understanding of fungi as etiological agents of disease requires knowledge of their form and function as biological entities. A detailed exposition is beyond the scope of the present text, but a very brief summary of relevant information would place in perspective the relationship of fungi to other microorganisms, and, in particular, set the stage for the role played by *Coccidioides immitis*. Those seeking more extensive information about fungi should consult texts on mycology.[1-4]

2. CHARACTERISTICS OF FUNGI

2.1. Definition

A precise definition of such a large and diverse group is difficult. Nevertheless, the fungi can be distinguished in a general sense from other large groups (e.g., bacteria, algae, protozoa, animals, plants), recognizing that there are exceptions to the definition and some overlapping among the groups. Fungi differ from bacteria and actinomycetes in several fundamental characteristics. The fungus nucleus is bound by a structurally organized membrane and divides by mitosis (eukaryotic). In addition, the fungal cell contains mitochondria and the principal structural component of the cell wall is chitin (cellulose in one group). Absence of chlorophyll distinguishes the fungi from plants and most algae. The presence of a cell wall and lack of motility (except for a single stage in the life cycle of one group) differentiate fungi from protozoa and animals. It is for these reasons that modern taxonomists have erected a separate kingdom which includes the fungi (e.g., reference 5).

2.2. Physiology

Since fungi lack photosynthetic mechanisms, they are dependent upon their chemical environment for nutrition, growth, and reproduction. With the exception of molecular oxygen and carbon dioxide obtained from the atmosphere, the essential nutrients must be in solution because uptake in fungi is absorptive. There is no universal medium for all fungi; a medium sufficient for one may mean starvation for another, or a medium supporting vegetative and sporulating growth for one fungus may result only in vegetative growth for another. Nevertheless, almost all of the fungi pathogenic for humans and animals grow satisfactorily in an aqueous environment containing partially digested substrates of biological origin as utilizable sources of organic carbon, vitamins, nitrogenous compounds, and inorganic ions. The limits of pH and temperature are also rather broad. Although optimal conditions may be narrowly defined, human pathogens with few exceptions will grow satisfactorily within a pH range of 5–8 and temperatures varying from below ambient to 37.5°C. Therefore, isolation of fungi from pathological material can be accomplished on a culture medium containing dextrose and peptone, adjusted to an appropriate pH, and incubated at either room or incubator temperatures.

2.3. Vegetative Structures

It is convenient to consider the fungi pathogenic for humans as composed of two groups: the yeasts and the filamentous molds. This distinction, however, applies only to the most common form usually seen in the laboratory, since a species in which the yeast form is predominant may appear as a mold, and vice versa, depending upon nutritional and environmental conditions.

Yeasts are unicellular fungi varying in size and in shape from rounded forms to elongated and even rectangular shapes. They reproduce either by budding or by fission.

In contrast to the unicellular structure of yeasts, molds grow by extension to form tubular structures, and septation without separation results in an apparent multicellular structure. This may be initiated by a single viable cell (e.g., conidium) which germinates by extension from one or more sites at the cell wall surface. Elongation occurs primarily at the tip (i.e., apical growth), with elaboration of a plastic cell wall structure covering the growing portion and gradual loss of plasticity as the cell wall is left behind. The resulting tubular filament is called a *hypha* (plural, hyphae). Branching usually occurs, and the mass of intertwined branching hyphae is known as *mycelium*. Hyphal growth is accompanied by repetitive nuclear divisions and by septum formation in older portions of the hyphae. Among some fungi, septation occurs only in the very oldest sections of hyphae or when cutting off reproductive structures, so that the majority of the mycelium contains aseptate

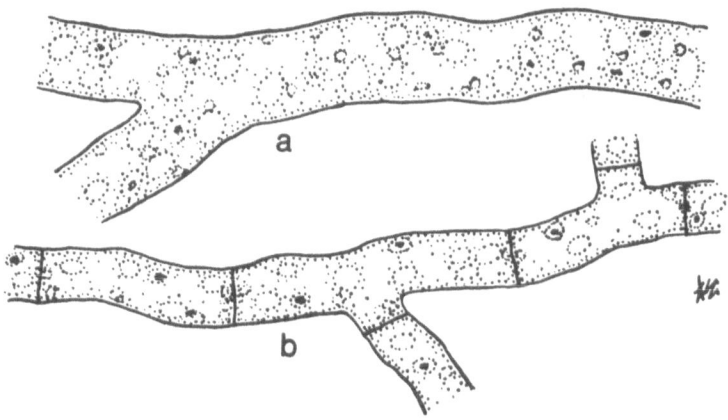

Figure 1. Aseptate coenocytic hyphae (a) and septate hyphae (b).

multinucleated protoplasm (coenocytic) as in species of *Mucor* and *Phycomyces* (Fig. 1a). Among the remaining molds, septum formation occurs regularly and at a relatively shorter distance from the growing tip so that the majority of mycelium appears as hyphae separated at intervals into individual cells (Fig. 1b). There is, however, a pore in each septum, and a strand of cytoplasm passing through this pore connects adjacent cells. Thus, even septate mycelium is functionally coenocytic. This functional coenocytic condition makes it possible for molds to grow above (i.e., aerial hyphae) their supporting medium, since nutrients can be transported throughout the mycelium. In addition, when a cell in the hypha is injured, the central pore of the septum is plugged by Woronin bodies (electron-dense round structures) allowing survival of adjacent cells. Therefore, when a portion of mycelium is cut away and transferred to fresh media, viable cells remain and grow to perpetuate the species.

2.4. Propagating Structures

The fungi have evolved many types of structures serving either for survival during unfavorable conditions or for propagation, adaptation, and dissemination of the species. Furthermore, each type of sporulating structure has many variations in size, shape, pigmentation, and morphogenesis. Some develop within a protective stroma of vegetative hyphae, but others are borne naked on hyphae which may or may not be differentiated from vegetative cells. Here we can consider only the general and most common types. Propagating structures may be considered as either sexual, in that two haploid nuclei fuse to form a diploid, or asexual, with nuclear fusion absent.

2.4.1. Asexual Conidia

During the nineteenth century, the collection, description, and classification of fungi was a new and exciting occupation. The great variety of organisms and their many forms of growth and reproduction led to a plethora of descriptive terms based on superficial morphological structures, and the field of mycology was littered with a debris of confusing terminology. In the twentieth century, beginning with Vuillemin, studies of the fungi focused increasingly on the ontogeny of these morphological structures as valid taxonomic criteria but with little effect on terminology. A serious and authoritative attempt to simplify and define terminology was undertaken at the First International Specialists'

Workshop-Conference on Criteria and Terminology in the Classification of Fungi Imperfecti, meeting in Kananaskis, Canada, in 1969. The proceedings of this conference have been published,[6] and the new terminology will be used in the following discussion (simplified considerably), with relationships to older terminology indicated. It should be recognized that continuing studies employing more sophisticated methods may require further modifications of terminology and definitions in the future. In addition, as stated by Carmichael, the methods of sporulation which have been described as separate and distinct are, in fact, "outstanding parts of a continuously intergrading and overlapping spectrum of methods for releasing propagative elements."[6]

A conidium is defined as "a specialized, non-motile, asexual propagule [i.e., a reproductive cell], usually caducous [i.e., a method of separation of cells analogous to a mature leaf dropping from a branch], not developing by cytoplasmic cleavage or free-cell formation."[6] Conidia may be produced singly or in chains. Since conidia may be unicellular or multicellular, pigmented or nonpigmented, and may occur in a wide variety of shapes and sizes, they have been used as differential characteristics for both species and genera among the Deuteromycotina (i.e., Fungi Imperfecti).

Some molds reproduce by forming arthroconidia (formerly arthrospores, a term which has been rejected). These may be either *blastic* when derived from part of a cell and recognizable as a conidium initially before being delimited by septa, or *thallic* when derived from an entire cell and recognizable as a conidium only after being delimited by septa. In addition, release of the arthroconidium may occur by fission at a double septum, or by fracture or disintegration of the cell wall of a nearby cell (i.e., not at a septum) as in *C. immitis*.

The definition of *aleuriospores*, although described clearly by Vuillemin, has been modified repeatedly and, therefore, has been rejected as a confusing term.

2.4.2. Sexual Reproduction

Many fungi are known to reproduce by a method involving mating of two compatible cells (plasmogamy), fusion of the two haploid nuclei (karyogamy) to produce a diploid nucleus within the single cell, followed by subsequent nuclear divisions, one of which reduces the diploid condition to haploid (meiosis). Eventually the haploid nuclei are incorporated into newly formed cells and released as spores. The sexual, or perfect, form of reproduction is in addition to asexual types.

3. TAXONOMY OF FUNGI

Various schemes have been proposed for taxonomic classification of the fungi. The older concept of only two kingdoms, plants and animals, has been found untenable by many modern taxonomists, who consider four or five kingdoms more realistic.[5,7] One of these is the Kingdom Fungi with eukaryotic organisms having an absorptive nutrition. This separates the fungi from bacteria and actinomycetes which are prokaryotic (i.e., a cell not containing membrane-bound genetic material) and from plants with photosynthetic nutrition and animals with ingestive nutrition. The characteristics of (1) presence or absence of plasmodial forms (an amoeboid multinucleate mass of protoplasm), (2) motile asexual conidia, and (3) morphogenesis among sexual forms are the primary bases for modern taxonomic classification of the fungi. The abbreviated taxonomic scheme in Table 1 is modified from Ainsworth.[7,8] More complete classifications of fungi can be found in several publications.[1,7,8]

The Kingdom Fungi contains two major groups. Organisms in the Division Myxomycota are plasmodial, those in the Division Eumycota are not. The fungi pathogenic for humans and animals are in Division Eumycota. Traditionally, the Eumycota had been divided into four classes, the *Phycomycetes, Ascomycetes,* and *Basidiomycetes,* based on types of sexual reproduction, and the Deuteromycetes or Fungi Imperfecti containing species for which sexual reproduction was unknown. The Phycomycetes, however, contained several groups of such diverse characteristics that modern taxonomic treatments have divided this class further, separating fungi which have motile asexual spores (Mastigomycotina) from those which have nonmotile asexual spores (Zygomycotina).

TABLE 1
Abbreviated Taxonomic Classification of Fungi[a]

Kingdom Fungi
   Division Myxomycota: plasmodial
   Division Eumycota: not plasmodial

Eumycota subdivisions	Asexual spores	Perfect spores
Mastigomycotina	Motile	Oospores
Zygomycotina	Nonmotile	Zygospores
Ascomycotina	Nonmotile	Ascospores
Basidiomycotina	Nonmotile	Basidiospores
Deuteromycotina	Nonmotile	Unknown

[a] Modified from Ainsworth.[7,8]

Further subdivision of the *Eumycota* is based on two characteristics, motility of asexual spores and type of sexual or perfect reproduction. The discussion here will be limited to the development of sexual forms among *Eumycota* subdivisions which contain species pathogenic for humans and animals.

3.1. Zygomycotina

Sexual, or perfect, reproduction is initiated when adjacent compatible hyphae grow lateral side branches toward each other. When contact is established, the advanced portions of each are cut off from their respective hyphae by septum formation and function as multinucleate gametangia (i.e., cells involved in sexual reproduction). The two gametangia fuse to form a *zygospore* encased in a thick, frequently pigmented wall derived from the gametangial walls. Nuclear fusion takes place within the zygospore, and meiosis occurs at a later stage after the zygospore has germinated to sooner or later develop saclike structures, called sporangia. *Zygomycotina* contains pathogenic species in several genera (e.g., *Mucor, Rhizopus, Mortierella, Absidia,* and *Basidiobolus*).

3.2. Ascomycotina

Within the Subdivision *Ascomycotina* (generally, the ascomycetes), there are many variations in the manner by which specialized hyphal mating branches containing haploid nuclei are joined and develop to form eventually a saclike structure, the ascus, containing endogenous *ascospores*.

The sexual stage of a number of human pathogens place them in *Ascomycotina*. For example, the perfect forms of many species of dermatophytes are in the genera *Nannizzia* and *Arthroderma,* the perfect form of *Blastomyces dermatitidis* is *Ajellomyces dermatitidis,* and that of *Histoplasma capsulatum* is *Emmonsiella capsulata.*

3.3. Basidiomycotina

Within the Subdivision *Basidiomycotina* (generally, the basidiomycetes), the general sequence of developmental stages to the perfect form is similar in principle to that in the *Ascomycotina*. The mechanism for maintenance of the dikaryotic stage (hyphal cell with two nuclei, prior to development of spores) differs for ascomycetes and basidiomycetes (which form basidiospores). The perfect form of *Cryptococcus neoformans* has been described recently as a basidiomycete comprising two species in the genus *Filobasidiella: F. neoformans* and *F. bacillispora*.[9,10]

3.4. Deuteromycotina

Fungi for which the perfect stage of reproduction is unknown are placed in the Subdivision *Deuteromycotina*. In the past, the *Deuteromycotina* contained most of the fungi pathogenic for humans. The numbers are being reduced gradually with the discovery of sexual reproductive forms. In most instances in the literature, the imperfect nomenclature has been retained for convenience.

4. MYCOLOGY OF *C. IMMITIS*

Several investigators have commented on the range of variations in cultural and morphological characteristics of *C. immitis*,[11-18] with some strains being so aberrant that recognition and identification in routine clinical laboratory practice would be unlikely.[11,14] Nevertheless, when a large number of strains are studied, there is a strong impression that these variations represent a continuous series within a broad spectrum of characteristics peculiar to *C. immitis*. Baker *et al.*[13] have stated that "strains appear to form an integrated series, each strain differing a little from the other." There is no justification at present for fragmenting the genus into more than one species. The majority of strains, about 80% according to Huppert *et al.*,[11] are quite consistent and comparable. Therefore, it is convenient to arbitrarily consider these as "typical" and those which are most different as "atypical."

4.1. Typical

Many species of fungi exhibit different colonial appearances and, to a lesser extent, microscopic morphology, depending on the composition of available nutrients. This occurs also with *C. immitis*. The following descriptions apply to growth on a dextrose–peptone agar (e.g., Sabouraud's dextrose) for two reasons. First, this would be the most common form seen in the clinical laboratory. Secondly, dextrose–peptone agar generally yields the best growth, and the more intense pigmentation.

Most strains of *C. immitis* grow more rapidly than other fungi causing systemic disease. In pure culture, the most rapidly growing strains may cover the surface of the medium in 2–3 weeks. Early growth is quite similar for typical strains. Colonies at 3–4 days appear flat, smooth, and gray. Attempts to transfer portions at this stage reveal a membranous texture. Development of aerial hyphae is apparent within the next few days. In some strains, erect and seemingly sturdy spicules rise from the surface at scattered points; in others a soft, velvety nap covers the membranous surface. The gray coloration persists through this stage. After approximately 1 week, aerial hyphae have become more abundant and the spicules are no longer obvious on colonies which developed them initially. At this point differences among strains are apparent, and these become more pronounced with continued incubation. During week 2, the aerial hyphae among some strains grow as grayish tufts with a wooly appearance, other colonies are overgrown with white to gray aerial hyphae of a cottony texture, and some develop only sparse, cobwebby, gray aerial growth. Frequently, the formation of aerial hyphae varies with time of incubation within a single colony, resulting in concentric rings of profuse aerial hyphae alternating with rings containing little or none. After 2 weeks, typical colonies are about 3–5 cm in diameter and are variably covered with white to gray aerial hyphae of differing texture. Pigmentation, if it occurs, usually is apparent at 2 weeks but only in the surface growth and therefore is observed best through the underside of the colony. In most of the typical strains which develop pigment, this is at first light brown in hue, confined to the area covered by the colony, and intensifies to darker brown with aging. It has not been established whether this type of pigment formation results from fungal metabolism or from dehydration of the agar with concentration of peptone. Occasional typical strains, however, elaborate a diffusible pigment varying from deep brown to almost black in hue. After 3–4 weeks, it is not unusual for the aerial hyphae to collapse onto the surface growth so that the colony now appears to be covered with a dark gray to brownish nap varying in texture from velvety to powdery or granular. Frequently, the colony has developed slight ridges and furrows radiating outward from the center.

Incubation at room temperature or at 37°C has relatively little effect on the sequential development of colonies. At the higher temperature, radial growth is somewhat more rapid, but aerial hyphae formation is delayed initially and less abundant ultimately. It should be noted that the optimal temperature for *C. immitis* (and most mycelial pathogenic fungi) is approximately 30°C.

Of all the routine primary isolation media used in the clinical laboratory, the most likely ones on which *C. immitis* may be encountered are liquid or gelled media containing blood, inspissated egg media, and various types of nutrient agars containing basically one or more carbohydrates and peptone or peptone digests. Typical *C. immitis* isolates appear similar on the nutrient agars at neutral or slightly alkaline pH to their growth on dextrose–peptone agar at pH 5.5. The rate of growth may be slightly faster and aerial hyphae a bit more profuse with a pH near neutrality. On inspissated egg media, which usually contain dyes that are slightly inhibitory for fungi, *C. immitis* may grow, but only poorly. The early membranous stage may be overlooked because of the restricted growth and opaque medium. If, and when, aerial hyphae develop, they are usually sparse, gray, and very loose and cobwebby in appearance. The white and cottony type of growth is rare on this medium in our experience. On blood agar at 37°C, *C. immitis* grows quite rapidly and the gray membranous stage may be apparent in 1–2 days. Development of aerial hyphae is usually less abundant than at temperatures of 30°C or less. On liquid media, aerobic conditions are required. The fungus grows on the surface and, if undisturbed, will form a grayish mat spreading over the liquid–air interface. Aerial hyphae are usually sparse with a tendency to grow up along the moist inner surface of the container. In liquid media aerated by continuous motion (rotary or reciprocating), *C. immitis* develops throughout the entire depth.

4.2. Atypical

A number of investigators in the past have commented about strains of *C. immitis* which exhibit cultural or morphological characteristics differing markedly from the usual, or typical, types encountered in the laboratory.[11–14,16,19,20] Some of these atypical cultures occur as primary isolates, and therefore the possibility for false negative results must be considered when these are not recognized as possible cultures of *C. immitis*. In our experience, growth on media containing 0.4 mg/ml cycloheximide is sufficient to consider the possibility of *C. immitis* until proven otherwise.

Atypical colonies may vary from typical types in rate of growth, pigmentation, production and texture of aerial hyphae, and topography of surface growth. Some colonies may never exceed a few centimeters in diameter even after several weeks. The surface may develop ridges and furrows, usually radiating outward from the center in an irregular pattern. Aerial hyphae may be absent, sparse, or dense, and in the latter case the texture may be powdery, granular, or velvety. Although aerial hyphae may be white or grayish in color, various shadings of pink, lavender, buff, yellow, and brown can occur. In addition, diffusible or nondiffusible pigmentation may be present in the agar, varying from hues of orange and brown to a very dark, almost black, color. Although a single isolate may appear different on several types of culture medium during the first 2 weeks of incubation, there is a tendency with increasing age for each strain to develop uniform characteristics regardless of culture medium. In contrast, differences among strains persist to a striking degree. Sectors with a gross appearance quite different from the remainder of the colony may occur with aging. Although there are strains which differ so much from typical cultures of *C. immitis* that they may not be recognized as pathogens, we agree with Baker *et al.*[13] that there is no reason to divide the genus *Coccidioides* into more than one species. If these cultures are arranged in a series from typical to the most atypical strains, they constitute a spectrum of gradual changes in appearance that is not sufficiently discontinuous at any point to justify separation into two or more species.

4.3. Fungi Resembling *C. immitis*

Accurate identification of an isolate is complicated not only by marked cultural variability among strains of *C. immitis*, but also by the fairly common occurrence of other species which resemble *C. immitis* culturally and morphologically.[19,21-23] Sigler and Carmichael[19] list 15 form genera with species having arthroconidial reproductive stages. These fungi are natural inhabitants of soil but may be encountered occasionally in the clinical laboratory. Many bear marked similarities to both typical and atypical cultures of *C. immitis*. Differentiation has required reproduction of coccidioidomycosis in laboratory animals with demonstration of endosporulating spherules. Simple recovery of the fungus from tissues of the inoculated animal is not sufficient for confirmation as *C. immitis*, since some of these nonpathogens can survive in animals for 30 days or more.[23] In this regard, the newer procedures for *in vitro* conversion of spores to endosporulating spherules[22,24,25] or the immunological test for antigens specific to *C. immitis*[26] may prove particularly useful for routine clinical laboratory service.

4.4. Mycelial Cycle

In the original reports of a fungus as the etiological agent of coccidioidomycosis, Ophüls[27] and Ophüls and Moffitt[28] described the formation of "highly refractile smaller bodies formed at the ends of the mycelium, mostly 3 or 4 in a row" which resembled oidia (i.e., a hyphal cell which separates from other hyphal cells through the septum).[27] Since then, there have been many morphological studies which, as noted by

Baker et al.[13] "have added little to Ophüls' description." Baker and his colleagues presented excellent descriptions of both the mycelial and spherule–endospore cycles. More recently, Kwon-Chung[29] and Sun and Huppert[30] have extended the cytological observations.

The principal stages in the mycelial cycle are illustrated in Figs. 2 (A–E) and 3 (A–E). (The shallow focal plane of photomicrographs in Fig. 3 is illustrated for detail by line drawings in Fig. 2.) Mycelial growth is initiated when spores are planted on suitable media and incubated at room temperature. Germination may occur at more than one point (Fig. 4), even through the side of the cylindrical conidium. Growth is apical, and nuclear divisions appear to be synchronous. Septa with a simple pore (Fig. 5) are formed behind the vigorously growing hyphal tips, delineating multinucleate cells. Since the septa contain a pore, the fungus is functionally coenocytic although morphologically septate. Eventually the hyphae branch to form a mycelium. Aerial hyphae destined to form spores are usually broader than nonfertile hyphae. Septa form simultaneously in the fertile hypha (Fig. 6) separating multinucleate cells of approximately equal size. Some of these, usually alternating on a single hypha, gradually lose cytoplasm as determined by staining, although nuclei are still apparent (Figs. 2E and 3E). The remaining cells close the septal pores and comprise the new generation of spores, which are released by fracture of the cell walls of the adjacent degenerating cells (Fig. 7). The formation of chains of spores separated by sterile segments and the release of these spores by disintegration of the adjacent sterile segments conforms to the description of arthroaleuriospores by Orr et al.,[31] i.e., alternate thallic arthroconidia according to recent generally accepted terminology.

Kwon-Chung[29] has described the nuclear cycle in the mycelial form. The resting nucleus is a round, dense, chromatinic mass which develops into a ring stage with apparently three chromatinic bodies. The ring opens to form a V stage which becomes rodlike and then extends into a filament. Longitudinal division occurs to form two daughter nuclei. Sun and Huppert[30] confirmed these observations but reported four pairs of chromosomes (Fig. 8) rather than the apparently three seen by Kwon-Chung. Both reports found a considerable degree of synchrony in nuclear division and septum formation producing arthroconidia.

4.5. Spherule–Endospore Cycle

A number of investigators have reported the occurrence of endo-sporulating spherules under in vitro conditions (reviewed in reference 13). These were not produced consistently, however, until Converse[32–34]

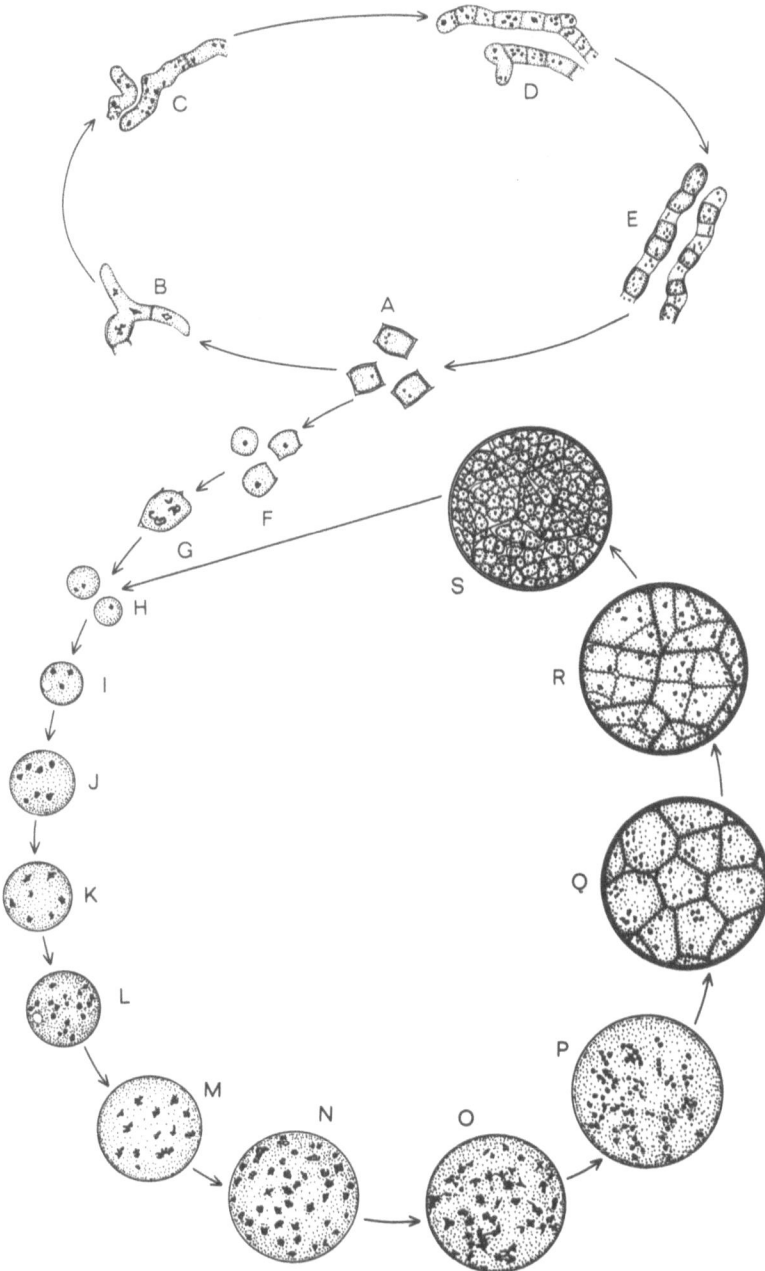

Figure 2. Saprobic (A–E) and parasitic (F–S) life cycles in *C. immitis*. Ink drawings of photomicrographs in Fig. 3 to illustrate detail. Reprinted with permission.[30]

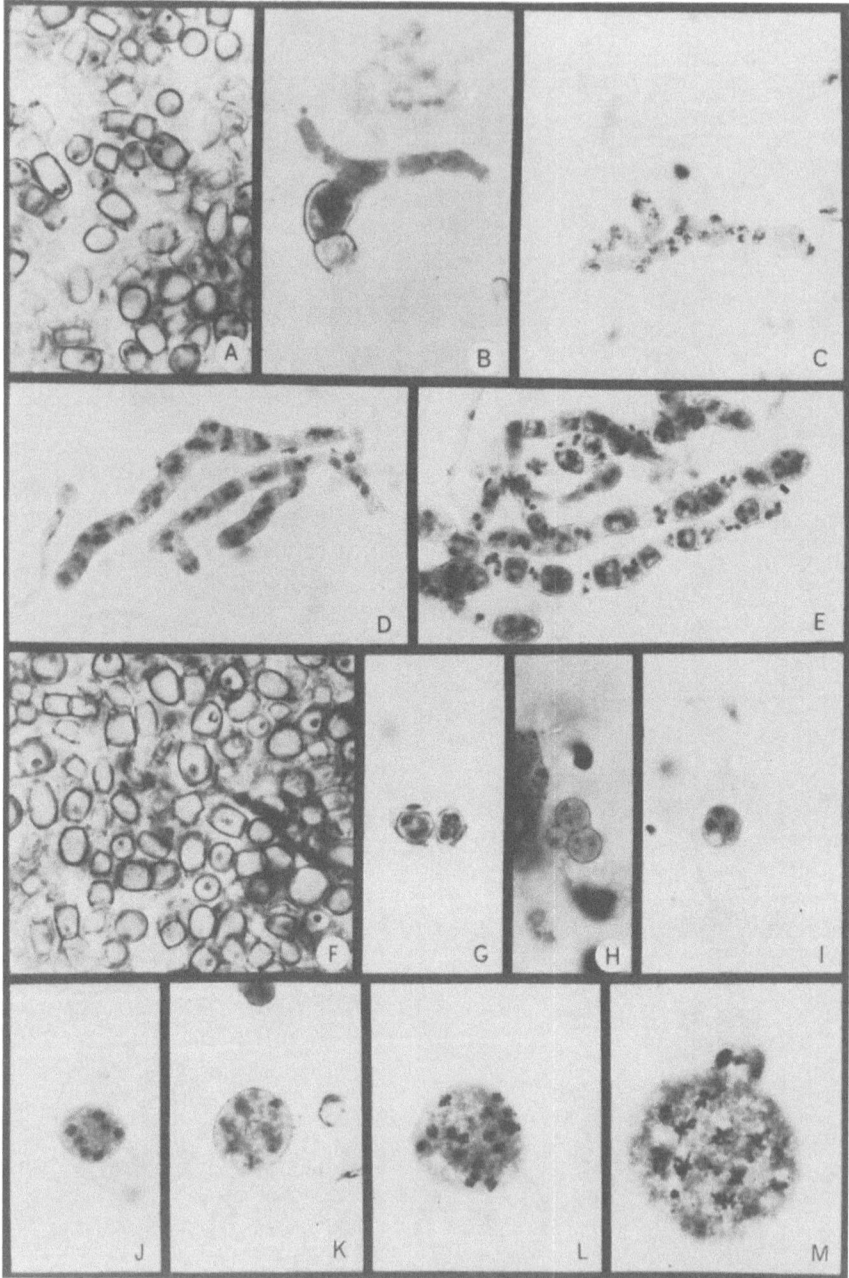

Figure 3. Photomicrographs illustrating successive morphological stages in the saprobic (A–E) and parasitic (F–S) life cycles of *C. immitis*. Reprinted with permission.[30]

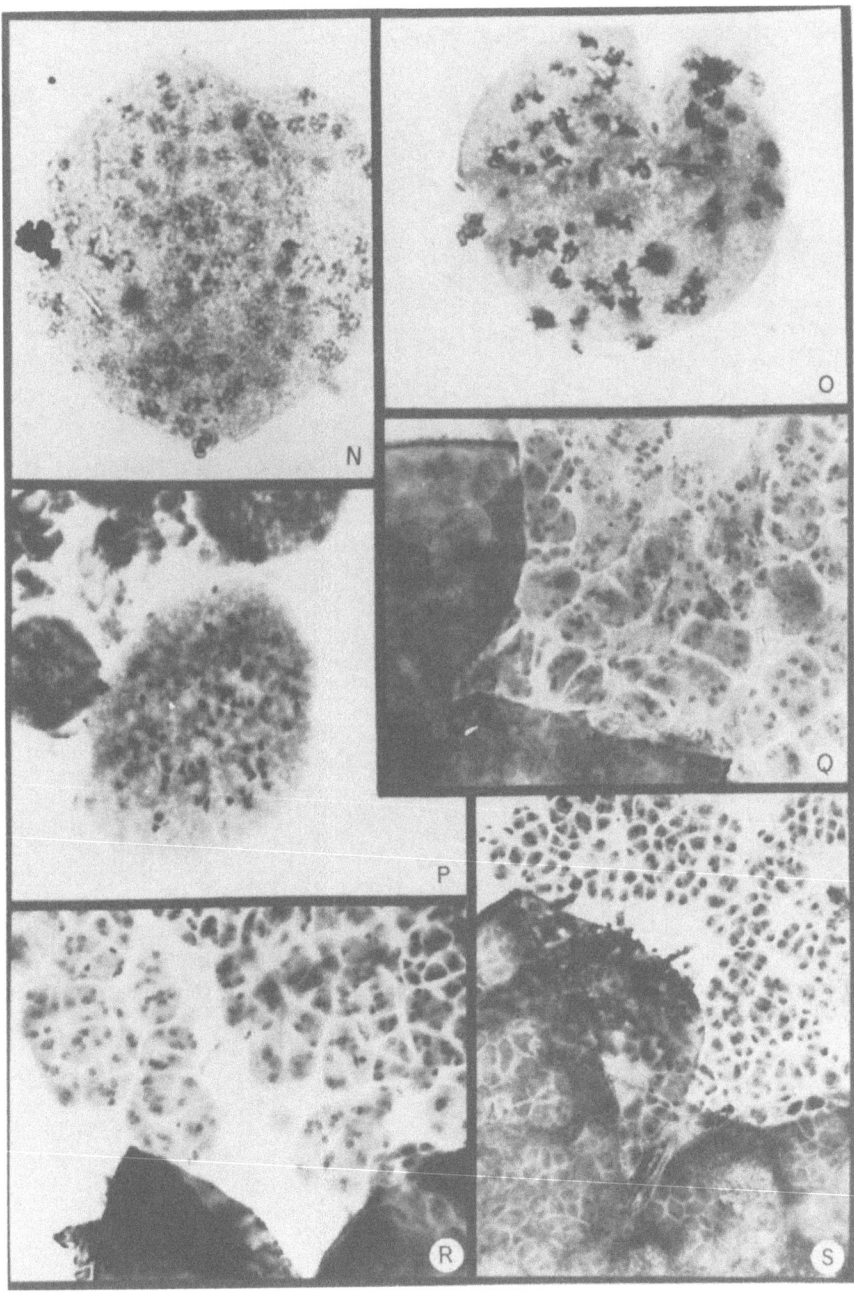

Figure 3. *(cont.)*

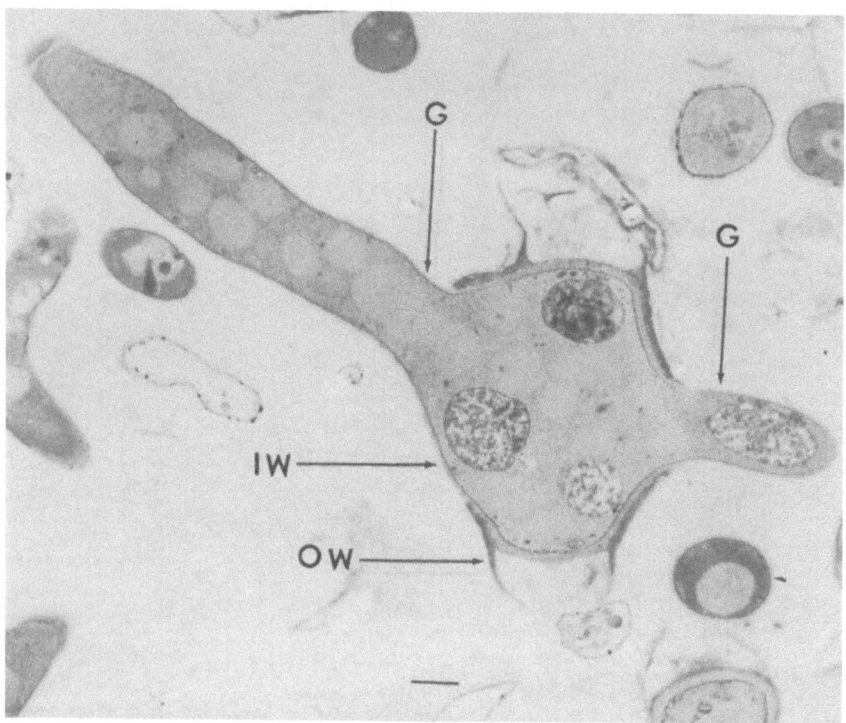

Figure 4. Arthroconidium germinating from both lateral sides. G, germ tube; IW, inner wall; OW, outer wall. (Bar represents 1 μm.)

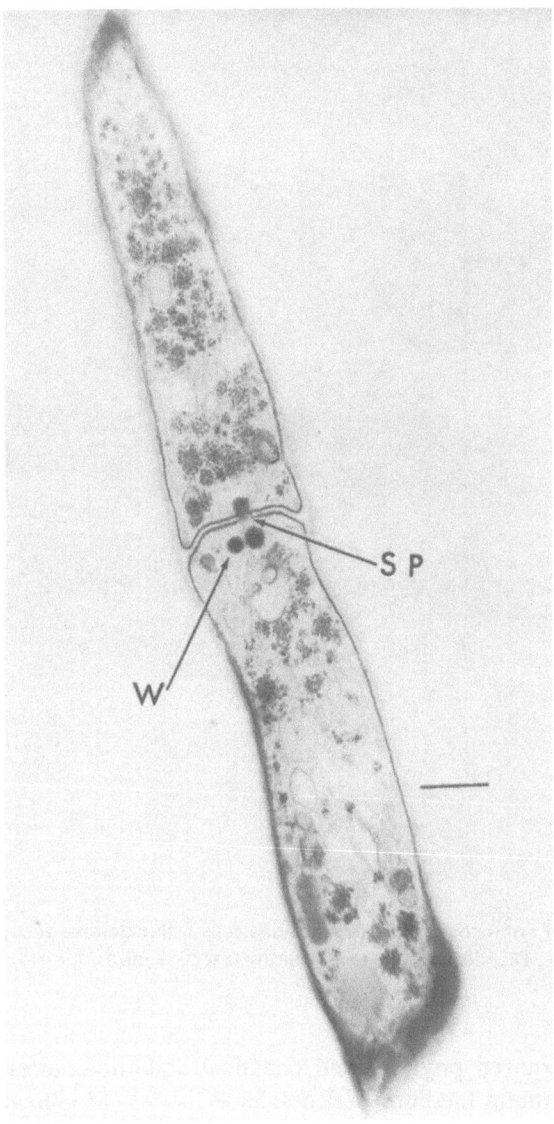

Figure 5. Apical hyphal growth with formation of septa and septal pore. SP, septal pore; W, Woronin body. (Bar represents 1 μm.)

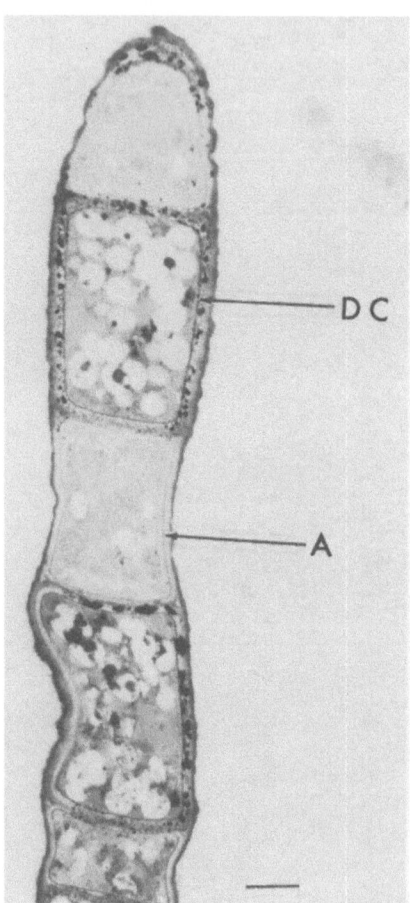

Figure 6. Chain of arthroconidia and degenerating cells with extensive vacuole formation. A, arthroconidium; DC, degenerating cell. (Bar represents 1 μm.)

defined the required physical and chemical conditions after modifying the liquid synthetic medium of Roessler *et al.*[35,36] Modifications introduced by Levine *et al.*[37] and Levine[38] made the procedure even more reproducible, and the incorporation of this into an agar gel by Brosbe[25] and by Sun *et al.*[22] made cytological studies feasible.

The spherule–endospore cycle under *in vitro* conditions is initiated with arthroconidia incubated in the modified medium of Roessler *et al.*[35,36] at 39–40°C in the presence of 20% CO_2–80% air. The thick-walled, multinucleate spores develop into round cells which for a short period (about 8 hr) appear to have only a single large, faintly stained nucleus (Figs. 2F and 3F). Progressive growth and enlargement of the

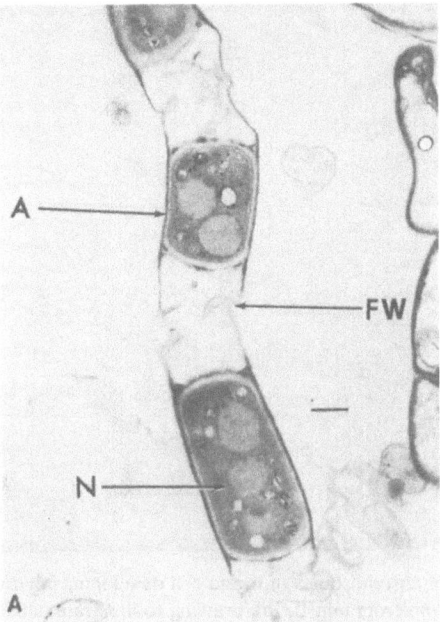

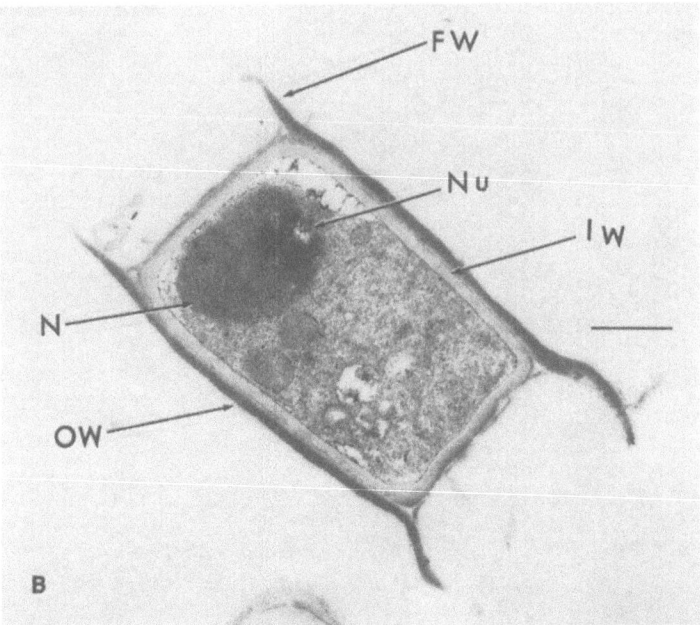

Figure 7. Release of arthroconidia by fracture of wall of degenerating cell (A) and fully developed free arthroconidium (B). A, arthroconidium; FW, fracturing wall; IW, inner wall; N, nucleus; Nu, nucleolus; OW, outer wall. (Bar represents 1 μm.)

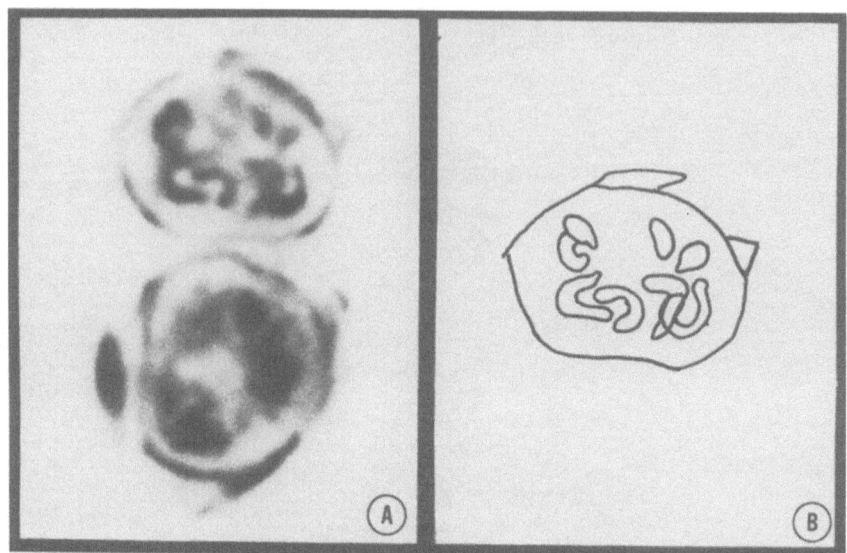

Figure 8. Four pairs of chromosomes in round cell developing *in vitro* from arthroconidum in first 24 hr. A, photomicrograph; B, ink drawing to illustrate detail.

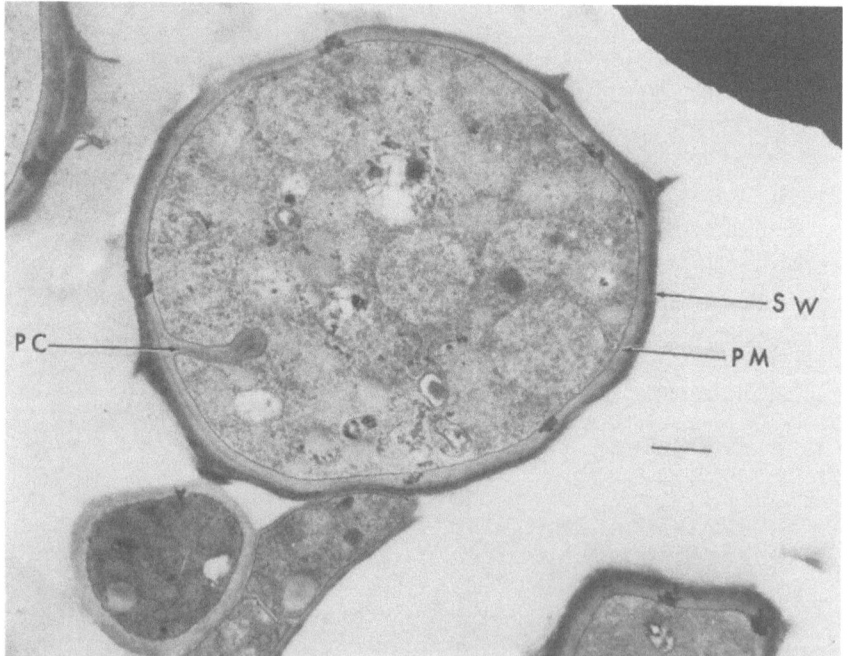

Figure 9. Initial progressive cleavage in immature spherule (*in vitro*). PC, primary cleavage; PM, plasma membrane; SW, spherule wall. (Bar represents 1 μm.)

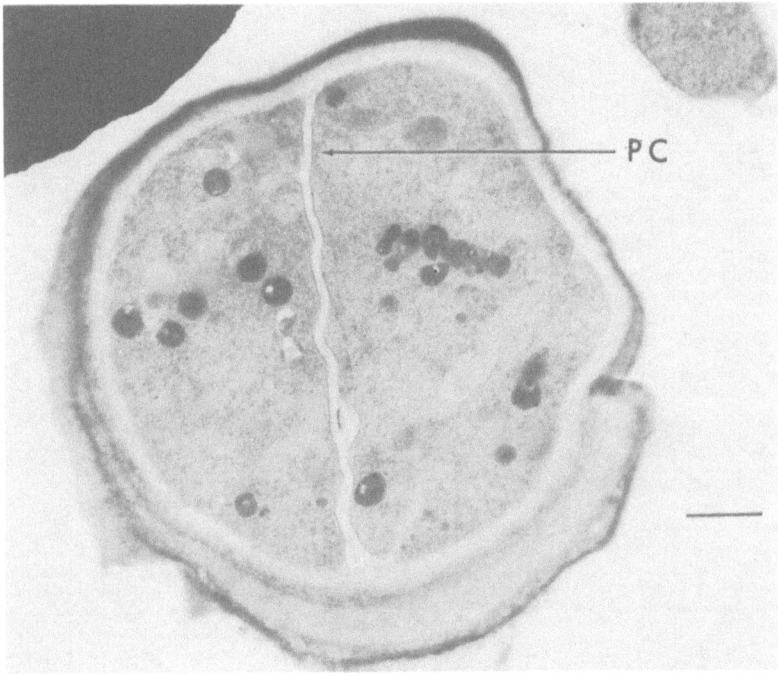

Figure 10. Primary progressive cleavage plane separating large masses of protoplasm (*in vitro*). PC, primary cleavage. (Bar represents 1 μm.)

round cell occur during 24–72 hr accompanied by successive, synchronous, nuclear divisions and thickening of the cell wall [Figs. 2 (G–P) and 3 (G–P)]. At approximately 3 days, cleavage of the protoplasm is apparent. This originates as invaginations of the cytoplasmic membrane (Fig. 9) accompanied by new wall formation, and proceeds until fusion of the several cleavage planes have separated the protoplasm into relatively large, multinucleate sections (Fig. 10). This process is continued by apparently secondary cleavage planes originating from the primary (Fig. 11) until ultimately single, apparently uninucleate endospores fill the mature, thick-walled spherule [Figs. 2 (Q–S), 3 (Q–S), and 12)]. The precise sequence resulting in release of endospores is not quite clear as yet. A ruptured wall with endospores spilling out is seen most frequently. Yet on occasion we have found what appears to be an ostiolar type of structure, i.e., an opening, from which endospores emerge. Negroni had depicted a similar structure.[39] Even though this ostiolar structure has not been demonstrated consistently, one must consider the

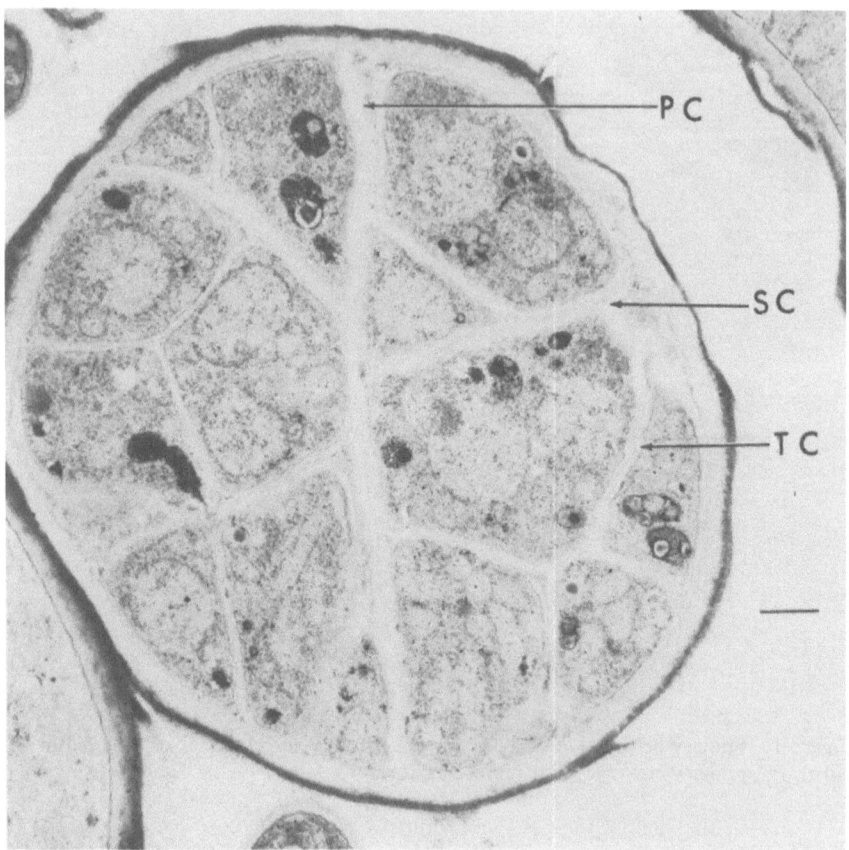

Figure 11. Secondary and tertiary cleavage planes separating smaller masses of protoplsm (*in vitro*). PC, primary cleavage; SC, secondary cleavage; TC, tertiary cleavage. (Bar represents 1 μm.)

possibility that initial release of endospores is through a pore in the spherule wall, but that increasing internal pressures generated by growing endospores eventually rupture the rigid wall.

4.6. Morphology and Morphogenesis by Electron Microscopy

Several investigators have studied finer structural details of *C. immitis* by electron microscopy.[40–43] In the hyphal form the wall is thin and apparently double layered.[40] Lipid granules and mitochondria are prominent, the latter frequently elongate. Finely granular, homogeneous nuclei are bounded by a double membrane with pores measuring about

50 nm.[41] Nucleoli can be demonstrated by their greater electron opacity relative to the nuclear substance. These are located usually adjacent to the nuclear membrane. Septum formation begins with invagination of the plasma membrane that proceeds centripetally. According to O'Hern and Henry,[41] the septal wall appears first near the lateral walls, and after the septal membrane splits, new wall material is formed between the two resulting membranes. Apparently, the septal wall derives from the inner layer of the lateral wall and the outer layer remains intact along the hyphae. Septum formation is associated with electron-dense rounded structures, presumably Woronin bodies. As noted above, the septum of hyphal cells contains a simple pore (Fig. 5), but septal wall formation is complete when arthroconidia are formed. Spores, transforming into spherules, round up, and the walls thicken and become lamellar.[40] Double-membraned nuclei containing nucleoli are present as in hyphal forms. Mitochondria are numerous and spherical in contrast to the common elongate form seen in hyphae. In addition, endoplasmic reticu-

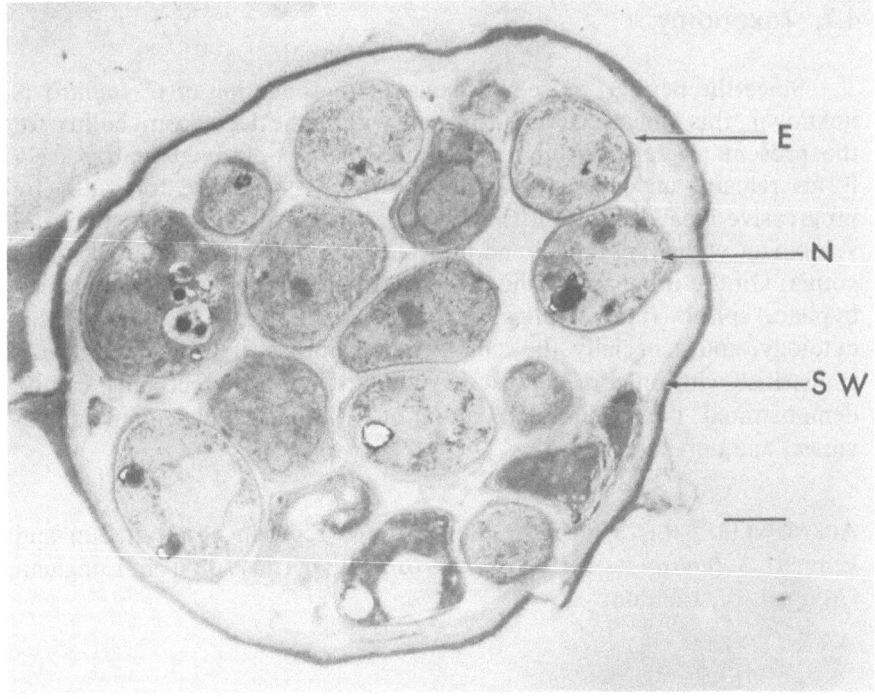

Figure 12. Mature endosporulating spherule (*in vitro*). E, endospore; N, nucleus; SW, spherule wall. (Bar represents 1 μm.)

lum is more obvious than in the mycelial form. Growth of the young spherule is accompanied by successive synchronous divisions of the nuclei and by thickening of the cell wall. Cleavage of the cytoplasm is accomplished by ingrowth of the plasma membrane at the spherule wall (Fig. 9). As the cleavage furrows advance to segment the cytoplasm into irregular packets, the membrane appears to split behind the advancing edge, and new wall material is formed between the split membrane. It appears to us that the primary cleavage furrows fuse to enclose irregular masses of cytoplasm (Fig. 10) and that secondary cleavage furrows complete the formation of endospores (Figs. 11 and 12). Baker *et al.*[13] also observed cleavage into relatively few irregular segments which could enlarge to form a spherule with a few large endospores or be followed by additional cleavage furrows to form many small endospores. The initially thin endospore wall thickens prior to liberation from within the spherule. Although it is our impression that young endospores are uninucleate (also reference 17), others have described them as both uninucleate and multinucleate.[13,40]

4.7. Taxonomy

Since the perfect, or sexual, stage of reproduction of *C. immitis* is unknown, this fungus must be placed within the Deuteromycotina for the present. A relationship to other subclasses of fungi with perfect forms remains an enigma. On the one hand, endospore formation by progressive cleavage within the spherule resembles sporangiospore development within sporangia and indicates a relationship to the Zygomycotina. On the other hand, the presence of arthroconidia, racket-shaped hyphae, spirals (i.e., hyphae coiled in a spiral shape), the nuclear cytology, and especially the simple septal pore structure, have strong similarities with fungi in the Ascomycotina. Until a perfect stage can be demonstrated, the taxonomic position of *C. immitis* will remain controversial and unresolved.

ACKNOWLEDGMENTS.   Figures 2, 3, and 8 reproduced from Sun and Huppert, *Sabouraudia* 14:185–198 (1976), with permission from Longman Group, Ltd., London.

REFERENCES

1. G. C. Ainsworth and A. S. Sussman, *The Fungi. An Advanced Treatise*, Academic Press, New York, Vol. I (1965); Vol. II (1966); Vol. III (1968); Vol. IVA and IVB (1973).

2. C. J. Alexopoulos, *Introductory Mycology,* 2nd ed., John Wiley, New York (1962).
3. E. A. Bessey, *Morphology and Taxonomy of Fungi,* Hafner, New York (1961).
4. J. H. Burnett, *Fundamentals of Mycology,* St. Martin's Press, New York (1968).
5. R. H. Whittaker, New concepts of kingdoms of organisms, *Science* **163**:150–160 (1969).
6. B. Kendrick, *Taxonomy of Fungi Imperfecti,* University of Toronto Press, Toronto (1971).
7. G. C. Ainsworth, A general purpose classification for fungi, *Bibl. Syst. Mycol.* **1**:1–4 (1966).
8. G. C. Ainsworth, *Ainsworth and Bisby's Dictionary of the Fungi,* 6th ed., Commonwealth Mycological Institute, Kew, Surrey, England (1971).
9. K. J. Kwon-Chung, A new genus, *Filobasidiella,* the perfect state of *Cryptococcus neoformans, Mycologia* **67**:1197–1200 (1975).
10. K. J. Kwon-Chung, A new species of *Filobasidiella,* the sexual state of *Cryptococcus neoformans* B and C serotypes, *Mycologia* **68**:942–946 (1976).
11. M. Huppert, S. H. Sun, and J. W. Bailey, Natural variability in *Coccidioides immitis,* in: *Coccidioidomycosis. Proceedings of the 2nd Symposium on Coccidioidomycosis* (L. Ajello, ed.), University of Arizona Press, Tucson (1967), pp. 323–328.
12. C. L. Spaur, Atypical cultures of *Coccidioides immitis, Am. J. Clin. Pathol.* **26**:689–690 (1956).
13. E. E. Baker, E. M. Mrak, and C. E. Smith, The morphology, taxonomy, and distribution of *Coccidioides immitis,* Rixford and Gilchrist, 1896, *Farlowia* **1**:199–244 (1943).
14. L. Friedman, D. Pappagianis, R. J. Berman, and C. E. Smith, Studies on *Coccidioides immitis*: Morphology and sporulation capacity of forty-seven strains, *J. Lab. Clin. Med.* **42**:438–444 (1953).
15. L. Friedman and C. E. Smith, The comparison of four strains of *Coccidioides immitis* with diverse histories, *Mycopathol. Mycol. Applic.* **8**:47–53 (1957).
16. O. A. Plunkett, L. Walker, and M. Huppert, An unusual isolate of *Coccidioides immitis* from the Los Baños area of California, *Sabouraudia* **3**:16–20 (1963).
17. C. W. Emmons, Biology of Coccidioides, in: *Biology of Pathogenic Fungi* (W. J. Nickerson, ed.), Chronica Botanica, Waltham, Mass. (1974), pp. 71–82.
18. L. Bogliolo and J. A. Neves, Researches on the etiological agents of the American blastomycosis. II. Morphology and systematic of the agent of Posadas-Wernicke's disease, *Mycopathol. Mycol. Applic.* **6**:137–160 (1952).
19. L. Sigler and J. W. Carmichael, Taxonomy of Malbranchea and some other hyphomycetes with arthroconidia, *Mycotaxon* **4**:349–488 (1976).
20. P. Negroni, Estudios sobre el *Coccidioides immitis.* III. Estudio micologico comparativo de las cepas Argentinas y Norteamericanas, *Rev. Argent. Dermatosifilol.* **32**:219–231 (1948).
21. C. W. Emmons, Fungi which resemble *Coccidioides immitis,* in: *Coccidioidomycosis. Proceedings of the 2nd Symposium on Coccidioidomycosis* (L. Ajello, ed.), University of Arizona Press, Tucson (1967), pp. 333–337.
22. S. H. Sun, M. Huppert, and K. R. Vukovich, Rapid *in vitro* conversion and identification of *Coccidioides immitis, J. Clin. Microbiol.* **3**:186–190 (1976).
23. G. F. Orr, Some fungi isolated with *Coccidioides immitis* from soils of endemic areas in California, *Bull. Torrey Bot. Club* **95**:424–431 (1968).
24. J. A. Roberts, J. M. Counts, and H. G. Crecelius, Production *in vitro* of *Coccidioides immitis* spherules and endospores as a diagnostic aid, *Am. Rev. Resp. Dis.* **102**:811–813 (1970).
25. E. A. Brosbe, Use of refined agar for the *in vitro* propagation of the spherule phase of *Coccidioides immitis, J. Bacteriol.* **93**:497–498 (1967).
26. P. G. Standard and L. Kaufman, Immunological procedure for the rapid and specific identification of *Coccidioides immitis* cultures, *J. Clin. Microbiol.* **5**:149–153 (1977).

27. W. Ophüls, Further observations on a pathogenic mould, formerly described as a protozoan *(Coccidioides immitis, Coccidioides pyogenes), J. Exp. Med.* **6**:443–485 (1905).

28. W. Ophüls and H. Moffitt, A new pathogenic mould (formerly described as a protozoan), *Coccidioides immitis, Coccidioides pyogenes.* Preliminary report, *Philadel. Med. J.* **51**:1471–1472 (1900).

29. K. J. Kwon-Chung, *Coccidioides immitis:* cytological study on the formation of the arthrospores, *Can. J. Genet. Cytol.* **11**:43–53 (1969).

30. S. H. Sun and M. Huppert, A cytological study of morphogenesis in *Coccidioides immitis, Sabouraudia* **14**:185–198 (1976).

31. G. F. Orr, H. H. Kuehn, and O. A. Plunkett, The genus *Myxotrichum* Kunze, *Can. J. Bot.* **41**:1457–1480 (1963).

32. J. L. Converse, Growth of spherules of *Coccidioides immitis* in a chemically defined liquid medium, *Proc. Soc. Exp. Biol. Med.* **90**:709–711 (1955).

33. J. L. Converse, Effect of physico-chemical environment on spherulation of *Coccidioides immitis, J. Bacteriol.* **72**:784–792 (1956).

34. J. L. Converse, Effect of surface active agents on endosporulation of *Coccidioides immitis* in a chemically defined medium, *J. Bacteriol.* **74**:106–107 (1957).

35. W. G. Roessler, E. J. Herbst, W. G. McCullough, R. C. Mills, and C. R. Brewer, Studies with *Coccidioides immitis.* I. Submerged growth in liquid mediums, *J. Infect. Dis.* **79**:12–22 (1946).

36. W. G. Roessler, E. H. Herbst, W. G. McCullough, R. C. Mills, and C. R. Brewer, The nutrition of *Coccidioides immitis* in submerged culture, *J. Bacteriol.* **51**:572 (1946).

37. H. B. Levine, J. M. Cobb, and C. E. Smith, Immunity of coccidioidomycosis induced in mice by purified spherule, arthrospores, and mycelial vaccines, *Trans. N.Y. Acad. Sci.* **22**:436–449 (1960).

38. H. B. Levine, Purification of the spherule-endospore phase of *Coccidioides immitis, Sabouraudia* **1**:112–115 (1961).

39. P. Negroni, Estudios sobre el *Coccidioides immitis* Rixford y Gilchrist. IX. Ciclo evolutivo, *An. Soc. Cient. Argent.* **149**:254–266 (1950).

40. A. M. Breslau, T. J. Hensley, and J. O. Erickson, Electron microscopy of cultured spherules of *Coccidioides immitis, J. Biophys. Biochem. Cytol.* **9**:627–637 (1961).

41. E. M. O'Hern and B. S. Henry, A cytological study of *Coccidioides immitis* by electron microscopy, *J. Bacteriol.* **72**:632–645 (1956).

42. E. M. O'Hern and B. S. Henry, An electron microscope study of *Coccidioides immitis,* in: *Proceedings of the Symposium on Coccidioidomycosis, U.S. Public Health Serv.* Publ. No. 575 (1957).

43. C. M. Koh, T. J. Choi, Y. K. Deung, and J. Lew, Electron microscopic observations of the mycelial and tissue phase of *Coccidioides immitis, Korean J. Microbiol.* **9**:169–174 (1971).

3

Mycological Diagnosis of Coccidioidomycosis

M. Huppert and S. H. Sun

1. DEFINITION

Coccidioides immitis, (Stiles) Rixford and Gilchrist, 1896, is a dimorphic fungus. In nature and on common laboratory media, *C. immitis* grows as a mycelial fungus developing alternate thallic arthroconidia (formerly arthrospores or arthroaleuriospores) (see Chapter 2). In infected hosts, *C. immitis* maintains a spherule–endospore cycle which can be reproduced consistently in the laboratory only with special physicochemical conditions.

2. PROCESSING SPECIMENS

Although coccidioidomycosis is primarily a pulmonary infection, the fungus may cause lesions in almost any tissue, i.e., disseminated disease. Therefore, the type of specimen for laboratory study will depend upon the clinical disease and accessibility of lesions. The success of the laboratory may be determined by the quality of the specimen received, and therefore both clinical and laboratory personnel should collaborate closely. In addition, distinct advantages are gained from cooperative patients who have received appropriate explanations and instructions with regard to why the specimen is required and how it is to be obtained.

2.1. Fluid Specimens

C. immitis has been recovered from pulmonary excretions, urine, blood, gastric lavage specimens, and spinal fluid and exudates into pleural, peritoneal, and synovial spaces. In addition, purulent material aspirated from accessible lesions or draining from sinus tracts is among the most rewarding specimens for microscopic demonstration and culture of the fungus (Tables 1 and 2).

2.1.1. Sputum

The most common specimen received in the laboratory is sputum. Unfortunately, it is also one of the most difficult for obtaining successful isolations. Many specimens are unsatisfactory because they represent only superficial oral secretions, and even properly collected sputum contains many transient and endogenous microorganisms from which the etiological agent must be separated. In addition, the differential diagnosis may include both mycobacterial and fungal infection as possibilities, and the customary processing procedures for the former severely reduce the chance of demonstrating the latter. For these reasons, more complicated procedures have been recommended for obtaining pulmonary specimens (e.g., bronchoscopy, transtracheal aspiration), and these have been employed successfully.

Nevertheless, sputum can be useful for isolating pathogenic fungi when it is obtained and processed properly. The best specimen is the one collected soon after the patient awakes in the morning; cumulative

TABLE 1
Results of Direct Microscopic Study of Specimens from
Patients with Coccidioidomycosis[a]

Specimens	Number positive	Number negative	Percent positive
Sputum	44	79	36
Bronchial	1	15	6
Gastric	0	9	0
Draining sinus	20	1	95
Tissues[b]	87	16	84
Fluids[c]	2	7	22
Unspecified	14	66	18
TOTALS:	168	193	47 (average)

[a] Data from Veterans Administration-Armed Forces Coccidioidomycosis Cooperative Study, 1955–1958 series.
[b] Scrapings, biopsies, surgical specimens.
[c] Cerebrospinal, pleural, ascitic, and peritoneal.

TABLE 2
Results of Cultures on Specimens from Patients with
Coccidioidomycosis[a]

Specimens	Number positive	Number negative	Percent positive
Sputum	133	125	52
Bronchial	9	22	29
Gastric	7	16	30
Draining sinus	22	1	96
Tissues[b]	60	26	70
Fluids[c]	12	15	44
Unspecified	23	70	25
TOTALS:	266	275	49 (average)

[a] Data from the Veterans Administration-Armed Forces Coccidioidomycosis Cooperative Study, 1955–1958 series.
[b] Scrapings, biopsies, surgical specimens.
[c] CSF, pleural, ascitic, peritoneal.

collections over 12-hr or longer periods are virtually useless for recovering pathogenic fungi. A small volume, even only 10 ml, of early morning sputum on successive days is far superior to a large volume of accumulated expectorant. If possible, the specimen should be obtained after cleansing the mouth thoroughly by brushing and rinsing with a mouthwash to minimize contamination with resident oral microorganisms. An informed and cooperative patient is most helpful at this point. A sterile, wide-mouth, screw-cap glass jar of 2- to 4-ounce capacity makes an excellent container. Although a clean sterile container does not seem to be an absolute requirement for collecting a naturally contaminated specimen, it is definitely preferable. There would be no justification for further complicating an already difficult procedure. Labeling on the specimen jar should indicate whether the pulmonary excretion had been induced with mucolytic agents, since liquefied material may be mistaken for saliva by laboratory personnel and rejected as unsatisfactory. The collected specimen should be transported immediately to the laboratory. Excessive delay favors bacterial multiplication and complicates processing unnecessarily.

Several techniques have been employed for selecting material from sputum. Regardless of the method used, material for demonstrating the presence of pathogenic fungi must be obtained prior to the digestion procedures employed for recovery of mycobacteria, since these kill a large portion of the fungus population present.[1,2] The classical approach has been to spread the specimen in a petri dish and select caseous, purulent, or granular flecks for examination and culture. Experienced personnel have used this method with variable success, but better procedures have been developed. We considered that homogenization of the sputum would distribute organisms more uniformly and that this would increase the chance of recovering fungi by sampling from the homogenate. This was achieved by preparing the screw-cap jars prior to use with a layer of glass beads (3- to 4-mm diameter) in the bottom. Since homogenization might produce dangerous aerosols, the screw cap was modified by removing the pulp liner, drilling a 6-mm hole through the cap, and cementing a rubber diaphragm into the cap. After collecting the specimen and securing the cap, the jars were shaken vigorously by machine for 30 min and samples were removed by aspiration with a syringe and needle through the hole in the cap. Comparative studies demonstrated not only an increased frequency of positive cultures, but also greater numbers of fungus colonies on each culture medium. An even better method has been reported by Reep and Kaplan.[2] They treated sputum samples with mucolytic agents (0.5% solution in 2.94% sodium citrate) for 5–10 sec in a vortex mixer followed by standing at room temperature for 15 min. Phosphate buffer (M/15, pH 6.8) was added, mixed by inversion, and centrifuged (950g, 15 min). The supernate was decanted and cultures made from the sediment. In 20 tests with sputa seeded with *C. immitis*, at least 95% recovery was achieved with mucolytic agents compared to 30% by decontamination–digestion with alkali. Dithiothreitol and *N*-acetyl-1-cysteine worked equally well as mucolytic agents. This Reep and Kaplan method should be readily adaptable into clinical laboratory routine with the advantages of rapid processing and high recovery of fungi from sputum.

2.1.2. Spinal Fluid

A diagnosis of coccidioidal meningitis is difficult to establish by demonstration of the fungus and in most cases, can be only inferred from serological results, albeit with a high level of confidence. Nevertheless, attempts to recover the fungus from spinal fluid are justified for two reasons: Success establishes the diagnosis unequivocably, and positive serology with cerebrospinal fluid may occur in nonmeningitic coccidioidomycosis. Pappagianis *et al.*[3] have reported that patients with juxtadural lesions or with comparatively high serum antibody levels occasionally yield positive spinal fluid serology, particularly if the spinal fluid is concentrated in an attempt to detect low levels of antibody. Additional justification for attempting recovery of the fungus derives from the fact that a spinal fluid specimen can be used for both mycological and serological studies.

Three principal methods have been used for demonstrating *C. immitis* in spinal fluid. With either of these, when the specimen is obtained aseptically, extreme care must be exercised to avoid inclusion of blood. If the patient should have a high level of serum antibody, this might be detected in serological tests with spinal fluid and lead to a possibly erroneous diagnosis of meningitis.

The simplest method is to remove a small volume for serology and to incubate the remainder. If viable fungus is present, it often will appear on the surface of the fluid as a cottony growth, but this may require up to one month. In the second and usually more successful procedure, the spinal fluid is centrifuged and the supernatant removed for serology. Portions of the sediment can be examined microscopically and cultured on suitable media. The third method is based on the demonstration by Wayne and Juarez[4] that *C. immitis* grows well on molecular filter membranes placed on culture media after filtration of the spinal fluid. Huppert et al.[5] showed that these filtrates yielded the same complement fixation titers as the unfiltered specimen, even though some protein was adsorbed to the membrane.[6] The filtration procedure has certain advantages to recommend it. When membranes with a pore size of 0.45 μm or less are used, one would expect to trap 100% of any fungal elements present, an efficiency which centrifugation is not likely to achieve. In addition, all viable fungus would have been removed from the filtrate sent to serology, thereby avoiding potential accidental infections.

2.1.3. Pus and Exudates

C. immitis can be found frequently in purulent material. Specimens should be aspirated with a syringe and needle from closed abscesses withdrawing as much volume as possible. Strict aseptic technique should be used when obtaining empyema specimens by percutaneous aspiration, not only to avoid contamination, but also to prevent introduction of surface microorganisms into the pleural space. An open abscess or a draining sinus tract probably is contaminated with surface and airborne microorganisms. The lesions should be cleansed thoroughly and specimens obtained by curetting. Swabbings are generally unsatisfactory because only small amounts of material are obtained, reducing opportunities for success by direct examination and culture.

2.1.4. Others

These may include bronchial washings, gastric lavage, blood, and urine, which can be processed by centrifugation or by membrane filtration if the volume is not too great.

2.2. Solid Lesions

Surgically removed tissues offer the best opportunity for obtaining diagnostic results (Tables 1 and 2). Specimen selection is more accurate and frequently contains a higher concentration of fungi than found in fluid specimens. Nevertheless, the degree of success in attaining efficient and accurate results will depend on the internist, surgeon, pathologist, and microbiologist cooperating as a unit rather than as individuals. Under these circumstances, any fungus recovered may be significant provided careful handling has excluded the possibility of contaminating the specimen.

Solid specimens should be divided into portions for histopathology and mycology laboratories. The division should be careful and selective rather than random to assure each laboratory a sample containing lesions. A portion of the lesion and any caseous material present should be transferred to sterile containers for the mycology laboratory. If multiple lesions are present, each should be handled separately since it is possible that more than one species of microorganism may be found in a single lesion or in different areas of the tissue. If suppurative material is present, a sample should be removed for immediate direct examination by microscopy. Tissues can be minced with sterile scissors or homogenized with a manually operated apparatus such as a mortar and pestle or in a Ten-Broeck-type tissue grinder. The latter is preferred because sterile mineral oil can be layered over the tissue to prevent dispersion of aerosols. If high-speed homogenizers are used, this should be done in a safety hood because of the danger of aerosol formation. Since these blenders generate high temperatures quickly, they should be operated for only short periods, alternating with cooling.

3. LABORATORY IDENTIFICATION

Three principal operations are involved in attempts by laboratory personnel to demonstrate and identify *C. immitis*: direct examination by microscopy, growth of the fungus on culture media, and reproduction of the disease in laboratory animals. The last is required when characteristic endosporulating spherules are not demonstrable. Even cultures which appear to be *C. immitis* must be tested for pathogenicity, because there are many species of saprobic fungi which resemble *C. immitis* in culture.[7,8]

3.1. Direct Microscopic Study

Ideally, every specimen should be examined microscopically. Heavy workloads, however, may necessitate a compromise between the time spent on a specimen and the chance of obtaining rewarding results. One can judge from the results in Table 1 the type of specimens most likely to be productive. It is obvious also that a negative result never excludes a diagnosis of coccidioidomycosis, since these patients (Table 1) all had proven coccidioidomycosis.

Pathological materials should be searched for the characteristic endosporulating spherule of *C. immitis* (Fig. 1). This appears as a thick-walled, nonbudding, large round ball containing spores within the outer shell. The mature spherule may be 20–60 μm in diameter and the endospores 2–5 μm. The spherule may be filled completely with endo-

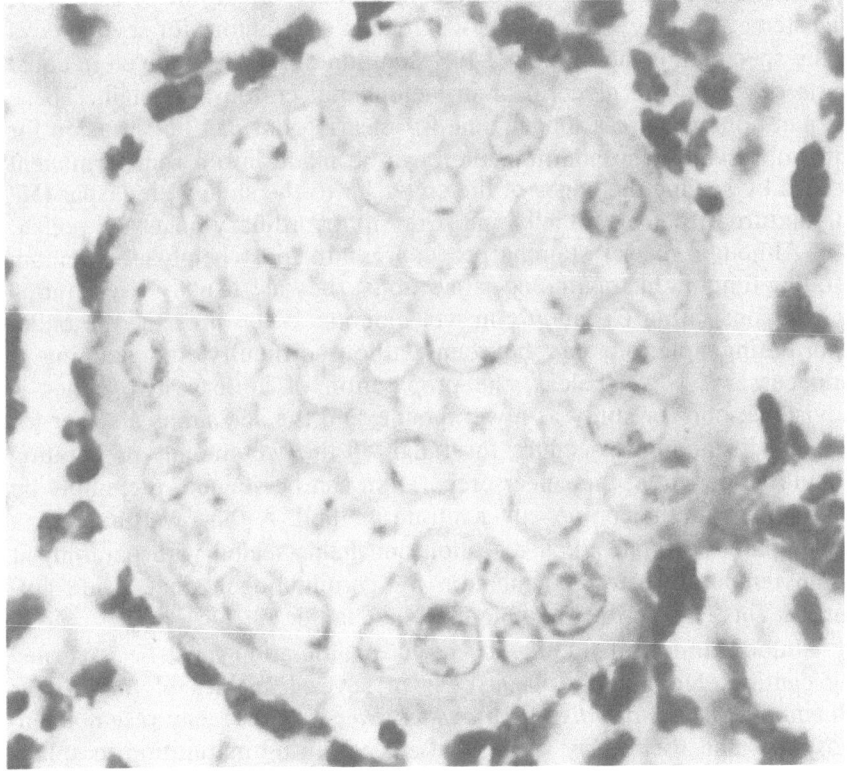

Figure 1. Endosporulating spherule.

spores or may have a central vacuole with endospores lining the inner side of the spherule wall. In the latter case, the endospores usually appear more rectangular than round and are probably immature. In the natural parasitic cycle, the spherule wall ruptures releasing the endospores into the surrounding tissue, and each endospore carries the potential for developing into a new endosporulating spherule. In addition to spherules, hyphae and even alternating arthroconidia may be found in 70–75% of specimens from cavitary lesions and in about 30% from granulomatous lesions of the lung.[9–11]

Specimens for direct examination can be prepared as either wet mounts or stained preparations. In the wet mount method, a small portion of the specimen is placed in one or two drops of alkali (10–20% NaOH or KOH) on a glass slide. A glass coverslip is placed on top and the slide is warmed gently to drive out air bubbles and to hasten the clearing process. Almost all host tissues will be dissolved, but fungi are quite resistant because of their chitinous cell wall. This type of preparation must be examined within a few hours, since all cells will be digested eventually. Wet mounts will remain satisfactory for several days if the specimen is mounted in a 10% solution of alkali dissolved in equal parts of water and glycerin or in lactophenol cotton blue stain. These preparations require a longer time for clearing but can be set aside for later observation; in addition, they can be made into a semipermanent record by sealing the edges of the coverslip to the slide with vaspar (50/ 50 mixture of petroleum jelly and paraffin) or ordinary fingernail polish.

Although special staining procedures are most helpful for demonstrating fungi in histopathological sections, they are usually not required for demonstrating *C. immitis* in wet mounts. When present, the endosporulating spherule can be seen without difficulty and staining is unnecessary. Nevertheless, the preparation of at least two slides is advisable: one for study as a wet mount, and the second as a smear for a special staining procedure for fungi. If the wet mount preparation should be negative, the smear preparation can be stained, preferably by the Gomori methenamine–silver nitrate method. A third wet mount can be prepared without alkali digestion and held (sealed with paraffin) at room temperature for examination for germinating hyphae (slide cultures). This is described and pictured in Chapter 13.

Interpretation of findings by direct examination must be governed by caution. Nonbudding yeast cells of several species of fungi (e.g., *Blastomyces dermatitidis, Cryptococcus neoformans*) may resemble endospores and their early successive stages during maturation to spherules. Occasionally, several endospores overlying one another may resemble budding yeast cells. Hyphal elements are not sufficiently characteristic to justify interpretation as *C. immitis*. Therefore, one must search for mature endosporulating spherules, and even these may not be definitive in sputum or gastric specimens, since some pollens (e.g., elm) may superficially resemble the endosporulating spherule. Structures seen in material from mucocutaneous lesions must be differentiated from *Rhinosporidium seeberi*. The mature endosporulating spherules of *R. seeberi* are much larger (up to 350 μm), but collapsed forms of younger immature stages resemble the shells of *C. immitis* spherules which have released their endospores. Mucicarmine stains *R. seeberi* but not *C. immitis*. Differential diagnosis of fungi seen in tissue specimens is also discussed in Chapter 7.

3.2. Cultures

The fungi which are pathogenic for humans and animals grow well on aqueous media containing digests of biological origin, and a variety of culture media can be used. Most of these fungi, however, grow slowly, and if the specimen contains bacteria, the fungi either may never develop or may be inapparent and overlooked. Therefore, primary culture media used in medical mycology have been selected for ability to support growth of fungi while restricting development of bacteria. Basically, these media are either quite acid (e.g., Sabouraud's dextrose agar, pH 5.5) or contain substances which strongly inhibit bacteria with relatively little effect on pathogenic fungi (e.g., broad spectrum antibacterial antibiotics such as chloramphenicol or gentamicin). Furthermore, the inclusion of cycloheximide adds a second dimension, since this antibiotic inhibits most of the common contaminating fungi. Media containing cycloheximide should never be used as the only culture media for two reasons. First, this antibiotic does inhibit some species of pathogenic yeasts. Second, many of the opportunistic infections among immunologically compromised patients are caused by fungi sensitive to cycloheximide.

Since cultures of *C. immitis* are an infection hazard for laboratory personnel (discussed below), special safety precautions are required. The use of petri dishes for mycological media should be discouraged, and if fungus colonies grow on bacteriological media in petri dishes, these should be taped completely and opened only in a safety hood. Media for culturing fungi should be contained in prescription-type glass bottles or test tubes. Several modifications have been described for handling potentially dangerous fungus colonies with safety.[12-14] Basically, these involve modification of the closure so that aeration and access to the culture is accomplished through a self-sealing rubber diaphragm. After specimens have been planted and the container closed, it need never be opened again.

Although the cultural characteristics of *C. immitis* are extremely variable,[15-18] the majority of strains (about 80%) at primary isolation are quite consistent. After 3–4 days at either room or incubator temperatures, colonies appear as a grayish membranous growth. Within the next few days, aerial hyphae develop, varying in color from white to grayish and in texture from loose and cobwebby to dense and cottony. These "typical" colonies do not usually develop any marked pigmentation either on the surface or underside. Many of these strains grow quite rapidly and, on uncontaminated media, a single colony may overgrow the entire surface of the culture medium in 2–3 weeks, frequently with concentric rings of cottony to wooly aerial hyphae separated by rings of sparse growth. In contrast, "atypical" colonies can be extremely variable with respect to rate and extent of growth, color and texture of aerial hyphae, and pigmentation in the agar (see Chapter 2, Section 4.2).

Since the cultural characteristics of *C. immitis* are variable and since there are many species of saprobic fungi which culturally resemble *C. immitis*,[7,8] the selection of colonies from a primary isolation culture can be a problem. Fortunately, a culture medium containing cycloheximide can be helpful.[19-21] All strains of *C. immitis* grow well on media containing 0.4 mg/ml cycloheximide, and this concentration of antibiotic inhibits most saprobic fungi. Therefore, growth on the antibiotic media could be considered a screening test for selection of colonies to be studied, and the corollary to this premise would be that any fungus growing in the presence of 0.4 mg/ml cycloheximide should be considered potentially *C. immitis* until proven otherwise.

Cultural characteristics alone are too variable for identification of a fungus to the species level, but typical microscopic structures are more significant. These can be demonstrated either in wet mount preparations or slide cultures. The most common strains of *C. immitis* produce septate hyphae approximating 2 μm in width, and cylindrical, thick-walled arthroconidia generally 3–4.5 μm in width and 3–12 μm in length.[15] The conidia along a strand of hypha usually are separated from each other by an apparently empty cell, but occasionally two or more conidia are contiguous (Fig. 2). Although the morphology of these microscopic structures is quite consistent among most primary isolates, variations do occur just as in cultural characteristics.

Since these conidia are infectious, it is most important for laboratory personnel to recognize the potential hazard of any fungus colony and especially those growing in the presence of cycloheximide. The empty cells interspersed among the arthroconidia are very fragile and readily

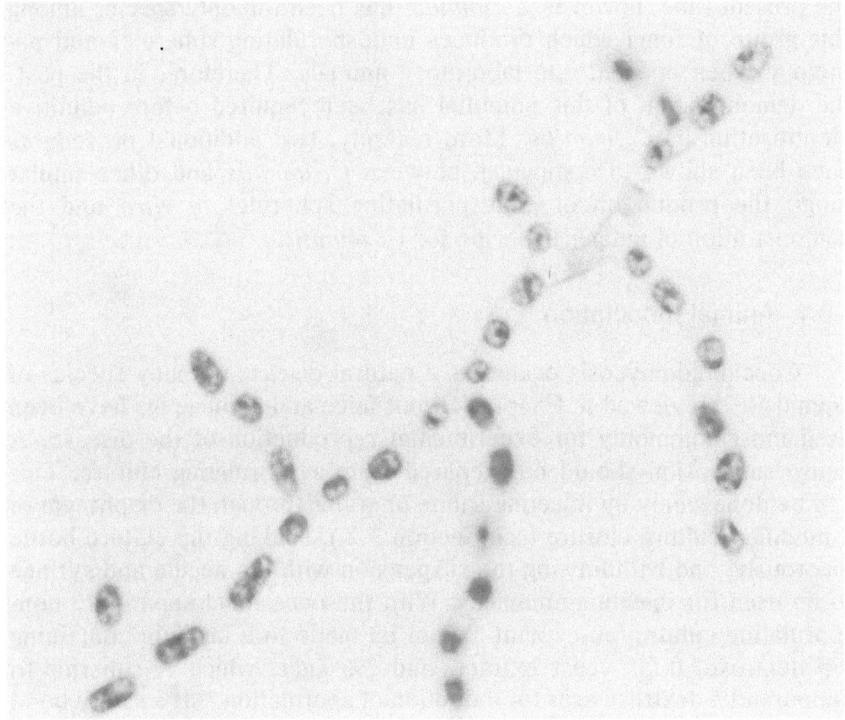

Figure 2. Branched chain of developing arthroconidia.

fractured. Any manipulation of these cultures can create a conidia-bearing aerosol. *C. immitis* is one of the most common causes of laboratory infections.[22,23] Wedum and Kruse[22] reported that laboratory-acquired infections of *C. immitis* ranked ninth in frequency among 2912 infections caused by 111 etiological agents. Hence, appropriate safety precautions must be instituted and adhered to meticulously.

Results with DTM (dermatophyte test medium), which is often used in diagnosis of dermal lesions, are discussed in Chapter 13.

3.3. Confirmation of Identification

The colony characteristics and morphology of microscopic structures are not so distinctive that an isolate can be categorically identified as *C. immitis*. As mentioned already, there is sufficient variation in these properties among proven strains of *C. immitis* so that differentiation from other species of fungi with similar characteristics is required. Up to the present time, however, *C. immitis* has been the only species among this group of fungi which produces endosporulating spherules and pathology when injected into laboratory animals. Therefore, in the past, the demonstration of this potential has been required before definitive identification as *C. immitis*. More recently, two additional procedures have been shown to distinguish between *C. immitis* and other similar fungi: the production of endosporulating spherules *in vitro* and the demonstration of antigens specific for *C. immitis*.

3.3.1. Animal Inoculation

Coccidioidomycosis occurs as a natural disease in many species of animals[24,25] (reviewed in Chapter 4), but mice and guinea pigs have been used most commonly for experimental reproduction of the disease. A dense suspension should be prepared from a sporulating culture. This can be done safely by injecting saline or water through the diaphragm of a modified culture closure (see Section 3.2.), shaking the culture bottle vigorously, and withdrawing the suspension with the needle and syringe to be used for injecting animals.[12] With the occasional apparently non-sporulating culture, an explant should be made to a medium containing 1% dextrose, 0.5% yeast extract, and 2% agar, which is superior to Sabouraud's dextrose agar for induction of sporulation.[18] If a safety hood is available, a small portion of the suspect colony can be cut out and transferred to a sterile bottle (with modified closure) containing a layer of glass beads and 1–2 ml of sterile saline or water. Vigorous mechanical shaking for 15–30 min will produce a fairly uniform suspension, additional diluent (about 4 ml) can be added, and the suspension withdrawn into a syringe. Mice should be injected intraperitoneally (0.5 ml) and male guinea pigs intratesticularly (0.5–1.0 ml). At least three animals should be used for sacrificing at 1, 2, and 3 weeks to obtain confirmation of pathogenicity as early as possible. It is not unusual to find extremely large (up to 200 μm in diameter) endosporulating spherules in these experimentally infected animals.

3.3.2. Culture Spherules

Although *in vitro* methods for inducing endosporulating spherules have been reported by several investigators (reviewed in reference 24), the most successful and reproducible procedures are based on the Roessler liquid medium[26,27] as modified by Converse[28–30] or by Levine *et al.*[31,32] Both of the latter investigators inoculated the liquid cultures with arthroconidia, incubated them at 40°C or 37°C with shaking, and obtained endosporulating spherules in 2–5 days. Roberts *et al.*[33] adapted this method as a diagnostic aid using stationary cultures at 40°C and found that all of 201 strains of *C. immitis* converted to endosporulating spherules in 1–8 days with maximum frequency at 2–3 days incubation. Brosbe[34] incorporated the nutrients into refined agar and reported conversions with incubation at 37°C or 40°C in an environment of 20% CO_2–80% air. Sun *et al.*[35] confirmed the results of Brosbe and added (1) that conversion occurred equally well in a simple candle jar incubated at 37° or 40°C, (2) that 40°C incubation was preferable because mycelial development was inhibited, while at 37°C mycelia and a new generation of potentially hazardous arthroconidia developed, and (3) that six species of fungi resembling *C. immitis* did not develop endosporulating spherules. This last observation is critical for confirming the identification as *C. immitis*. The relatively simple conversion procedure on agar media should be readily adaptable into the routine of clinical microbiology laboratories.

3.3.3. Immunological

Standard and Kaufman[36] considered that if *C. immitis* produced species-specific antigens these could be identified with appropriate reference antisera to confirm the identity of a suspect culture. Heavily inoculated duplicate broth cultures were incubated at 25°C with shaking, and killed after 3 and 6 days with thimerosal. Supernatants were concentrated rapidly (10-fold and 25-fold) and tested in an agar gel double diffusion system against a reference antigen–antibody system that produced three lines of precipitate. All of 66 isolates, identified later as *C. immitis*, developed one or more lines of identity with the reference system; three strains of *Auxarthron* species produced a single band of precipitate, but this differed from the three in the reference system; and 97 additional cultures which were not *C. immitis* failed to react with the antiserum. It is important to recognize that 10 of the latter, in addition to the 3 strains producing bands of nonidentity, were fungi that most resemble *C. immitis*; i.e., *Arachniotus, Auxarthron, Malbranchea, Myxotrichum,* and *Pseudoarachniotus.* In an extensive and currently continuing evaluation of this method (unpublished results), we have confirmed the results reported by Standard and Kaufman: all strains of *C. immitis* were identified, and none of the species resembling *C. immitis* produced lines of identity, although four strains of *Malbranchea* species have developed rather weak lines of nonidentity. If the 100% record for identifying *C. immitis* continues, this should be the simplest and most useful method for the clinical laboratory to confirm the identity of a culture as *C. immitis*.

REFERENCES

1. L. Ajello, V. Q. Grant, and M. A. Gutske, The effect of tubercle bacillus concentration procedures on fungi causing pulmonary mycoses, *J. Lab. Clin. Med.* **38**:3–8 (1951).
2. B. R. Reep and W. Kaplan, The use of *N*-acetyl-l-cysteine and dithiothreitol to process sputa for mycological and fluorescent antibody examinations, *Health Lab. Sci.* **9**:118–124 (1972).
3. D. Pappagianis, M. Saito, and K. H. Van Hoosear, Antibody in cerebrospinal fluid in non-meningitic coccidioidomycosis, *Sabouraudia* **10**:173–179 (1972).
4. L. G. Wayne and W. J. Juarez, Isolation of *Coccidioides immitis* from spinal fluid by molecular filter membrane technic, *Am. J. Clin. Pathol.* **25**:1209–1211 (1955).
5. M. Huppert, L. J. Walker, and J. W. Bailey, Complement fixation for coccidioidomycosis on spinal fluids filtered through molecular membranes, *J. Bacteriol.* **83**:692 (1962).
6. L. G. Wayne and G. C. Kidd, Adsorption of chemical constituents of cerebrospinal fluid by molecular filter membrane, *Am. J. Clin. Pathol.* **28**:495–497 (1957).
7. C. W. Emmons, Fungi which resemble *Coccidioides immitis*, in: *Coccidioidomycosis. Proceedings of the 2nd Symposium on Coccidioidomycosis* (L. Ajello, ed.), University of Arizona Press, Tucson (1967), pp. 333–337.
8. L. Sigler and J. W. Carmichael, Taxonomy of *Malbranchea* and some other hyphomycetes with arthroconidia, *Mycotaxon* **4**:349–488 (1976).
9. D. Salkin and B. H. Evans, in: *Coccidioidomycosis. The Treatment of Mycotic and Parasitic Diseases of the Chest* (J. Steele, ed.), Charles C. Thomas, Springfield, Ill. (1964), pp. 55–119.
10. T. F. Peckett, Hyphae of *Coccidioides immitis* in tissues of the human host, *Am. Rev. Tuberc.* **70**:320–327 (1954).
11. W. D. Forbus and A. M. Bestebreurtje, Coccidioidomycosis: A study of 95 cases of the disseminated type with special reference to the pathogenesis of the disease, *Mil. Surg.* **99**:653–719 (1946).
12. M. Huppert, A technique for the safe handling of *Coccidioides immitis* cultures, *J. Lab. Clin. Med.* **50**:158–164 (1957).
13. R. H. Kruse, Potential aerogenic laboratory hazards of *Coccidioides immitis*, *Am. J. Clin. Pathol.* **37**:150–161 (1962).
14. D. T. Omieczynski, Safe isolation of *Coccidioides immitis* from clinical specimens, *Health Lab. Sci.* **7**:227–232 (1970).
15. M. Huppert, S. H. Sun, and J. W. Bailey, Natural variability in *Coccidioides immitis*, in: *Coccidioidomycosis. Proceedings of the 2nd Symposium on Coccidioidomycosis* (L. Ajello, ed.), University of Arizona Press, Tucson (1967), pp. 323–328.
16. C. L. Spaur, Atypical cultures of *Coccidioides immitis*, *Am. J. Clin. Pathol.* **26**:689–690 (1956).
17. E. E. Baker, E. M. Mrak, and C. E. Smith, The morphology, taxonomy, and distribution of *Coccidioides immitis*, Rixford and Gilchrist, 1896, *Farlowia* **1**:199–244 (1943).
18. L. Friedman, D. Pappagianis, R. J. Berman, and C. E. Smith, Studies on *Coccidioides immitis:* morphology and sporulation capacity of forty-seven strains, *J. Lab. Clin. Med.* **42**:438–444 (1953).
19. M. Huppert and L. J. Walker, The selective and differential effects of cycloheximide on many strains of *Coccidioides immitis*, *Am. J. Clin. Pathol.* **29**:291–295 (1958).
20. L. K. Georg, L. Ajello, and M. A. Gordon, A selective medium for the isolation of *Coccidioides immitis*, *Science* **114**:387–389 (1951).
21. L. K. Georg, L. Ajello, and C. Papageorge, Use of cycloheximide in the selective isolation of fungi pathogenic to man, *J. Lab. Clin. Med.* **44**:422–428 (1954).

22. A. G. Wedum and R. H. Kruse, Assessment of risk of human infection in the microbiology laboratory, Dept. of the Army, Fort Detrick, Misc. Publ. No. 30 (1969), pp. 1–89.
23. J. E. Johnson, J. E. Perry, F. R. Fekety, P. J. Kadull, and L. E. Cluff, Laboratory-acquired coccidioidomycosis. A report of 210 cases, *Ann. Intern. Med.* **60**:941–956 (1964).
24. M. J. Fiese, *Coccidioidomycosis,* Charles C. Thomas, Springfield, Ill. (1958).
25. K. T. Maddy, Coccidioidomycosis in animals, *Vet. Med.* **54**:233–242 (1959).
26. W. G. Roessler, E. J. Herbst, W. G. McCullough, R. C. Mills, and C. R. Brewer, Studies with *Coccidioides immitis.* I. Submerged growth in liquid mediums, *J. Infect. Dis.* **79**:12–22 (1946).
27. W. G. Roessler, E. H. Herbst, W. G. McCullough, R. C. Mills, and C. R. Brewer, The nutrition of *Coccidioides immitis* in submerged culture, *J. Bacteriol.* **51**:572 (1946).
28. J. L. Converse, Growth of spherules of *Coccidioides immitis* in a chemically defined liquid medium, *Proc. Soc. Exp. Biol. Med.* **90**:709–711 (1955).
29. J. L. Converse, Effect of physico-chemical environment on spherulation of *Coccidioides immitis*, *J. Bacteriol.* **72**:784–792 (1956).
30. J. L. Converse, Effect of surface active agents on endosporulation of *Coccidioides immitis* in a chemically defined medium, *J. Bacteriol.* **74**:106–107 (1957).
31. H. B. Levine, J. M. Cobb, and C. E. Smith, Immunity of coccidioidomycosis induced in mice by purified spherule, arthrospores, and mycelial vaccines, *Trans. N.Y. Acad. Sci.* **22**:436–449 (1960).
32. H. B. Levine, Purification of the spherule-endospore phase of *Coccidioides immitis*, *Sabouraudia* **1**:112–115 (1961).
33. J. A. Roberts, J. M. Counts, and H. G. Crecelius, Production *in vitro* of *Coccidioides immitis* spherules and endospores as a diagnostic aid, *Am. Rev. Resp. Dis.* **102**:811–813 (1970).
34. E. A. Brosbe, Use of refined agar for the *in vitro* propagation of the spherule phase of *Coccidioides immitis*, *J. Bacteriol.* **93**:497–498 (1967).
35. S. H. Sun, M. Huppert, and K. R. Vukovich, Rapid *in vitro* conversion and identification of *Coccidioides immitis*, *J. Clin. Microbiol.* **3**:186–190 (1976).
36. P. G. Standard and L. Kaufman, Immunological procedure for the rapid and specific identification of *Coccidioides immitis* cultures, *J. Clin. Microbiol.* **5**:149–153 (1977).

4

Epidemiology of Coccidioidomycosis

Demosthenes Pappagianis

1. GEOGRAPHIC

Coccidioidomycosis is primarily a disease of the New World in which certain soil foci harbor *Coccidioides immitis* (Fig. 1). However, the disease, acquired by inhalation of airborne arthroconidia from the soil, may lead to infections in persons outside the endemic foci either because the individuals have traveled or lived in the endemic areas, or more rarely, because the arthroconidia are transported on some product (fomites), e.g., cotton contaminated in the endemic areas or on the wind. The endemic areas have remained relatively well delimited. While it is true that new endemic foci have been demonstrated over the past several years, e.g., in Northern California, these have been within or near the established outlines of endemicity. The endemic area extends from approximately 40° N 120° W in California to the north to 40° S 65° W in Argentina to the south.

1.1. Endemic Areas

1.1.1. North America

1.1.1.1. United States. The states in which coccidioidomycosis is endemic are California, Arizona, New Mexico, Texas, Nevada, and Utah, in which some 20% of the population of the United States resides. The areas affected in Nevada, New Mexico, and Utah are not well defined. Some patients from the Las Vegas area of Nevada apparently

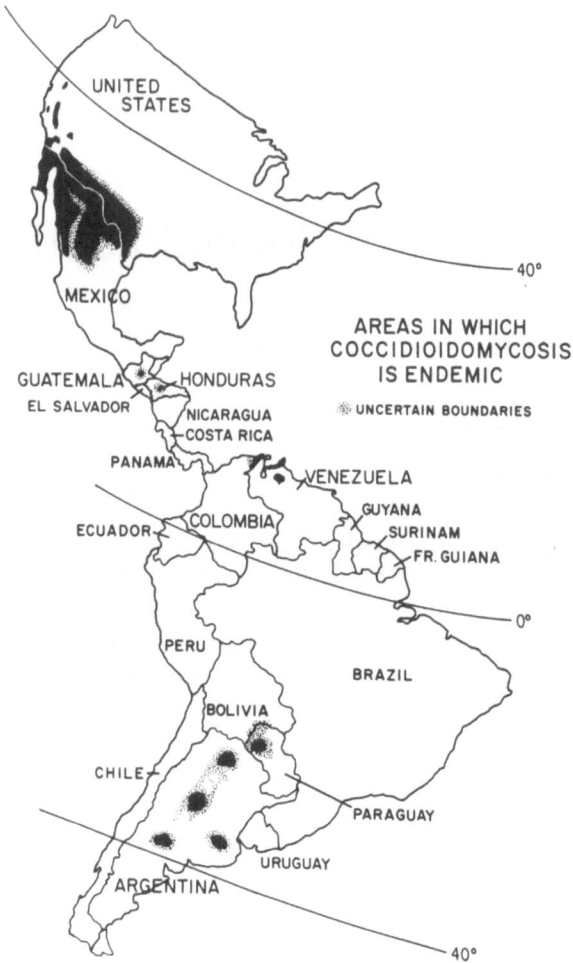

Figure 1. Geographic distribution of *C. immitis* and sites where coccidioidomycosis is usually acquired.

acquired coccidioidal infections near there, but precisely where is unknown. From skin test surveys in humans and from isolation of *C. immitis* from local rodents, the southwest corner of Utah (near St. George) appears endemic. The southern portion of New Mexico appears to be endemic.

In California, infections have been acquired from as far north as Tehama County near Red Bluff to as far south as San Diego County near Chula Vista (Fig. 2). Most affected areas are inland, e.g., along the San

Joaquin River and the Sacramento River Valleys enclosed between the Sierra Nevada range of mountains to the east and the Coast Range to the west. However, there are endemic foci west of the Coast Range, e.g., Camp Roberts in San Luis Obispo County; and San Diego County was the locus of a small outbreak of the disease approximately one mile from the Pacific Ocean. More recently, a sea otter with coccidioidomycosis was found on the shore of Morro Bay, San Luis Obispo County (*C. immitis* has been isolated from the soil in several inland sites in San Luis

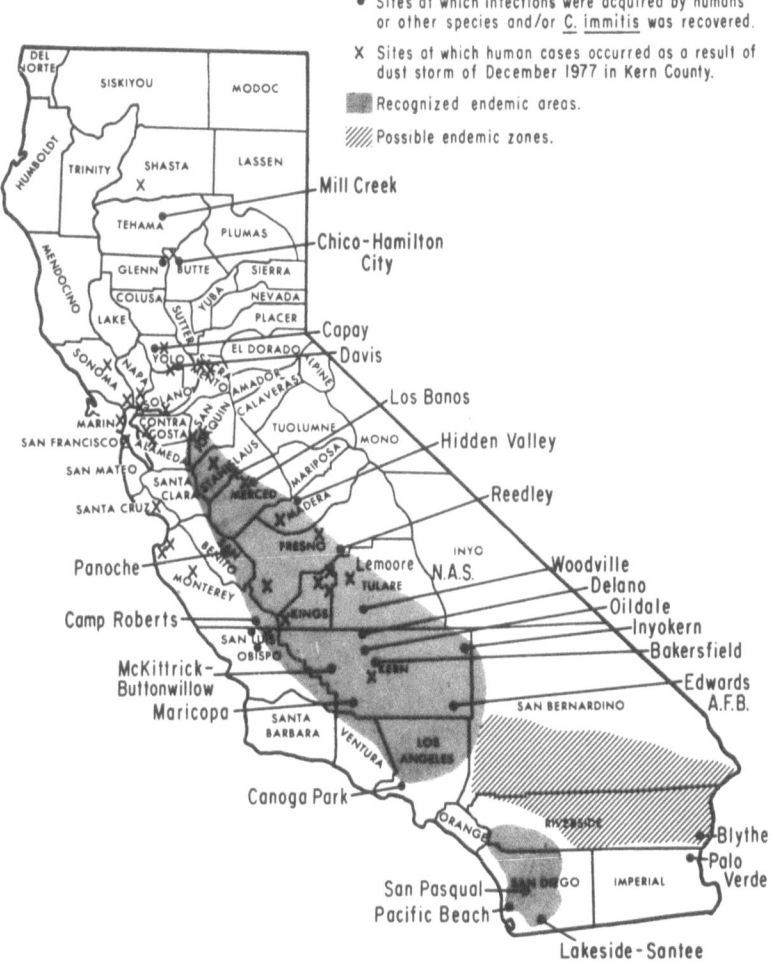

Figure 2. Sites of occurrence of *C. immitis* or of acquisition of coccidioidomycosis in California.

Obispo County by R. J. Cano). Interestingly, Imperial County, although showing ecologic characteristics of other endemic areas, appears generally nonendemic, except at its northeast corner area near Palo Verde (though Maddy[1] indicated that cattle presumably acquired coccidioidal infections in the Imperial Valley). Those counties identified with endemicity largely fall in the geological zone known as the Lower Sonoran Life Zone (more about this later), but many of the infections in California have occurred in local outbreaks with several individuals becoming infected at a single site of exposure, e.g., where digging by children or archeologists has taken place. Thus, *C. immitis* may be distributed in the soil in pockets rather than diffusely throughout the state.

On December 20, 1977, prior to advent of any significant recent rainfall, California experienced a tremendous wind and dust storm. Soil raised by this dust storm from the lower San Joaquin Valley was deposited as far north as 300 miles from Bakersfield, and as far west as the coast. As a result of this, spores of *C. immitis* were transported in considerable numbers, as reflected by a tremendous upsurge in acute primary coccidioidomycosis (Table 1).[2] Northern California cases occurred in Sacramento and Davis to the north, Marin County, San Francisco, and Salinas to the west. A similarly remarkable movement of spores in the past may have led to the spotty distribution in northern and west central California. The storm of 1977 may thus provide new sites of acquisition of infection in the future.

Although coccidioidomycosis was described in Arizona first in 1937, some 43 years after its discovery in California, Arizona is recognized as being an important coccidioidal region. During the time that the disease was "reportable" to the Arizona State Department of Health, more cases were reported annually than in California. The endemicity of coccidioidomycosis appears to be largely in the southern half of Arizona, though the northwest county of Mohave may also have provided a substantial number of infections. The areas around Tucson (Pima County) and Phoenix (Maricopa County) are endemic. Florence, which lies roughly between Tucson and Phoenix, appeared to have the highest attack rate of any area studied (with the exception of intense local outbreaks). Thus, 50% of susceptible individuals were infected within 6 months of arrival at Florence.

Infections among Arizonans occur not only in the expanding group of immigrants but also the relatively stable population of American Indians. Many of the latter reside on reservations, some of which lie within the endemic counties.

The southwestern quarter of Texas is endemic. Specific localized outbreaks of infection have been described in El Paso in the western

TABLE 1
New Cases of Coccidioidomycosis[a]

	1975	1976	1977	1978	
				12 weeks	Total
CSDH	442	500	375	359	1095
UC Davis	411	363	406	379[b]	1015
	Disseminated		22	23(16)[b]	
	Meningeal		8	13(9)[b]	

[a] New cases of coccidioidomycosis reported to the California State Department of Health or detected through the coccidioidomycosis serology laboratory, Department of Medical Microbiology, School of Medicine, University of California, Davis. The large increase in cases in 1978 resulted from a dust storm in Kern County that contaminated many areas of California with arthroconidia of *C. immitis*.
[b] Dust-storm-related.

most part of Texas, and Beeville that lies between San Antonio and Corpus Christi in southern Texas.[3] Interestingly, the latter endemic area lies east of a recognized locus of endemicity for *Histoplasma capsulatum* (at Concan near Uvalde), and thus there is overlapping of endemic areas for the two fungi.[4]

1.1.1.2. Mexico. Endemic zones of Mexico were mapped by Gonzalez Ochoa.[5] Three zones, based largely on results from coccidioidin skin tests, were recognized: (1) Northern Zone, including the northern half of Baja California, Sonora, Chihuahua, Coahuila, Nuevo Leon, and Tamaulipas, adjacent to the endemic southwestern United States, with skin test reactivity decreasing from west to east; (2) Pacific Littoral Zone, extending as far south as Guerrero and including parts of Sonora, Sinaloa, Nayarit, Jalisco, and Michoacan; (3) the Central Zone, beginning in Coahuila, extending into Nuevo Leon and southward into Durango and San Luis Potosi. Most of these areas are arid, and the presence of *Larrea tridentata,* the creosote bush, in much of the area is coincident with distribution of coccidioidin reactors. However, two areas with tropical character also provided notable numbers of coccidioidin reactors. One of these areas, part of the Pacific Littoral Zone, lay in Colima (Tecoman Valley) and Michoacan (Apatzingan Valley) and yielded 10 to 30% reactors; the other with lower rates of coccidioidin reactivity (5 to 10%) was further south and inland in Guerrero (Arcelia Valley). Cases of coccidioidomycosis were noted from Sonora, Baja California, Chihuahua, Coahuila, Nuevo Leon, San Luis Potosi, Jalisco, and Nayarit, in the tropical areas between Michoacan and Colima, and in Guerrero. Thus "autochthonous" cases of the disease appeared to support the skin test findings with coccidioidin. Two areas where there is some overlap of endemicity with that of histoplasmosis are in Nayarit and Coahuila.

1.1.2. Central America

The clinically recognized cases of coccidioidomycosis from Central America have been few. Mayorga[6] summarized six cases in humans— four from Guatemala, two from Honduras (and eight in other mammals), seven from Guatemala, and one from Nicaragua. Skin testing with coccidioidin yielded reaction rates as high as 25.5% in the towns of Zacapa and Gualan in northeast Guatemala in the Motagua River Valley.

In Honduras, skin test reactivity yielded 15.7% reactors in the Comayagua Valley, and in other areas from 1 to 4%.

Reactivity to coccidioidin in Panama was less than 1%, and even lower in Costa Rica.

With a population greater than 13 million, Central America appears to have an ill-defined but minor problem with clinical coccidioidomycosis.

1.1.3. South America

Despite the original description of coccidioidomycosis in Argentina in 1892, it was not until 35 years later that the second case was described from that country. By 1965, Negroni[7] had summarized a total of 27 diagnosed cases of coccidioidomycosis. (However, one of these was a laboratory-acquired infection, and another had been acquired in Paraguay). Presumed isolation of *C. immitis* from the soil has been reported from sites in Central Argentina in the provinces of San Luis and Mendoza.[8] However, confirmation of identity of these isolates by spherule formation apparently was not achieved.

Paraguay was the site of at least two cases of illness apparently coccidioidal (deduced from skin test results); and skin testing revealed 16 to 44% coccidioidin reactors among persons in the drier south- and northwestern Chaco regions. The wetter and more verdant southern Chaco yielded very few coccidioidin reactors.[9]

Venezuela, recognized as an endemic focus since 1949, has yielded a variety of clinical forms of coccidioidomycosis, most from the northwest states of Zulia, Falcon, and Lara. As many as 46% of individuals in one area of Lara were reactive to coccidioidin.[10]

Evidence that coccidioidomycosis may be endemic in Colombia was indicated by reports of 2 cases (1 poorly documented) of coccidioidomycosis in humans and demonstration of 3.3 to 6.3% reactivity to coccidioidin (with a high of 18% among adults) in the area of Guajira y Magdalena.[11] However, no case of coccidioidomycosis was included in a clinicopathologic study of 162 cases of systemic mycotic infections.[12]

1.2. Infection Acquired or Recognized Outside the Endemic Areas

Reports of presence of indigenous *C. immitis* outside the New World have had no mycologic confirmation. Coccidioidal infections that have been confirmed outside the endemic areas of the New World can usually be traced to a contaminated product from the known endemic area, to the prior presence of a patient in the endemic areas, or to exposure of laboratory workers to cultures. For example, infections reported from Naples, Italy, could have been acquired from some imported farm products from the endemic area. Rothman *et al.*[13] reviewed cases of coccidioidomycosis acquired by such apparent contact with *C. immitis* on contaminated materials outside the endemic area. Albert and Sellers[14] summarized the various cases apparently acquired from exported, contaminated fomites and added one of their own. The latter was an infection in a native of Georgia, never in the endemic area, who had been employed in a waste cotton processing plant that had handled cotton from the endemic Tulare, California, and from Los Angeles County. Subsequently a fatal coccidioidal infection occurred in a North Carolinian who had also handled cotton from the San Joaquin Valley.[15] Unfortunately in most instances *C. immitis* was not recovered from the putative sources to establish unequivocally the source of the infecting *C. immitis*.

Descriptions of 12 cases each from Michigan[16] and Iowa[17] exemplify the need to consider coccidioidomycosis in the differential diagnosis of varied illnesses outside the endemic zones.

Two cases were reported from Belgium in military men who had been assigned to Fort Bliss, Texas, for training and then returned to Belgium.[18] Similar cases among military personnel assigned from other nations for training in the U.S. have been recognized, as have numerous civilian cases. The hazard represented by working with *C. immitis* in the laboratory has also been recognized by infections acquired outside the endemic area, e.g., in Wuppertal-Eberfield, West Germany.[19,20]

2. ECOLOGIC

2.1. Distribution of Infections

While certain areas, e.g., Kern County, California, or the environs of Florence, Arizona, are recognized areas of heavy endemicity, newly diagnosed infections are generally from widespread loci. Sporadic concentrated outbreaks are detected among individuals with a recognized heavy exposure to dust (Canoga Park, Pacific Beach, and Chico, all in

California). However, single cases among humans and other species[21] suggest occurrence of microendemic foci.

While "Valley Fever" is often associated with lower elevations, e.g., the San Joaquin Valley (Bakersfield, elevation 421 ft) and Sacramento River Valley, (Red Bluff, elevation 304 ft), *C. immitis* has caused infections at higher altitudes. Thus, Plunkett and Swatek[22] isolated *C. immitis* from the soil at 3200 ft above sea level from a site near Inyokern, California, where anthropology students had previously acquired coccidioidal infection. The endemic zones of Tucson, elevation 2300 ft, El Paso, elevation 3710 ft, and Phoenix, elevation 1083 ft, also reflect the presence of *C. immitis* at relatively high altitudes.

2.2. Natural Distribution of *C. immitis*

Maddy[23] pointed to the general conformity of distribution of *C. immitis* in nature and the bioclimatic zone recognized as the Lower Sonoran Life Zone (LSLZ). This zone is typified by "arid or semiarid climates, with hot summers and few winter freezes, low altitude [see above] and alkaline soil." The creosote bush *L. tridentata* is a conspicuous member of the flora of much of the LSLZ. Maddy summarized the probable environmental desiderata for the development of *C. immitis* in nature: mean temperatures in July of 26°C to 32°C and in January of 4°C to 12°C, and an annual rainfall of 5 to 20 inches. Lacy and Swatek[24] have added to this by pointing out that recovery of *C. immitis* from the soil of American Indian middens (primitive habitation site) was related to sandy texture and alkalinity (more than to organic content), and that presence of the creosote bush was not significantly correlated with recovery of the fungus. They indicate, moreover, that some endemic sites are found in "mediterranean woodland"-type areas with characteristics different from the LSLZ.[25] These workers suggested that "the limiting factor may be the competitive saprophytic ability of the fungus," a concept propounded by Egeberg *et al.*[26] and Elconin *et al.*[27] The latter have proposed that increased salinity (e.g., $CaCl_2$ and NaCl) of surface soil would enhance growth of *C. immitis* especially at 40°C while inhibiting or killing microbial antagonists of *C. immitis*, e.g., *Bacillus subtilis* and *Penicillium janthinellum*.

A possibly unique selective advantage to *C. immitis* in the soil may be provided by borate, for at a concentration of 0.25%, $Na_2B_4O_7$ permitted growth of *C. immitis* (some growth was also noted at 0.5 and 1% concentrations) but not of several other pathogenic fungi.[28]

In the laboratory, *C. immitis* can be found to grow in a pH range of 3.5 to 9.0. The arthroconidia (of one strain of *C. immitis*) manifested great hardiness, surviving 6 months at 4°C and 25°C in saturated NaCl solution.[29] Dry arthroconidia died in 2 weeks at 50°C but survived well at temperatures of –15°C to 37°C for at least 6 months. At 10% relative humidity and 37°C there was a significant loss of viability, but at higher relative humidities (up to 95%) the dry arthroconidia survived at temperatures from –15°C to 37°C.

Despite this hardiness, Egeberg and Ely[30] found that recovery of *C. immitis* from the soil at the end of the *dry* season (January) was only 4.2%, while at the end of the wet season (April) 16% of soil samples were positive. All of the latter were recovered from the surface while only one of six positive cultures at the end of the dry season was from the surface; the other five were from 4- to 12-inch depths. Thus, the *surface* exposure to ultraviolet rays and exposure to temperatures as high as 60 to 67°C for 5 hr at 0.5 inch below the surface would likely overpower even *C. immitis*.[31] In the soil, it appears that the "blooms" (growth) of *C. immitis* require 56 to 90% humidity for several weeks (Lacy, cited by Swatek).[32] Evidently rodent holes do not provide a specific or unique site for development of *C. immitis* in the soil other than can be provided in other soil sites.[32] It was shown that burying infected canine, murine, or bovine tissues in the soil near Phoenix permitted recovery of *C. immitis* for at least 7 years, though soil obtained 200 ft away remained negative during the same period save for one specimen.[33] Emmons[34] had earlier shown the natural occurrence of coccidioidal infection of rodents, and this could lead to recycling of growth of *C. immitis* in the soil. Also, *C. immitis* has persisted in Indian middens in which the remains of Indians had been buried. However, it is likely that *C. immitis* can survive and grow in the soil in the absence of contribution to the soil of mammalian cadavers. After all, growth of *C. immitis* in the laboratory can be achieved in a medium so simple that ammonium acetate can provide carbon, nitrogen, and energy. Nevertheless, the presence of colloidal material in blood may permit survival of *C. immitis* from infected tissues long enough for germination of endospores into the more hardy mycelial phase with formation of arthroconida.[28]

The role of water (the requirement for certain levels of humidity has been mentioned above) in the growth of *C. immitis* in nature can be inferred from certain studies. Smith *et al.*[35] demonstrated that following winters of heavy rainfall, in the San Joaquin Valley there would be increased numbers of cases of coccidioidomycosis the following dry season. Elconin *et al.*[27] showed a direct correlation between the recovery of *C. immitis* from the soil in Kern County and the concentration of salts in the upper levels of soil—the latter increasing with the leaching effect of heavy rains and subsequent deposition of salts by capillarity from the deeper layers to the surface layers. Maddy[36] observed visible mycelial growth of *C. immitis* at the surface of soil in nature; Sorensen[28] observed it in soil previously intentionally inoculated with spores and moistened several months later. The isolation of *C. immitis* from the air at Camp Roberts, California,[37] was made near a dry stream bed, and Swatek *et al.*[38] indicated that positive soil samples in three loci in California were from "virgin desert soil along washes." It is likely that stream beds or their banks would provide a moist environment for a longer period for growth and arthroconidia formation (which takes about 5 days *in vitro*) than well-drained sites.

Seasonal variation in infection is likely tied to rainfall in at least two ways: first, the provision of the necessary aqueous cultural environment, and second, the diminution of the airborne dust including arthroconida. In California, the number of cases increases markedly during the dry dusty period from summer to late fall.[35] In Arizona, there are often two periods of precipitation, with a peak in January and very little rain in May and June, and a second peak in July–August, followed by two peaks in incidence of coccidioidal infections, respectively, one in the late spring, the other in the fall.[31,39] One must be alert, however, to the occurrence of coccidioidomycosis at any time of the year.

Despite the recognized association of certain environmental factors with development of *C. immitis* and with cases of coccidioidomycosis, the spottiness of the distribution of the fungus and its failure to become established outside apparently well-defined zones is not satisfactorily explained. It is of interest that several outbreaks of infections have occurred following excavation of "virgin," or at least long undisturbed, uncultivated soils.[22,40,41] Microbial competitors in regularly cultivated soils may inhibit *C. immitis*. Perhaps the increase in cases of primary coccidioidomycosis in *late* summer and fall, rather than during the *earlier* springtime cultivating disturbances of the soil, occur at a time when there has been restriction of the competitors, and sporulation–disarticulation of *C. immitis* has become extensive.

Fungicides have been used to temporarily rid small soil foci of *C. immitis*.

2.3. Occupationally Associated Infection

Despite the foregoing allusion to infections related to uncultivated soils, there is a conspicuous association of infection and employment in agricultural field work and other activities related to tillage of the soil.[42,43] To the list offered by Gifford *et al.*[44] of "agricultural workers, cattle and sheep men, oil riggers, telephone post diggers . . ." may be added anthropologists, archeologists, construction workers, baseball players, and children in their playful pursuits in the soil. Schmelzer and Tabershaw[45] provided the following breakdown of 106 cases of "occupational coccidioidomycosis": agriculture 32; construction 39; professional (engineer, scientist, geologist) 22, "other and unknown 13." Still, a sizable fraction of patients is derived from persons with no usual soil-centered occupation, and some with only a brief traveler's exposure in the endemic area.

The marked problem in terms of efficiency and person-days lost from military bases in endemic areas has been referred to in Chapter 1.

2.4. Laboratory-Acquired Infection

The high degree of infectivity of *C. immitis* has been amply borne out by numerous infections among laboratory workers.[46,47] Despite the recognition of this hazard for many years, recent cases have occurred.[19,20] Even knowledge of the risk must be accompanied by adequate technical facilities, e.g., biological containment hoods, to prevent exposure to the airborne arthroconidia. However, at least four cases of infection in laboratory workers have resulted from hypodermic injection of suspensions of *C. immitis* (summarized by Sorensen and Cheu).[48]

The colonial variability of *C. immitis* noted by Huppert *et al.*[49] makes it imperative that laboratory workers use the greatest caution, even with cultures that may not seem to fit the usual picture of *C. immitis*.

2.5. Infection of Nonhuman Species

2.5.1. Domestic

Domestic animals that have undergone natural infection with *C. immitis* are the dog, cat (rare),[50] horse, burro, cattle, sheep, and swine. Cattle, sheep, and swine appear to be quite resistant, focalizing their infections to the bronchial or mediastinal lymph nodes. Some serious disseminated infections have been recognized in horses. The range of disease in dogs is from very mild to severe disseminated. Boxers and Doberman Pinschers appeared to undergo dissemination of their infections more often than other breeds.[51,52]

2.5.2. Zoo

Zoo (or captive) animals naturally infected with *C. immitis* include the following: aardvark, chinchilla, gorilla, kangaroo, llama, monkey (tropical American, and sooty mangabey), sea lion, tapir (South African), and tiger (Bengal).

2.5.3. Feral

Rodents—deer mice, pocket mice, kangaroo rat, ground squirrels[34]—and a sea otter have been found infected with *C. immitis* in nature.

3. MODES OF TRANSMISSION

Infection with *C. immitis* usually results from inhalation of arthroconidia. The infective dose of arthroconidia for humans is unknown. Assuming that the arthroconidium is a 5-μm cube, 1 mm^3 would contain over 10^6 spores. Thus a large dose of spores (10 suffice to infect a dog, monkey, or mouse) can be contained in a very small volume of dust. There have been a small number of cases of coccidioidomycosis acquired by direct percutaneous inoculation.[53] Animal-to-animal (including humans) infection has not been demonstrated, with one possible exception: Castleberry *et al.*[54] reported a pulmonary lesion with an immature spherule in an infant monkey that had been born and lived for 2 months with its mother, which had been previously inoculated subcutaneously with *C. immitis*. The mother had a draining purulent lesion on the forearm all the while the infant monkey was housed with her. The infant was apparently in good health until it incurred an injury at the age of 5 months, at which time it was euthanatized and necropsied. (Borelli and Marcano[55] have reported the unusual transmission of *C. immitis* by necrophagia to rats fed cadavers of infected mice. The usual sites of involvement in the rats were cervical lymph nodes. Possibly this resulted from trauma and inoculation through oropharyngeal mucosa by ingested bones of the mice.)

The arthroconidia of *C. immitis* in the laboratory are often difficult to wet, and although their dimensions are about 2 × 5 μm, their settling rate in air was that of a particle 0.1 to 0.2 μm (R. L. Dimmick, personal communication). Because the arthroconidia could be suspended in an aqueous environment more readily after subjecting them to a vacuum, their "hydrophobic" (floating) nature may be due to entrapped air. What influence this would have on their retention after inhalation is not clear, though if the spores behave as particles 0.1 to 0.2 μm in size, then retention in the alveoli would be less than if they behaved as 2 × 5-μm particles.

Another influence, as yet of incompletely explored significance, on the transmission and infectivity of *C. immitis* in nature is that of air ions. Positively charged air ions led to earlier illness and higher cumulative mortality of mice inoculated intranasally with spores of *C. immitis* than was observed in mice kept in the usual laboratory air.[56]

4. DEMOGRAPHIC

4.1. Attack Rate

In the localized exposures among archeology students or children digging in the same area, attack rates of 60 to 93% have been noted.[57-59] In such outbreaks symptomatic infection is more frequent than was detected in more generalized exposure.[42] Thus, approximately 60% of persons infected with *C. immitis* have an asymptomatic or inconspicuous encounter usually reflected only by a positive coccidioidin skin test.[60] (This proportion may actually be higher, as suggested by detection of more reactors with spherulin than with coccidioidin. Spherulin, an antigenic extract from the spherule phase of the organism, appears to detect about one-third more skin test reactors in several surveys, without loss of specificity.[61]) Of the 40% of individuals who do develop symptoms, most develop a benign disease, though 5 to 10% may be left with pulmonary sequelae, e.g., cavity or granuloma. Estimates based on skin test surveys suggest 25,000–100,000 new infections in the U.S. annually. In endemic areas recognized cases are notoriously under-reported. It has been shown that the illness in recognized symptomatic cases in otherwise healthy individuals necessitates an average of 33 to 35 missed days from work (or school).[62] The estimated cost to the U.S. is almost a million person-days of labor and $9 million in medical expenses annually. The medical expenses of the 1977 dust storm mentioned are estimated at $2 million alone.

4.2. Influence of Race on Infection

There is limited information suggesting possible differences among various races in the development of *symptomatic primary* coccidioido-mycosis, but there are marked differences in response to infection. Among those individuals with symptomatic infections, approximately 1/100 adult white males will develop extrapulmonary spread of the infec-tion. In adult males of Filipino ancestry, the rate of dissemination is higher than in any other group. This was estimated as 175 times the rate among whites, and in blacks it is 10 to 20 times the rate among whites.[44,63] This difference also was reflected in more recent data on coccidioidal meningitis.[64] Thus, males of Filipino ancestry represented 4.2% of cases of coccidioidal meningitis, while representing approximately only 0.4% of the total population of California and Arizona. Black males constituted 16% of the cases of coccidioidal meningitis, while their representation in California and Arizona is 3.4% of the population. White males contributed 43% of the cases of meningitis and represent approximately 44% of the population. Of 19 deaths due to coccidioidomycosis in Arizona in 1976, 5 (4 males, 1 female) were in blacks (data provided by Ben Chaiken, Arizona Lung Association). Of 45 cases of fatal coccidioidal pneumonia, 28 were in blacks (18 males, 10 females).[65] These were patients who had been hospitalized in five hospitals in four California counties.

Iger[66] compiled data on 112 cases of coccidioidal osteomyelitis in Kern County. Black patients represented 50.9% of the total (34% black males, 17% black females), persons of Filipino ancestry 9.8% (all males), whites 28.6% (17% male, 12% female), persons of Mexican ancestry 9.8% (5% males, 4.8% females). Most of these were drawn from the patient population of the Kern County General Hospital (Kern Medical Center) for the years 1949–1976, and unfortunately the baseline of *total* coccidioidal infections and their racial distribution was not presented. In addition, the racial distribution of the Kern Medical Center population was not presented. However, the disproportionate involvement of blacks and persons of Filipino ancestry whose representation in the population of Kern County was approximately 5.7% and 0.6%, respectively, was suggested when compared with patients of Mexican ancestry, whose 9.8% representation was considerably less than the approximately 14% representation (of Spanish surnames) in the population of Kern County. Johnson,[67] in studying morbidity and mortality of coccidioidomycosis in Arizona, pointed out the difficulty in studying the influence of racial background because of the influence in his population group of underlying diseases and immunosuppressant drugs. Nevertheless, his data for 1968–1975 indicated that while blacks represented 3.0% of the population of Arizona, their deaths from coccidioidomycosis represented approximately 15% of the total. Mexican-Americans made up 19% of the population and only 9% of the deaths due to coccidioidomycosis. Whites, making up 72% of the population, contributed 66% of the deaths.

The racial difference in response to coccidioidal infection does not appear to be environmentally influenced. Smith et al.[63] showed that in military personnel living under the same conditions, dissemination occurred in 12% of clinically apparent cases in black males versus 1% dissemination in white males, and a similar difference was reported by Willett and Weiss.[63a] Gifford et al.[44] indicated that in 70% of the cases of coccidioidal granulomas there was a history of "outside work or work involving soil, vegetation, animals and general outdoor labor." The lesser rate of dissemination for persons of Mexican ancestry in the report of Gifford et al., and their lesser representation among the cases of disseminated coccidioidomycosis in the report of Iger,[66] Huntington,[65] and Johnson[67] cited above, indicate that environmental exposure does not account for the differences in rates of dissemination, since the

Mexican-American group is heavily represented in the agricultural labor effort. Furthermore, Sievers[68] has shown that the rate of dissemination among some American Indian tribes in Arizona is the same (3.5 times that in whites) as that reported 40 years earlier for the Mexican-American group by Gifford *et al.*, a group closely related to them ethnically. The high attack rate among archaeologists suggests substantial exposure to arthroconidia of *C. immitis*. Yet clinically apparent dissemination has been infrequent in these groups of largely white individuals.

Two additional sets of data affirm the ethnic differences in response to coccidioidal infection. In Table 2 are shown the numbers of diagnosed cases (clinically apparent) among the military personnel and their dependent families at the Lemoore Naval Air Station, California. Occupational exposure and housing were not significantly different for the different ethnic groups, yet the rate of dissemination for blacks and persons of Filipino ancestry was some 10-fold greater than that for whites. Another opportunity to study ethnic differences in response to infection was provided by the aforementioned dust storm of Kern County, California, that led to infections in early 1978 in nonendemic areas of northern and coastal California. Since the duststorm was followed within 24 to 48 h by rain, exposure to the arthrospores deposited in nonendemic areas was brief. Of 230 patients with clinically apparent coccidioidomycosis whose ethnic background was reported to us, blacks disseminated at some five times the rate noted in whites, and patients of Asian ancestry similarly seemed to have a greater tendency to disseminate than whites (Table 3).

TABLE 2
Coccidioidomycosis at Lemoore U.S. Naval Air Station, 1961–1977

Ethnic derivation known	Number of patients[a]	%	Disseminated Number	%
"Caucasian"	173	77	4	2.3
Black	17	7.5	4	23.5
Filipino	19	8.4	4	21
Mexican	6	2.7		
Asian	4	1.8		
Guamanian	2	0.9		
"Caucasian"/Indian	1	0.4		
Filipino/Italian	1	0.4	1	
Hawaiian	1	0.4		
Spanish	1	0.4		
TOTAL:	225	100	13	5.7

[a] A total of 231 cases were detected, but the ethnic background of 6 was not known. The calculations are based on the 225 cases.

TABLE 3
Coccidioidomycosis Resulting from a Dust Storm in December 1977, among
Various Ethnic Groups in Nonendemic Areas[a]

Ethnic derivation known	Number of patients[b]	%	Disseminated	
			Number	%
"Caucasian"	169	73.5	19	11.2
Black	26	11.3	14	53.8
Filipino	3	1.3	2	66.6
Mexican	17	7.4	3	17.6
Asian[c]	14	6.1	5	38.4
Pakistani	1	0.4		
TOTAL:	230	100	43	18.7

[a] Included, among others, the following cities or towns and environs: Sacramento, San Francisco, San Rafael, Santa Cruz, Salinas, Santa Rosa, Stockton, Redding, and Vallejo.
[b] A total of 272 cases were detected, but the ethnic background of 42 had not been ascertained at the time of this writing.
[c] Chinese 7, Japanese 5, Korean 1, Vietnamese 1.

4.3. Influence of Sex

Nonpregnant adult white females appear most likely to develop Valley Fever with erythema nodosum and the least likely to undergo dissemination of their primary infection. Thus, Smith et al.[63] indicated that dissemination would occur in 1/100 clinical cases of coccidioidomycosis in white males and in 1/500 clinical cases in white females. Black females appear to share the heightened likelihood of dissemination with black males.

4.4. Influence of Age

In general, there is an impression that children are better able to cope with coccidioidal infection than are adults. However, Sievers,[68] who studied coccidioidomycosis in Indians in Arizona, reported that the likelihood of dissemination was greater in children under 5 years of age and in adults over 50. Richardson et al.[69] noted one dissemination during 5 years' experience with a pediatric clinic population, and concluded that dissemination was rare. However, from the data they provided we estimated that the rate of dissemination among their population group was 1/121 patients, not greatly different from what would be expected in adults.[70] Furthermore, in a compilation of 240 cases in children 12 years old and under (1974–1978), we estimated an overall dissemination rate of 2.9% (Table 4). The sites of dissemination in children reported by us in 1970 are shown in Table 5. (See also Chapter 18.)

4.5. Influence of Intercurrent Conditions

A number of reports have indicated that the natural history of coccidioidomycosis is influenced by superimposed diseases or therapy.[67,71–76] Rowland et al.[75] reviewed 25 cases of fatal coccidioidomycosis in one hospital in Phoenix. Twenty-one (84%) of these patients had some underlying compromising disease and/or therapeutic state. These included malignant neoplasms, collagen vascular diseases, diabetes mellitus, renal failure, and pregnancy. The latter alters the otherwise favorable response of adult white females, a particular hazard resulting when a primary coccidioidal infection develops during the third trimester of pregnancy[77–84] (Table 6). (It is unlikely from present data that pregnancy has an untoward effect on preexisting coccidioidomycosis. See also Chapter 17.)

Conditions that alter immune competence, e.g., Hodgkins disease or intentional immunosuppression for renal transplantation, may reactivate an old arrested coccidioidal infection, pushing the patient into the disseminated category. (See also Chapter 19.)

4.6. Influence of Other Factors

Recent data suggest blood group and/or transplantation antigen allelic type (HLA type) may be related to rates of dissemination.[85]

TABLE 4
Extrapulmonary Dissemination of Coccidioidomycosis in Children 12 Years of Age and under

Ethnic group	Total infected number of children	Number disseminated	Dissemination rate, %
"Caucasian"	93	3	3.3
Mexican-American	29	2	7.0
American Indian	42	2	4.8
Black	2	0	
Filipino	1	0	-
Black/Mexican	1	0	-
Not given	72	0	0
TOTAL:	240	7	2.9

TABLE 5
Sites of Involvement in Serologically Proven Cases of
Coccidioidomycosis in Children 12 Years of Age and
under[a]

Total	158 cases
Extrapulmonary dissemination	33 (21% of total)
Osteomyelitis	13
Meningitis	13
Soft tissue—cutaneous abscess, lymph node abscess	6
Peritonitis	1
Deaths	4
Age of youngest infected	5 weeks
Age of youngest with dissemination	3 months
Disseminated group, racial derivation	
8 Black	
13 Mexican	
3 American Indian	
9 "Caucasian"	

[a] From Pappagianis.[70]

5. RESISTANCE TO NATURAL REINFECTION

Smith[42] concluded that second attacks of Valley Fever (with coccidioidal erythema nodosum), if they do occur, must be exceedingly rare.
In addition, Smith et al.[46] added that of 6000 serologically diagnosed
primary coccidioidal infections and hundreds of coccidioidin reactors,
none developed a second diagnosable coccidioidal infection. While 4
instances of second exogenous infections have been recorded (1 by
respiratory route, 3 by injection into the skin or deeper), these were
among laboratory workers accidentally exposed (and probably to a

TABLE 6
Influence of Time of Pregnancy on Outcome of
Coccidioidomycosis[a]

Infection acquired	Number		
	Cases	Disseminated	Fatal
First trimester	16	2	1 (or 2)
Second trimester	12	6	5
Third trimester	22	20	19
TOTAL:	50	28	25

[a] Data from references 77–84, one unpublished case of S.
Schwartzman and L. Kaufman (1971), and 15 cases from
our own files.

substantial inoculum). All 4 were able to focalize their infections successfully.

A positive coccidioidin skin test in a healthy individual denotes
resistance to reinfection with *C. immitis*. Under natural conditions,
therefore, new exogenous infections will occur only in those not previously infected with *C. immitis* (with the possible exception of immunocompromised individuals). The resistance acquired by humans has been
demonstrated experimentally in other animal species. This significant
fact and the relative infrequency of serious coccidioidal disease explain
why long-term residents need not flee from the endemic areas for fear of
having repeated infections.

6. SUMMARY

C. immitis has a limited distribution in the soil and airborne dust in
the New World. Its general ecologic preferences have been established,
but these include a variety of climates, vegetation, and elevation.
Coccidioidomycosis can be acquired by the resident human and other
fauna, those who merely visit the endemic areas, or, rarely, by those
exposed to contaminated products. It is not transmitted from human to
human. Acquisition of infection is more likely in the dry periods of the
year, and in those persons occupationally exposed to soil dust. The
response to infection varies with age, sex, and race and with presence of
some immunocompromising states. Recovery from infection leads to
resistance to reinfection.

REFERENCES

1. K. T. Maddy, Coccidioidomycosis of cattle in the southwestern United States, *J. Am.
   Vet. Med. Assoc.* **124**:456–464(1954).
2. D. Pappagianis and H. Einstein, Tempest from Tehachapi takes toll, *West. J. Med.*
   129:527–530 (1978).
3. K. W. Teel, M. D. Yow, and T. W. Williams, Jr., A localized outbreak of coccidioidomycosis in Southern Texas, *J. Pediatr.* **77**:65–73 (1970).
4. C. W. Emmons, P. D. Klite, G. M. Baer, and W. B. Hill, Jr., Isolation of *Histoplasma
   capsulatum* from bats in the United States, *Am. J. Epidemiol.* **84**:103–109 (1966).
5. A. Gonzalez Ochoa, Coccidioidomycosis in Mexico, in: *Coccidioidomycosis* (L. Ajello,
   ed.), University of Arizona Press, Tucson (1967), pp. 293–299.
6. R. Mayorga, Coccidioidomycosis in Central America, in: *Coccidioidomycosis* (L.
   Ajello, ed.), University of Arizona Press, Tucson (1967), pp. 287–291.
7. P. Negroni, Coccidioidomycosis in Argentina, in: *Coccidioidomycosis* (L. Ajello, ed.),
   University of Arizona Press, Tucson (1967), pp. 273–278.
8. A. L. Borghi, M. S. R. de Benetti, and B. J. C. de Bracalenti, *Coccidioides immitis:*

Su aislamiento de muestras de suelos de las provincias de San Luis y Mendoza, *Sabouraudia* **15**:51–57 (1977).

9. R. F. Gomez, Endemism of coccidioidomycosis in the Paraguayan Chaco, *Calif. Med.* **73**:35–38 (1950).

10. H. Campins, Coccidioidomycosis in Venezuela, in: *Coccidioidomycosis* (L. Ajello, ed.), University of Arizona Press, Tucson (1967), pp. 278–285.

11. M. Robledo, A. Restrepo, M. Restrepo, S. Ospina, and F. Gutierrez, Encuesta epidemiologica sobre coccidioidomycosis en algunas zonas aridas de Colombia, *Antioquia Med.* **18**:505–522 (1968).

12. C. E. Pena, Deep mycotic infections in Colombia. A clinico-pathologic study of 162 cases, *Am. J. Clin. Pathol.* **47**:505–520 (1967).

13. P. E. Rothman, R. G. Graw, Jr., J. C. Harris, Jr., and J. M. Anslow, Coccidioidomycosis-possible fomite transmission, *Am. J. Dis. Child.* **118**:792–801 (1969).

14. B. L. Albert and T. F. Sellers, Coccidioidomycosis from fomites, *Arch. Intern. Med.* **112**:253–261 (1963).

15. S. H. Gehlbach, J. D. Hamilton, and N. F. Conant, Coccidioidomycosis—an occupational disease in cotton mill workers, *Arch. Intern. Med.* **131**:254–255 (1973).

16. E. R. Harrell and W. M. Honeycutt, Coccidioidomycosis: A traveling fungus disease, *Arch. Dermatol.* **87**:188–196 (1963).

17. G. F. Key and I. M. Smith, Coccidioidomycosis in Iowa: 12 cases in a nonendemic area, *J. Iowa Med. Soc.*, pp. 531–535 (October 1972).

18. J. Williot, Apropos de deux observations de coccidioidomycose, *J. Franc. Med. Chir. Torac.* **20**:545–555 (1966).

19. T. Weymann and M. Plempel, Das Krankheitsbild der Coccidioidomycose, *Deutsche Med. Wochenschr.* **99**:1653–1656 (1974).

20. F. G. Aguilar-Torres, L. J. Jackson, J. E. Ferstenfeld, D. Pappagianis, and M. W. Rytel, Counterimmunoelectrophoresis in the detection of antibodies against *Coccidioides immitis, Ann. Intern. Med.* **85**:740–744 (1976).

21. D. Pappagianis, J. Vanderlip, and B. May, Coccidioidomycosis naturally acquired by a monkey, *Cercocebus atys,* in Davis, California, *Sabouraudia* **11**:52–55 (1973).

22. O. A. Plunkett and F. E. Swatek, Ecological studies of *Coccidioides immitis,* in: *Proceedings of the Symposium on Coccidioidomycosis,* U.S. Public Health Serv. Publ. No. 575, pp. 158–160 (1957).

23. K. Maddy, Ecological factors possibly relating to the geographic distribution of *Coccidioides immitis,* in *Proceedings of the Symposium on Coccidioidomycosis,* U.S. Public Health Serv. Publ. No. 575, pp. 144–157 (1957).

24. G. H. Lacy and F. E. Swatek, Soil ecology of *Coccidioides immitis* at Amerindian middens in California, *Appl. Microbiol.* **27**:379–388 (1974).

25. F. E. Swatek, The epidemiology of coccidioidomycosis, in : *The Epidemiology of Human Mycotic Diseases* (Y. Al-Doory, ed.), Charles C. Thomas, Springfield, Ill. (1975), pp. 74–102.

26. R. O. Egeberg, A. E. Elconin, and M. C. Egeberg, Effect of salinity and temperature on *Coccidioides immitis* and three antagonistic soil saprophytes, *J. Bacteriol.* **88**:473–476 (1964).

27. A. E. Elconin, R. O. Egeberg, and M. C. Egeberg, Significance of soil salinity on the ecology of *Coccidioides immitis, J. Bacteriol.* **87**:500–503 (1964).

28. R. H. Sorensen, Survival characteristics of diphasic *Coccidioides immitis* exposed to the rigors of a simulated natural environment, in: *Coccidioidomycosis* (L. Ajello, ed.), University of Arizona Press, Tucson (1967), pp. 313–317.

29. L. Friedman, C. E. Smith, D. Pappagianis, and R. J. Berman, Survival of *Coccidioides*

immitis under controlled conditions of temperature and humidity, *Am. J. Public Health* **46**:1317–1324 (1956).

30. R. O. Egeberg and A. F. Ely, *Coccidioides immitis* in the soil of the southern San Joaquin Valley, *Am. J. Med. Sci.* **23**:151–154 (1956).

31. K. T. Maddy, A study of a site in Arizona where a dog apparently acquired a *Coccidioides immitis* infection, *Am. J. Vet. Res.* **20**:642–646 (1959).

32. F. E. Swatek, Ecology of *Coccidioides immitis*, *Mycopathol. Mycol. Applic.* **40**:3–12 (1970).

33. K. T. Maddy and G. T. Crecelius, Establishment of *Coccidioides immitis* in negative soil following burial of infected animals and animal tissues, in: *Coccidioidomycosis* (L. Ajello, ed.), University of Arizona Press, Tucson (1967), pp. 309–312.

34. C. W. Emmons, Isolation of *Coccidioides* from soil and rodents, *Public Health Rep.* **57**:109–111 (1942).

35. C. E. Smith, R. R. Beard, H. G. Rosenberger, and E. G. Whiting, Effect of season and dust control on coccidioidomycosis, *J. Am. Med. Assoc.* **132**:833–838 (1946).

36. K. T. Maddy, Observations on *Coccidioides immitis* found growing naturally in soil, *Ariz. Med.* **22**:281–288 (1965).

37. M. D. Hoggan, J. P. Ransom, D. Pappagianis, G. E. Donald, and A. D. Bell, Isolation of *Coccidioides immitis* from the air, *Stanford Med. Bull.* **14**:190 (1956).

38. F. E. Swatek, D. T. Omieczynski, and O. A. Plunkett, *Coccidioides immitis* in California, in: *Coccidioidomycosis* (L. Ajello, ed.), University of Arizona Press, Tucson (1967), pp. 255–264.

39. P. Hugenholtz, Climate and coccidioidomycosis, in: *Proceedings of the Symposium on Coccidioidomycosis,* U.S. Public Health Serv. Publ. No. 575, pp. 136–143 (1957).

40. S. B. Werner and D. Pappagianis, Coccidioidomycosis in northern California—an outbreak among archeology students near Red Bluff, *Calif. Med.* **119**:16–20 (1973).

41. B. Joffe, An epidemic of coccidioidomycosis probably related to soil, *N. Engl. J. Med.* **262**:720–722 (1960).

42. C. E. Smith, Epidemiology of acute coccidioidomycosis with erythema nodosum, *Am. J. Public Health* **30**:600–611 (1940).

43. M. J. Fiese, *Coccidioidomycosis,* Charles C. Thomas, Springfield, Ill. (1958).

44. M. A. Gifford, W. C. Buss, and R. J. Douds, Data on coccidioides fungus infection, Kern County, 1900–1936, *Kern County Health Dept. Ann. Rep.* 1936–1937, pp. 39–54 (1937).

45. L. Schmelzer and I. R. Tabershaw, Exposure factors in occupational coccidioidomycosis, *Am. J. Public Health* **58**:107–113 (1968).

46. C. E. Smith, D. Pappagianis, and M. Saito, The public health significance of coccidioidomycosis, in: *Proceedings of the Symposium on Coccidioidomycosis,* U.S. Public Health Serv. Publ. No. 575, pp. 3–9 (1957).

47. J. E. Johnson, J. E. Perry, F. R. Fekety, P. J. Kadull, and L. E. Cluff, Laboratory acquired coccidioidomycosis, *Am. Intern. Med.* **60**:941–956 (1964).

48. R. Sorensen and S. Cheu, Accidental cutaneous coccidioidal infection in an immune person, *Calif. Med.* **100**:44–47 (1964).

49. M. Huppert, S. Sun, and J. W. Bailey, Natural variability in *Coccidioides immitis,* in: *Coccidioidomycosis* (L. Ajello, ed.) pp. 323–328, University of Arizona Press, Tucson (1967).

50. R. E. Reed, R. S. Hoge, and R. J. Trautman, Coccidioidomycosis in two cats, *J. Am. Vet. Med. Assoc.* **143**:953–956 (1963).

51. R. E. Reed, Diagnosis of canine coccidioidomycosis, *J. Am. Vet. Med. Assoc.* **128**:196–201 (1956).

52. K. Maddy, Disseminated coccidioidomycosis of the dog, *J. Am. Vet. Med. Assoc.* **132**:483–489 (1958).
53. D. Pappagianis, Coccidioidomycosis, in: *Clinical Dermatology,* Vol. 3 (D. J. Demis, R. L. Dobson, and J. McGuire, eds.), Harper and Row, Hagerstown, Md. (1973), Unit 17–18, 11 pp.
54. M. W. Castleberry, J. L. Converse, and J. E. Del Favero, Coccidioidomycosis transmission to infant monkey from its mother, *Arch. Pathol.* **75**:459–461 (1963).
55. D. Borelli and C. Marcano, Transmisión experimental de micosis profunda por "predación," *Med. Cutanea* **VI**:193–198 (1972).
56. A. P. Krueger and H. B. Levine. The effect of unipolar positively ionized air on the course of coccidioidomycosis in mice, *Int. J. Biometeorol.* **11**:279–288 (1967).
57. D. W. Gilman, P. F. Wehrle, and H. Cowper, Coccidioidomycosis—Canoga Park, California, *Morbid. Mortal. Weekly Rep.,* U.S. Public Health Service, Atlanta, pp. 302–303 (1965).
58. S. B. Werner, D. Pappagianis, I. Heindl, and A. Mickel, An epidemic of coccidioidomycosis among archeology students in northern California, *N. Engl. J. Med.* **286**:507–512 (1972).
59. G. H. Lacy and F. E. Swatek, Film: Coccidioides in California, in: *Coccidioidomycosis: Current Clinical and Diagnostic Status* (L. Ajello, ed.), Symposia Specialists, Miami (1977), pp. 79–90.
60. C. E. Smith, E. G. Whiting, E. E. Baker, H. G. Rosenberger, R. R. Beard, and M. T. Saito, The use of coccidioidin, *Am. Rev. Tuberc.* **57**:330–360 (1948).
61. D. A. Stevens, H. B. Levine, S. C. Deresinski, D. R. Ten Eyck, and A. Restrepo-M., Epidemiological and clinical skin testing studies with spherulin, in: *Coccidioidomycosis: Current Clinical and Diagnostic Status* (L. Ajello, ed.), Symposia Specialists, Miami (1977), pp. 107–114.
62. J. T. Scogins, Comparative study of time loss in coccidioidomycosis and other respiratory disease, in: *Proceedings of the Symposium on Coccidioidomycosis, U.S. Public Health Serv. Publ.* No. 575 (1957), pp. 132-135.
63. C. E. Smith, R. R. Beard, E. G. Whiting, and H. G. Rosenberger, Varieties of coccidioidal infection in relation to the epidemiology and control of the diseases, *Am. J. Public Health* **36**:1394–1402 (1946).
63a. F. M. Willett and A. Weiss, Coccidioidomycosis in southern California; report of a new endemic area with review of 100 cases, *Ann. Int. Med.* **23**:349–375 (1945).
64. D. Pappagianis and R. Crane, Survival in coccidioidal meningitis since introduction of amphotericin B, in: *Coccidioidomycosis: Current Clinical and Diagnostic Status* (L. Ajello, ed.), Symposia Specialists, Miami (1977), pp. 223–237.
65. R. W. Huntington, Acute fatal coccidioidal pneumonia, in: *Coccidioidomycosis: Current Clinical and Diagnostic Status* (L. Ajello, ed.), Symposia Specialists, Miami, (1977), pp. 127–137.
66. M. Iger, Coccidioidal osteomyelitis, in: *Coccidioidomycosis: Current Clinical and Diagnostic Status* (L. Ajello, ed.), Symposia Specialists, Miami (1977), pp. 177–190.
67. W. M. Johnson, Coccidioidomycosis mortality in Arizona, in: *Coccidioidomycosis: Current Clinical and Diagnostic Status* (L. Ajello, ed.), Symposia Specialists, Miami (1977), pp. 33–44.
68. M. Sievers, Disseminated coccidioidomycosis among southwestern American Indians, *Am. Rev. Resp. Dis.* **109**:602–612 (1974).
69. H. B. Richardson, J. A. Anderson, B. M. McKay, Acute pulmonary coccidioidomycosis in children, *J. Pediat.* **70**:376–382 (1967).
70. Pappagianis, D., Epidemiology of coccidioidomycosis, *Proceedings of the International Symposium on Mycoses, Pan Am. Health Organ. Sci. Publ.* No. 205, pp. 195–201, (1970).

71. S. C. Deresinski and D. A. Stevens, Coccidioidomycosis in compromised hosts, *Medicine* **54**:377–395 (1974).

72. L. Krulig, P. H. Jacobs, and D. Loeffel, *Pemphigus vulgaris* and disseminated coccidioidomycosis, *Sabouraudia* **14**:5–9 (1976).

73. D. Pappagianis, Opportunism in coccidioidomycosis, in: *Opportunistic Fungal Infections* (E. W. Chick, A. Balows, and M. L. Furcolow, eds.), Charles C. Thomas, Springfield, Ill. (1975), pp. 221–234.

74. P. L. Roberts, J. H. Knepshield, and R. F. Wells, *Coccidioides* as an opportunist, *Arch. Intern. Med.* **121**:568–570 (1968).

75. V. S. Rowland, R. E. Westfall, and W. A. Hinchcliffe, Fatal coccidioidomycosis: analysis of host factors, in: *Coccidioidomycosis: Current Clinical and Diagnostic Status* (L. Ajello, ed.), Symposia Specialists, Miami (1977), pp. 91–106.

76. N. Smithline, D. A. Ogden, A. I. Cohn, and K. Johnson, Disseminated coccidioidomycosis, in: *Coccidioidomycosis: Current Clinical and Diagnostic Status* (L. Ajello, ed.), Symposia Specialists, Miami (1977), pp. 201–206.

77. L. E. Smale and J. W. Birsner, Maternal deaths from coccidioidomycosis, *J. Am. Med. Assoc.* **140**:1152–1154 (1949).

78. J. E. Vaughan and H. Ramirez, Coccidioidomycosis as a complication of pregnancy, *Calif. Med.* **74**:121–125 (1951).

79. R. L. Baker, Pregnancy complicated by coccidioidomycosis: report of 2 cases, *Am. J. Obstet. Gynecol.* **70**:1033–1038 (1955).

80. H. N. Harrison, Fatal maternal coccidioidomycosis, *Am. J. Obstet. Gynecol.* **75**:813–820 (1958).

81. E. S. Mongan, Acute disseminated coccidioidomycosis, *Am. J. Med.* **24**:820–822 (1958).

82. R. E. Harris, Coccidioidomycosis complicating pregnancy. Report of 3 cases and review of the literature, *Obstet. Gynecol.* **28**:401–405 (1966).

83. L. E. Smale and K. G. Waechter, Dissemination of coccidioidomycosis in pregnancy, *Am. J. Obstet. Gynecol.* **107**:356–361 (1970).

84. W. VanBergen, F. J. Fleury, and E. L. Cheatle, Fatal maternal disseminated coccidioidomycosis in a nonendemic area, *Am. J. Obstet. Gynecol.* **124**:661–663 (1976).

85. S. C. Deresinski, D. Pappagianis, and D. A. Stevens, Association of ABO blood group and outcome of coccidioidal infection, *Sabouraudia* **17**:261–264 (1979).

5

Immunology of Coccidioidomycosis

David A. Stevens

1. THE IMMUNE SEQUENCE

The arthroconidium is the optimum size (<10 mm) to breach the first lines of pulmonary defense: filtration, mucociliary transport in the upper airways, and the chemical inhibitors in the mucoid blanket. The initial response of the host to the arthroconidia in the lower airways is an ingress of macrophages and polymorphonuclear leukocytes.[1] The stimulus for this response may be a nonspecific irritation, but *in vitro* studies have suggested that *C. immitis* antigens activate the complement mechanism, generating chemotactic factors.[2] The function of this "ingress" response is presumed to be phagocytosis and intracellular killing. *In vitro* studies have shown killing of other fungi by polymorphonuclear leukocytes and macrophages.[3,4] In several days mononuclear cells are more in evidence.[1] This is coincident with the start of conversion of the fungus from the saprophytic to the parasitic phase. There is *in vitro* evidence that neutrophils may be important in this conversion.[5] Included among these mononuclear cells are presumed to be lymphocytes that are beginning to recognize the fungal antigens as foreign, and monocytes that are undergoing transformation to macrophages. The immediate origin of these mononuclear cells is as yet undefined—peripheral blood, the network of paratracheal, carinal and hilar nodes, broncho-aveolar cells, and bronchial-associated lymphoid tissue are possible sources.[6] Alveolar macrophages, presumably in the process of "activation," which appears so central for their defensive actions against microbial invaders, must also play a role in the mononuclear cells' attempts at phagocytosis and restriction of fungal growth and multiplication.[7] The relative contributions of the various cell types described, and their possible defensive mechanisms, has not been delineated in this infection. Speculation regarding such mechanisms arises from extrapolation from other host–parasite immunological interactions, including tumor immunology.

The mononuclear cells predominate for the remainder of the residence of the fungus in the body. The only exception to this occurs when a mature spherule ruptures, releasing its endospores.[8,9] At this time there is again a transient polymorphonuclear response, presumably sparked by some stimulating substance released by this fungal replication step.

A feature of the later mononuclear response must be the presence of specifically committed lymphocytes, the descendants of those cells which initially recognized the fungus as foreign. These memory cells likely include the descendants of B lymphocytes and T lymphocytes.[10–12] B lymphocytes originate in the marrow, and their descendants are found in the peripheral blood, in primary follicles and germinal centers of lymph nodes, and in tissues such as the lung. They can be identified by such markers as surface immunoglobulin, complement receptors, and receptors for the Fc portion of antibody, and are presumed to give rise to plasma cells. The B-cell family produces antibodies, their presumed principal defensive contribution. Six possible mechanisms by which antibodies may assist the defensive process are (1) as opsonins, which enhance the process of phagocytosis; (2) as agglutinins, which may facilitate phagocytosis; (3) as an arming mechanism for lytic mononuclear and polymorphonuclear cells (antibody-dependent cellular cytotoxicity)[13]; (4) direct inhibition of fungal growth and multiplication[14]; (5) prevention of attachment of the fungus to host structures, if this is important in invasion, persistence of infection, or metastasis[15]; and (6) by complexing with antigen, activating the complement sequence, which may generate components that are chemotactic and/or important in phagocytosis and killing.[16–18] Recently, depletion of complement activity in serum removed from patients with acute primary coccidioidal infection has been demonstrated.[18]

2. LYMPHOCYTE IMMUNITY

There is more evidence that the descendants of T lymphocytes are essential for a successful host defense. T lymphocytes arise from precursors which mature in the thymus. These cells can be found in the peripheral blood, in paracortical areas of lymph nodes, and in tissue such as the lung. They can be identified by such markers as the ability to form rosettes with sheep erythrocytes. The descendants of those T lymphocytes which initially recognized the fungus as foreign are capable of recognition and response when they confront these antigens again. Then several defensive roles are possible. T cells help B cells in the process of antibody production, and probably orchestrate and regulate the entire immune process. T cells also produce soluble products, lymphokines (B cells can produce some of these products, too).[19] One which has been characterized *in vitro* is migration inhibitory factor (MIF), which immobilizes macrophages. At the sites of infection, this would increase the local phagocytic cell population. Other lymphokines are involved in the killer function ascribed to T cells (and other lymphocyte subpopulations).[20] These lymphokines have been well characterized in relation to killing of mammalian cells,[21] but evidence has been provided that fungi may be killed in similar fashion.[22,23] Lymphokines can activate macrophages, setting in motion physiological changes and biochemical processes which enhance the phagocytic and killing function of these cells. Other lymphokines are chemotactic, attracting inflammatory cells to the sites of infection, thus amplifying all the processes described.

3. CORRELATIONS IN INFECTION

The utility of markers of the immune reaction in diagnosis of coccidioidal infection are discussed elsewhere in this book—i.e., the humoral antibody response as assayed in the complement-fixing (CF) and precipitin antibody tests, and the cellular immune response which precedes it, as assayed by dermal delayed hypersensitivity.

It has also been noted that these immune reactions correlate with the course of the illness. Patients with dissemination of their infection commonly have a negative skin test and high CF antibodies,[24] in contrast to patients who successfully resolve the infection within the chest. It was shown in the era before therapy was available that patients with negative coccidioidin skin tests, for example, are more likely to die of their disease than those with positive tests.[24] It was indicated that the transition, in the course of disease from a negative to a positive skin test, is a favorable prognostic sign, and that the reverse is also true. However, recent studies[25] have indicated poor correlation of skin test status with outcome in patients with disseminated disease at the outset of therapy, although a correlation was suggested in patients with pulmonary disease (these same comments apply to lymphocyte transformation to coccidioidal antigen, techniques discussed in the next section). Moreover, conversions to positive reactions on treatment didn't always correlate with a favorable outcome.

4. *IN VITRO* AND *IN VIVO* STUDIES

Cellular immunity to *C. immitis* can be demonstrated in other ways than by skin testing: lymphocyte transformation using mycelial phase soluble antigen,[26-28] spherule phase soluble antigen[29] or fungal elements[30] (endospores appear to be the most potent of these); MIF production[31]; and possibly leukocyte migration inhibition.[32,33] With the soluble antigens, the substances responsible for the activity appear to be nondialyzable.[29] It is not uncommon to find patients with active disease with negative skin tests who are reactive in one or more of these *in vitro* assays. Possible explanations for this include differences in cell populations involved, presence of subpopulations of cells or serum factors which suppress reactivity in some tests and not in others, and absent capabilities in some necessary sequences in assays requiring multiple steps for a positive response. Often the defects are selective, i.e., patients with coccidioidal disease and negative coccidioidal skin tests will have intact skin test reactivity to other antigens, and when the *in vitro* measures of coccidioidal reactivity are negative in such patients, they may have intact *in vitro* reactivity to mitogens and other antigens.[28,31,34-37] The patients usually have normal numbers of circulating lymphocytes and percentage of erythrocyte-rosetting cells.[35,36] Decreased ability to develop cutaneous sensitization to dinitrochlorobenzene has been noted to occur in patients with disseminated disease with high titers of CF antibodies.[38]

Studies[39,40] have suggested that the mechanism of such unreactivity to coccidioidal antigens may be due to antigen overload. Guinea pigs sensitized to coccidioidin with killed hyphal cells could be desensitized by daily injections of coccidioidin or killed hyphae. This was reversible; reactivity returned after discontinuation of the injections. The desensitization was specific; reactivity to an unrelated antigen was unaffected. The loss of reactivity could be demonstrated in skin testing or *in vitro*. The desensitizing activity in coccidioidin was dialyzable. Intraperitoneal administration of antigen was more efficient in desensitization than subcutaneous administration, and starting the desensitizing process shortly after birth was more efficient than later. Of significance to immunotherapy, reactivity could be restored to tolerant animals by cellular transfer.

Other experiments[35] suggest that the mechanism for the immunological perturbations is active suppression of antigen-committed lymphocytes. Whereas lymphokines produced *in vitro* by exposure to coccidioidin of lymphocytes of healthy, skin-test-positive subjects could produce a skin test response on injection into patients with disseminated coccidioidomycosis, lymphocytes transferred from the subjects to the patients could not respond in the transfer skin site to coccidioidal antigen. Two possible suppressive mechanisms that come to mind are serum factors (antibody subtype, immune complexes, antigenemia) or suppressor cells.[41,42] These same investigators reported that examination of the skin test site in disseminated coccidioidomycosis patients revealed a paucity of mononuclear cells. Others[43] reported no differences between test sites of skin-test-negative patients and positive sites in other subjects (ample mononuclears), whereas other investigations[34] reported no cellular response at all at test sites of skin-test-negative patients.

More information about a possible mechanism for the immunological abnormalities has been reported.[34,44] The plasma of some skin-test-negative disseminated coccidioidomycosis patients was found to block transformation by their lymphocytes induced by coccidioidin[34] or spherulin[44] *in vitro,* whereas the cells transformed normally in response to coccidioidal antigen in the absence of autologous plasma (and mitogen-induced transformation was normal even in autologous plasma). Moreover,[34] this plasma also specifically blocked *in vitro* transformation induced by coccidioidin in other skin-test-negative (but not skin-test-positive) patients. These investigators hypothesize that there are circulating humoral factors in some skin-test-negative disseminated coccidioidomycosis patients which block altered cellular receptors found in such patients.

5. IMPAIRMENT OF IMMUNITY

Animal studies have stressed the importance of cellular immunity in coccidioidal infection. Protection against infection can be transferred by immune cells, but not by immune serum.[1,45] Removal of T lymphocytes from the cell populations removes the ability to confer protection.[45] Thymectomy of rats enhances the disease,[46] as does thymectomy of mice.[45] Reconstitution of thymectomized mice with bone marrow does not enhance their resistance.[45] Genetically athymic ("nude") mice are more susceptible than heterozygote counterparts possessing a thymus.[45] Steroids have the same disease-enhancing effect in rats,[47,48] mice,[49] and humans,[50] but the locus of action is less clear than that with thymectomy, since steroids can potentially inhibit so many sites in the immune response: the number of circulating mononuclears,[51,52] leukocyte adherence,[53] chemotaxis,[54,55] primary sensitization,[56] intracellular killing,[57] reticuloendothelial function,[52,58] pulmonary macrophages,[59,60] complement levels,[61] and the expression of cellular immunity.[62,63]

In man, lymphocytopenia correlates with dissemination in the immunocompromised host. Other endogenous and exogenous factors also appear to inhibit the immune response and enhance coccidioidal disease.[50] For this reason, coccidioidomycosis in the immunocompromised patient is discussed in Chapter 19. Our present understanding of the relationship of the immune response to the disease has also led to attempts to influence the course of the disease by manipulating (boosting) the host immune response, discussed in Chapter 21.

6. DURABILITY OF IMMUNITY

In the normal host who has an unrecognized infection or an apparent but successfully resolved primary infection, the skin test reactivity generally persists for many years, perhaps for life, as demonstrated in persons who have long-term residence outside the endemic area. Once having been infected with *C. immitis,* exogenous reinfection will not occur except under unusual circumstances, such as the massive type of exposure that can occur in a laboratory accident.

REFERENCES

1. D. C. Savage and S. H. Madin, Cellular responses in lungs of immunized mice to intranasal infection with *Coccidioides immitis, Sabouraudia* **6:**94–102 (1968).
2. J. N. Galgiani, R. A. Isenberg, and D. A. Stevens, Chemotaxigenic activity of extracts from the mycelial and spherule phases of *Coccidioides immitis* for human polymorphonuclear leukocytes, *Infect. Immun.* **21:**862–865 (1978).
3. R. I. Lehrer, Antifungal effects of peroxidase systems, *J. Bacteriol.* **99:**361–365 (1969).
4. M. Territo and M. J. Cline, Monocyte function in man, *J. Immunol.* **118:**187–192 (1977).
5. O. Baker and A. I. Braude, A study of stimuli leading to the production of spherules in coccidioidomycosis, *J. Lab. Clin. Med.* **47:**169–182, 1956.
6. H. B. Kaltreider, Expression of immune mechanisms in the lung, *Am. Rev. Resp. Dis.* **113:**347–379 (1976).
7. M. Lundborg and B. Holma, *In vitro* phagocytosis of fungal spores by rabbit lung macrophages, *Sabouraudia* **10:**152–156 (1972).
8. W. D. Forbus and A. M. Bestebreurtje, Coccidioidomycosis: A study of 95 cases of the disseminated type with special reference to the pathogenesis of the disease, *Mil. Surg.* **99:**653–719 (1946).
9. J. E. Tarbet, E. T. Wright, and V. D. Newcomer, Experimental coccidioidal granuloma, developmental stages of sporangia in mice, *Am. J. Pathol.* **28:**901–917 (1952).
10. R. C. Seeger and E. R. Stiehm, T and B lymphocyte subpopulations, *Pediatrics* **55:**157–160 (1975).

11. M. Richter and D. Algon, The heterogeneity of lymphocytes, *Med. Clin. North Am.* **56**:305–317 (1972).

12. J. Wybran and H. H. Fudenberg, How clinically useful is T and B cell quantitation? *Ann. Intern. Med.* **80**:765–767 (1974).

13. R. P. Gale and J. Zighelboim, Modulation of polymorphonuclear leukocyte-mediated antibody-dependent cellular cytotoxicity, *J. Immunol.* **13**:1793–1800 (1974).

14. D. B. Louria, M. Buse, J. Hsieh, and J. K. Smith, The influence of serum anti-candida substances on experimental candida infections, in: *Recent Advances in Medical and Veterinary Mycology* (K. Iwata, ed.), University of Tokyo Press, Tokyo (1977), pp. 189–195.

15. W. H. Johnston and H. Latta, Acute hematogenous pyelonephritis induced in the rabbit with *Saccharomyces cerevesiae*, *Lab. Invest.* **29**:495–505 (1973).

16. S. V. Boyden, R. J. North and S. M. Faulkner, Complement and the activity of phagocytes, in: *Complement* (G. E. W. Wolstenholme and J. Knight, eds.), pp. 190–213, Little, Brown, Boston (1965).

17. L. M. Muschel, Immune bactericidal and bacteriolytic reactions, in: *Complement* (G. E. W. Wolstenholme and J. Knight, eds.), pp. 159–169, Little, Brown, Boston (1965).

18. J. N. Galgiani, L. D. Petz, D. A. Stevens, and P. L. Williams, Activation of complement by *Coccidioides immitis*: *in vitro* and clinical studies, *Clin. Res.* **27**:41A (1979).

19. J. R. David, Lymphocyte mediators and cellular hypersensitivity, *N. Engl. J. Med.* **288**:143–149 (1973).

20. C. S. Henney, Killer T cells, *N. Engl. J. Med.* **291**:1357–1358, 1974.

21. G. A. Granger, Mechanisms of lymphocyte-induced cell and tissue destruction *in vitro*, *Am. J. Pathol.* **60**:469–481 (1970).

22. N. N. Pearsall, J. S. Sundsmo, and R. S. Weiser, Lymphokine toxicity for yeast cells, *J. Immunol.* **110**:1444–1446 (1973).

23. D. E. Gorcyca and G. C. Cozad, Quantitation of lymphotoxin activity in murine blastomycosis, *Abstr. Annu. Meet. Am. Soc. Microbiol.* No. F30 (1977).

24. C. E. Smith, E. G. Whiting, E. E. Baker, H. G. Rosenberger, R. R. Beard, and M. T. Saito, The use of coccidioidin, *Am. Rev. Tuberc.* **57**:330–360 (1948).

25. A. Catanzaro, Development of immunologic and clinical staging for immunotherapy, in: *Coccidioidomycosis: Current Clinical and Diagnostic Status* (L. Ajello, ed.), Symposia Specialists, Miami (1977), pp. 325–334.

26. N. E. Levan, C. S. Korn, E. G. McNall, and L. Pineda, Coccidioidomycosis and lymphocyte transformation, in: *Proceedings of the Third Annual Leukocyte Culture Conference* (W. O. Rieke, ed.), Appleton-Century-Crofts, New York, (1969), pp. 533–538.

27. B. Zweiman, D. Pappagianis, H. Maibach, and E. A. Hildreth, Coccidioidin delayed hypersensitivity: skin test and *in vitro* lymphocyte reactivities, *J. Immunol.* **102**:1284–1289 (1969).

28. R. A. Cox, J. R. Vivas, R. Gross, G. Lecara, E. Miller, and E. Brummer, *In vivo* and *in vitro* cell-mediated responses in coccidioidomycosis, *Am. Rev. Resp. Dis.* **114**:937–943 (1976).

29. S. C. Deresinski, H. B. Levine, and D. A. Stevens, Soluble antigens of mycelia and spherules in the *in vitro* detection of immunity to *Coccidioides immitis*, *Infect. Immun.* **10**:700–704 (1974).

30. S. C. Deresinski, R. J. Applegate, H. B. Levine and D. A. Stevens, Cellular immunity to *Coccidioides immitis*: *In vitro* lymphocyte response to spherules, arthrospores and endospores, *Cell. Immunol.* **32**:110–119 (1977).

31. A. Catanzaro, L. E. Spitler, and K. M. Moser, Cellular immune response in coccidioidomycosis, *Cell. Immunol.* **15**:350–371 (1975).

32. S. H. Astor, L. E. Spitler, O. L. Frick, and H. H. Fudenberg, Human leukocyte migration inhibition in agarose using four antigens: Correlation with skin reactivity, *J. Immunol.* **110**:1174–1179 (1973).

33. G. Senyk and W. K. Hadley, *In vitro* correlates of delayed hypersensitivity in man: Ambiguity of polymorphonuclear neutrophils as indicator cells in leukocyte migration test, *Infect. Immun.* **8**:370–380, 1973.

34. G. Opelz and M. I. Scheer, Cutaneous sensitivity and *in vitro* responsiveness of lymphocytes in patients with disseminated coccidioidomycosis, *J. Infect. Dis.* **132**:250–255 (1975).

35. E. A. Petersen, J. A. Frey, J. R. Davis, M. Dinowitz, and D. Rifkind, Mechanism of anergy in disseminated coccidioidomycosis, *Clin. Res.* **24**:152A (1976).

36. R. A. Cox and J. R. Vivas, Spectrum of *in vivo* and *in vitro* cell-mediated immune responses in coccidioidomycosis, *Cell. Immunol.* **31**:130–141 (1977).

37. R. A. Cox, E. Brummer, and G. Lecara, *In vitro* lymphocyte responses of coccidioidin skin test-positive and -negative persons to coccidioidin, spherulin, and a coccidioides cell wall antigen, *Infect. Immun.* **15**:751–755 (1977).

38. T. H. Rea, H. Einstein, R. Johnson, and N. E. Levan, Further study of dinitrochlorobenzene responsivity in disseminated coccidioidomycosis, in: *Coccidioidomycosis* (L. Ajello, ed.), Symposia Specialists, Miami (1977), pp. 365–370.

39. A. Bin Ibrahim and D. Pappagianis, Experimental induction of anergy to coccidioidin by antigens of *Coccidioides immitis, Infect. Immun.* **7**:786–794 (1973).

40. Bin Ibrahim, A. Induction of tolerance to coccidioidin in newborn guinea pigs, *J. Immunol.* **112**:387–391 (1974).

41. R. K. Gershon, A disquisition on suppressor T cells, *Transplant Rev.* **26**:170–185 (1975).

42. J. D. Stobo, S. Paul, R. E. Van Scoy, and P. E. Hermans, Suppressor thymus-derived lymphocytes in fungal infection, *J. Clin. Invest.* **57**:319–328 (1976).

43. V. D. Newcomer, J. W. Landau, R. Lehman, and J. R. Rowe, The local cellular response in patients with coccidioidomycosis, *Arch. Dermatol.* **88**:799–808 (1963).

44. R. P. Harvey and D. A. Stevens, Cell-mediated immunity in disseminated coccidioidomycosis-evaluation of suppressive influences with parasitic phase antigen, *Abstr. Annu. Meet. Am. Soc. Microbiol.* No. F19 (1978).

45. L. Beamon, D. Pappagianis, and E. Benjamini, Significance of T cells in resistance to experimental murine coccidioidomycosis, *Infect. Immun.* **17**:580–585 (1977).

46. H. R. Hicks and W. T. Northey, Studies on the response of thymectomized mice to infection with *Coccidioides immitis,* in: *Coccidioidomycosis. Proceedings of the 2nd Coccidioidomycosis Symposium* (L. Ajello, ed.), University of Arizona Press, Tucson (1967), pp. 183–187.

47. C. Cavallero and G. Sala, Cortisone and infection, *Lancet* **1**:175 (1951).

48. V. D. Newcomer, T. W. Wright, J. E. Tarbet, L. H. Winer, and T. H. Sternberg, The effects of cortisone on experimental coccidioidomycosis, *J. Invest. Dermatol.* **20**:315–326 (1953).

49. P. Redaelle, C. Cavallero, M. Borasi, G. Sala, and A. Amira, Experimental *Coccidioides immitis* and the adrenocortical steroids, *Mycopathologia* **6**:7–14 (1951).

50. S. C. Deresinski and D. A. Stevens, Coccidioidomycosis in compromised hosts, *Medicine* **54**:377–395 (1975).

51. W. L. Ford and J. L. Gowans, The traffic of lymphocytes, *Semin. Hematol.* **6**:67–83 (1969).

52. J. Thompson and R. Van Furth, The effect of glucocorticoids on the kinetics of mononuclear phagocytes, *J. Exp. Med.* **131**:429–442 (1970).

53. R. R. MacGregor, P. J. Spagnuolo, and A. L. Lentnek, Inhibition of granulocyte adherence by ethanol, prednisone and aspirin, measured with an assay system, *N. Engl. J. Med.* **291**:642–646 (1974).

54. J. E. Balow and A. S. Rosenthal, Mechanisms of steroid suppression of cellular immunity, *Clin. Res.* **20**:506 (1972).

55. D. R. Boggs, J. W. Athens, G. E. Cartwright, and M. M. Wintrobe, The effect of adrenal glucocorticosteroids upon the cellular composition of inflammatory exudates, *Am. J. Pathol.* **44**:763–773 (1964).

56. W. J. Casey and C. E. McCall, Suppression of cellular interactions of delayed hypersensitivity by corticosteroids, *Immunol.* **21**:225–231 (1971).

57. G. Weissman, The effect of steroids and drugs on lysosomes, in: *Lysosomes in Biology and Pathology*, Vol. 3 (J. T. Dingle and H. B. Fell, eds.), Elsevier, New York (1969), pp. 276–295.

58. F. Allison and M. H. Adcock, The influence of hydrocortisone and certain electrolyte solutions upon phagocytic and bactericidal capacities of leukocytes obtained from peritoneal exudates of rats, *J. Immunol.* **92**:435–445 (1964).

59. G. L. Huber, F. M. LaForce, R. J. Mason, and A. P. Monaco, Impairment of pulmonary bactericidal defense mechanisms by immunosuppressive agents, *Surg. Forum* **21**:285–286 (1970).

60. L. P. Merkow, S. M. Epstein, H. Sidransky, E. Verney, and M. Pardo, The pathogenesis of experimental pulmonary aspergillosis, *Am. J. Pathol.* **62**:57–74 (1971).

61. J. P. Atkinson and M. M. Frank, Effect of cortisone therapy on serum complement components, *J. Immunol.* **111**:1061–1066 (1973).

62. D. C. Dale and R. G. Petersdorf, Corticosteroids and infectious disease, *Med. Clin. North Am.* **57**:1277–1287 (1973).

63. R. B. Zurier and G. Weissman, Anti-immunologic and anti-inflammatory effects of steroid therapy, *Med. Clin. North Am.* **57**:1295–1307 (1973).

6

Serology and Serodiagnosis of Coccidioidomycosis

Demosthenes Pappagianis

1. INTRODUCTION

Serologic tests have achieved great utility in the diagnosis and management of coccidioidomycosis. The use of information from serologic studies must of course be tempered by appropriate clinical data and other laboratory data. The latter include the *sine qua non* of diagnosis, i.e., demonstration of *Coccidioides immitis* in the tissues or its recovery in culture.

2. HISTORICAL DEVELOPMENT OF SEROLOGIC STUDIES

Cooke[1] in 1914 demonstrated a ring precipitin reaction using triturated preparations of mycelium and spherules. In 1924 Davis[2] reported the first successful coccidioidal complement fixation reaction utilizing a suspension of the fungus. However, no consistent use of serology was made at that time.

During the 1930s C. E. Smith[3] demonstrated fortuitously that serum from guinea pigs infected with *C. immitis* when mixed with coccidioidin, a culture filtrate of the mycelial phase, yielded a precipitate. This was followed by testing sera from infected animals and humans by the complement fixation (CF) test. This proved successful and set the stage for the important *quantitative* serologic results derived from the CF procedure.

3. NATURE OF ANTIGENS

Until the late 1950s it was only possible to culture the mycelial phase of *C. immitis* in any significant quantity and with regularity. Coccidioidin is a filtrate of culture of *C. immitis* mycelium grown in a liquid medium. As coccidioidin came to be prepared by C. E. Smith, various strains of *C. immitis* were grown together in a synthetic nonantigenic medium modified from the Bureau of Animal Industry medium for preparation of tuberculin.[4] Cultures were grown in static phase for several weeks, and it was evident that autolysis of the mycelium was occurring with the release of antigen.[4,5] Smith *et al.*[4] commented on the variability of coccidioidins, particularly the difficulty in producing satisfactory CF antigens. It was found that regularly satisfactory CF antigens could be prepared by lysing, in the presence of toluene, the mycelium that had grown for 3 days in an incubator-shaker.[6,7] Antigen was released very early.[8] Indeed, the culture medium in which the young mycelium was grown yielded antigen.[9] The toluene-induced lysates yield antigens reactive in the tube precipitin (TP), CF, immunodiffusion (ID), and counterimmunoelectrophoresis (CIE) assays, skin test (ST), and could coat latex particles (LP) for agglutination. The culture filtrates have been shown reactive in CF, ID, and CIE tests. Ajello *et al.*[10] prepared a coccidioidin by cultivating *C. immitis* in a peptone–glucose–yeast extract medium for 3 weeks and collecting the culture filtrate for use as a CF and ID antigen.[11]

These various antigens are utilized in different laboratories and with the different serologic techniques doubtless provide some differences in serologic results and interpretations.

With the development of techniques that yielded spherules *in vitro*,[12,13] preparation of antigens from this morphologic phase become feasible. Landay *et al.*[14] tested sonic extracts and culture supernates of spherules by ID and reported differences between such spherule preparations and arthroconidia and coccidioidin antigens. The spherule extract appeared more specific (was nonreactive with antisera to *Histoplasma capsulatum* that reacted with arthroconidia antigen) and reacted with antisera to killed spherules, whereas arthroconidia and mycelial antigens reacted to antisera prepared against all morphologic forms. The lysate of spherules incubated in distilled water for several days, spherulin, was found to provide a higher titer in CF tests with human sera than mycelial coccidioidin.[15] It has been suggested that the higher titer detected with spherulin may result from its reaction with precipitins that customarily do not react in the CF test with coccidioidin. This has not been demonstrated unequivocally. Such spherulin also proved reactive in the

CIE test (Aguilar-Torres *et al.*[16]), but did cross-react with serum from one patient with mucormycosis. Huppert *et al.*[17] provided evidence of markedly greater cross-reactivity of spherulin than of coccidioidin in the CF test. Our own experience indicates that spherulin may yield a slightly higher CF titer with some human sera than does coccidioidin, but coccidioidin used in the ID test has detected coccidioidal antibody in sera that were negative in the CF test with both spherulin and coccidioidin. At this time, therefore, it does not appear appropriate to substitute spherulin for coccidioidin in serologic tests.

Smith *et al.*[18,19] utilized coccidioidins pooled from several strains of *C. immitis,* though no convincing evidence had been brought forth to indicate that this was essential for adequate serologic versatility. Huppert[20] reported on variable production of four different antigens by nine different strains of *C. immitis* as detected by immunodiffusion.

4. SEROLOGIC METHODS

4.1. Preparation of Specimens

Serologic tests for coccidioidomycosis may be carried out using serum, cerebrospinal, pleural, ascitic, or joint fluids. The latter is often very viscous, and this makes it difficult to handle in precipitin tests. However, all these fluids should be collected aseptically and preserved with aqueous merthiolate (final concentration 1 : 10,000). Plasma should not customarily be used, as some anticoagulants may adversely affect certain serologic tests. Some laboratories accept whole blood instead of serum, but hemolysis may interfere with reactions in the TP and CF tests, perhaps by providing a milieu for microbial growth. Such microbial contamination may make a serum anticomplementary, i.e., leads to fixation of (or damage to) complement by serum in the absence of antigen. For example, production of NH_3 by certain bacteria could lead to damage of the C4 component of complement. Anticomplementariness may also result for other reasons, e.g., the taking of certain drugs. It is conceivable that certain drugs, e.g., amphotericin B in the serum, may adversely affect the sheep erythrocytes used in the hemolytic system of the CF test. Specimens should be placed in sterile screw-capped or other securely enclosed containers sealed with tape to prevent leakage.

Specimens not preserved with merthiolate and sent to a distant laboratory may be kept frozen, though transport through the mail usually leads to melting long before arrival at the destination.

4.2. Methods Involving Precipitation or Agglutination

4.2.1. Tube Precipitin

The original TP test of Smith et al.[18] consisted of addition of 0.2 ml of serum to each of four 7 × 75-mm tubes. To one tube (control) was added culture medium similar to that in which the coccidioidin had been prepared, and to the others was added 0.2 ml of "undiluted" antigen or 1 : 10, 1 : 40, or 1 : 100 dilution of antigen. (These dilutions were derived from a comparison with a reference coccidioidin.) This covered a sufficient range of antigen concentrations to permit detection of the early precipitins somewhere in the "zone of equivalence." Smith et al.[21] found that the 1 : 100 antigen was of little use and consequently removed this dilution from the testing, and recommended that the 1 : 40 dilution be omitted. In subsequent experience, we found that the 1 : 40 dilution rarely, if ever, yielded a positive reaction that was not also detected by the 1 : 10 or undiluted antigen. Despite the use of varying dilutions of antigen, the TP test is to be regarded as a qualitative test and has no clear value as a quantitative test. Antigen and serum are mixed (not layered) and incubated at 35 to 37°C for 4 days. Readings are made each day by flicking the tubes to dislodge an almost gelatinous-appearing precipitate from the bottom of the tube. Most reactive sera will yield a "button" of precipitate in 24 hr, but some will take 3 days, and infrequently 4 days.

With this test, Smith et al.[21] detected precipitins in some 91% of patients with primary nondisseminating coccidioidomycosis. The antigen reactive in the TP test is stable at 60°C, differentiating it from the heat labile CF component.

4.2.2. Latex Agglutination

The latex agglutination test evolved as a test to detect the early precipitins. The test relies on reaction of antibody with polystyrene latex particles (0.15 to 0.35 μm in diameter—more recently 0.8 μm) coated with antigen.[22] The latter is culture filtrate pooled from 15 strains of C. immitis grown in glucose–yeast extract broth that has been heated (to inactivate antigen active in the CF test). The reaction is read at 4 min. The test is qualitative. While the latex agglutination test appears more sensitive than the TP test, it has yielded false-positive reactions with serum (6% in the study of Huppert et al.[23]), particularly when sera are diluted, and with cerebrospinal fluid.[24]

4.2.3. Agar–Gel Diffusion

4.2.3.1. Two-Dimensional Double Diffusion. In early studies on ID tests for histoplasmosis, coccidioidal antibody reactivity of coccidioidal antigen and antibody was also demonstrated.[26] Multiple lines of reaction were demonstrated between human coccidioidal serum and various fractions of coccidioidal antigens.[27] The diagnostic usefulness of gel diffusion was set forth by Huppert and Bailey,[9,28] who demonstrated the detection of coccidioidal CF antibody particularly, but also of coccidioidal precipitins. Wells containing reactants were 4.5 mm in diameter separated (wall to wall) by 5.0 mm. The wells contained approximately 50 μl of serum or antigen solution. Huppert's method utilized careful selection of the appropriate dilution of antigen and prediffusion of serum for 2 hr prior to addition of antigen solution to the apposed well. Such prediffusion assured that the optimal concentration of antigen and antibody would lie somewhere close to the midpoint between wells simplifying the detection of antigen–antibody precipitates. Reactions could be read in 24 hr with 69% of positive sera (visible reactions are sometimes detected earlier); 84% were positive at 48 h, 100% at 72 hr. In our experience an occasional additional reaction may be detected up to 5 days. Huppert and Bailey[28] suggested a blending of optimal dilutions of antigens to detect both CF and precipitin antibody with a single preparation. However, we have observed that reaction of the precipitin–antigen combination may block or obscure the development of the line between CF antibody and antigen when the CF antibody is present at low titer (1 : 2 to 1 : 8 by complement fixation). Use of heated and unheated antigen assures detection and distinction of precipitins and CF antibody, respectively.

Concentrating the serum [or cerebrospinal fluid (CSF)] eight- to tenfold by evaporation has in our hands enhanced the detection of coccidioidal antibody.[25] This has been particularly useful in detecting precipitins, and CF antibody when present in very low titer as with coccidioidal pulmonary cavities.

4.2.3.2. Quantitative Immunodiffusion. Simple dilution of sera tested with the appropriately selected concentration of antigen can provide a titer often close to that of the CF test.[29] These authors reported, however, that approximately 20% of the titers differed from the CF titers by more than one tube of the twofold-dilution series, and that final readings should be made at 3 days. Krasnow and Huppert[30] made additional observations on the favorable comparability of the quantitative ID with CF.

The agar–gel precipitin inhibition test[31] is an indirect test that involves incubating serial dilutions of the test serum with an appropriate dilution of antigen, followed by diffusion of the serum–antigen mixture against a standard serum. Prior reaction of antibody in the test serum with antigen would thus bind antigen, precluding its precipitation by the standard serum. The end point of this more involved procedure was read at 48 hr and appeared to provide no particular advantage over the CF test.

4.2.3.3. Counterimmunoelectrophoresis. The application of an electrical potential across the immunodiffusion wells hastens the precipitation reaction by bringing antigen and antibody together quickly. The reaction may be read in 30 to 90 min. Studies (on relatively few specimens to date) have indicated that the method may be useful as a quantitative as well as qualitative method[16] for CF antibody. Both spherulin and coccidioidin have been utilized in CIE.

4.3. Complement Fixation

The CF method originally applied by Smith *et al.*[18,21] was the quantitative Kolmer method utilizing 0.25 ml of serum or other body fluid (twofold serial dilutions beginning with 1 : 2) with 2 units of complement. Primary incubation was for 2 hr at 37°C, and the hemolytic system was incubated for 1 hr. The 100% end point was used, i.e., the highest dilution of serum giving complete "4+" inhibition of hemolysis. Smith *et al.*[21] noted that overnight binding of complement at 4°C was more sensitive, i.e., yielded higher titers than incubation at 37° for 2 hr. This was therefore adopted for testing CSF. However, the significant clinical correlations established by Smith *et al.* with thousands of specimens were made with the 2-hr binding. Several other CF methods have been applied, including the microtiter method, and these offer only the advantage that they may require less than 0.5 ml of serum, but the disadvantage of not having had the extensive clinical correlation of Smith's method. It has been concluded erroneously by some[11] that CF titers less than 1 : 8 are not diagnostic of coccidioidal infection, and this has been adopted as the practice by some laboratories. Low CF titers may be detected in acute primary coccidioidal infections, in old, well-focalized pulmonary coccidioidomycosis (e.g., with a cavity or granuloma), with limited extrapulmonary dissemination, or from cross-reactivity, but a positive CF reaction at low titer must not be discarded as "not diagnostic."

As previously pointed out, spherulin yielded slightly higher titers than coccidioidin[15] but also provided greater cross-reactivity[17] (*vide infra*).

4.4. Immunofluorescence

Fluorescent antibody (FA) techniques have been used for the demonstration of cells of *C. immitis* in infected tissue, and by FA inhibition, the presence of coccidioidal antibody in sera.[32] Antisera were prepared by infecting rabbits with viable *C. immitis* or by injecting them with killed arthroconidia. Globulins precipitated from the rabbit sera were labeled with fluorescein isothiocyanate. These conjugates stained endospores and the contents but not the walls of spherules in infected tissues; however, the walls of spherules produced in culture were stained by the FA.

In the FA inhibition test, serum from patients suspected of having coccidioidomycosis was mixed with labeled rabbit antihuman globulin allowed to react with endospores obtained from infected mouse tissues. The intensity of staining was compared with that of the endospores treated with a mixture of *normal* human serum and fluorescent-labeled rabbit antiglobulin.

4.5. Sensitivity and Specificity of Serologic Methods

4.5.1. Cross-Reactivity of *C. immitis*, *H. capsulatum*, and *Blastomyces dermatitidis*

Infection with *C. immitis* leads to immunologic stimulation reflected both by development of delayed hypersensitivity to coccidioidin or spherulin and by production of detectable antibody. The production of detectable antibody in asymptomatic individuals who had become reactive to coccidioidin was infrequent, only 7% of such individuals developing antibody detected by the original tube precipitin and CF tests used by Smith *et al.*[18] Smith *et al.*[21] reported that less than 0.5% of disseminated infections were missed by TP and CF tests, including the use of the more sensitive overnight binding of complement at 4°C.

4.5.2. Cross-Reactivity with Other Fungi

In the studies of Campbell and Binkley,[33] Salvin *et al.*,[34] and Smith *et al.*,[21] coccidioidin cross-reacted irregularly by CF test with sera from patients with histoplasmosis, but did not react with sera from patients with blastomycosis or cryptococcosis. In the TP test, coccidioidin showed more cross-reactivity than in the CF test with sera from primary histoplasmosis and cutaneous (disseminated) blastomycosis. Toluene-induced autolysate of *C. immitis* did not show cross-reactivity in the CF test with pooled sera from human patients with histoplasmosis.[27]

Kaufman and Clark[11] reported cross-reactivity of their coccidioidal CF antigen with sera from patients with histoplasmosis, blastomycosis, and candidiasis. Coccidioidin and spherulin were reported to show cross-reactivity in the CF test with sera from patients infected with *Petriellidium (Allescheria) boydii, Aspergillus* species, *B. dermatitidis, H. capsulatum, Phialophora pedrosoi, Candida albicans, Candida parapsilosis, Cryptococcus neoformans,* and *Torulopsis glabrata.*[17] In this study, spherulin showed markedly greater cross-reactivity than coccidioidin.

Heiner[26] had demonstrated by immunodiffusion the sharing of a similar antigen by *C. immitis, H. capsulatum,* and *B. dermatitidis.*

4.5.3. "Cross-Reaction" in Nonmycotic Conditions

Patients with sarcoidosis who were found to yield some low-serum CF titers to *H. capsulatum* yeast phase antigen, gave no reactions with histoplasmin (mycelial phase) or coccidioidin.[35] Chapman[36] had demonstrated no reactivity of coccidioidin in immunodiffusion using sera from patients with sarcoidosis, though reactions were noted with sera from patients with cryptococcal, blastomycotic, and histoplasmal infections.

Sera from various nonmycotic diseases—some not even infectious conditions—have been reported by Schubert and Hampson[37] and Kaufman and Clark[11] to fix complement in the presence of coccidioidal antigen. Thus, sera from patients with tuberculosis, pneumococcal pneumonia, staphylococcal empyema, central nervous system malacia, macular degeneration, pulmonary carcinoma, and regional enteritis fixed complement at titers of 1 : 2 to 1 : 8. Kaufman and Clark[11] also demonstrated reaction of coccidioidal antigen in immunodiffusion with sera from one patient with reticulum cell sarcoma and one with "central chorioretinitis" (but see Chapter 15). The latter stated that CF titers of 1 : 2 and 1 : 4 with coccidioidin are not always of diagnostic significance, implying that titers of 1 : 8 or greater do have such significance. That this is an exaggeration is reflected by patients with established coccidioidomycosis who yield low titers (1 : 2 to 1 : 4) early in their disease (inclining titer), late (declining titer), when there is limited extrapulmonary spread, or with coccidioidal pulmonary residuals or cavities.[21] Huppert *et al.*[17] also included among their nonmycotic conditions showing cross-reaction with coccidioidin and spherulin infections or hypersensitivity states associated with actinomycetes, though Smith *et al.*[18] had not detected cross-reaction of coccidioidin with sera from actinomycosis patients.

The 16 to 20% "nonspecificity of coccidioidin" (and worse with spherulin) reported by Huppert *et al.*[17] suggests considerable difference from the previously held view that coccidioidin possesses a high degree of specificity. What contribution the different antigens made in the overall results of these various studies can only be established by well-controlled comparative studies. It is likely that in endemic areas and with appropriate selection of patients on historical or clinical grounds, one could lessen the problem of cross-reactivity. Immunodiffusion utilizing appropriate control-positive sera should enable one in most cases to determine if coccidioidal antibodies *per se* are present in a patient's serum.

5. APPLICATION OF SEROLOGY IN CLINICAL SETTING

5.1. Sequence of Antibody Response

The general response of patients who have a primary nondisseminating coccidioidal infection is to produce precipitins (likely IgM) early, followed by CF (IgG) antibodies[21] (Fig. 1). Thus, during the 1st week after onset of symptoms, 53% of patients have detectable precipitins, and this increases to a maximum of 91% during the 2nd and 3rd weeks, declining gradually thereafter. By the 5th month after onset, only 10% of patients still have detectable precipitins. (With the advent of the latex agglutination test and immunodiffusion using serum concentrated by evaporation, it is likely that these percentages would be somewhat higher, as the above percentages were obtained using the classical TP test.)

CF antibodies, slower to appear (only 9% during the 1st week of illness, and conversion of serum to CF-positive may continue up to the 3rd month after onset of illness), are more persistent. CF antibodies may be detected in approximately 90% of patients with primary nondisseminating coccidioidomycosis 7 months after onset of the illness[21] and may persist in low titer, e.g., 1 : 2 to 1 : 4, for some years after recovery from primary coccidioidomycosis. Of course, with disseminated coccidioidomycosis that remains chronically active, CF antibody can be present at substantial levels for years.

The precise antigen(s) that induces the precipitin and CF antibodies is not known. However, precipitins but not CF antibodies are adsorbed

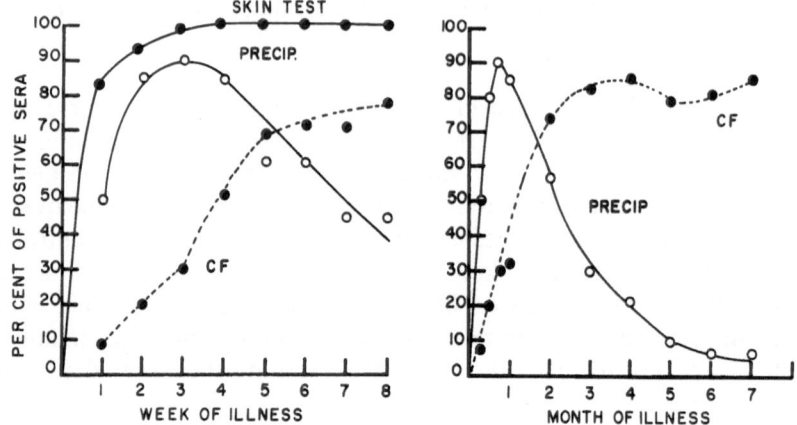

Figure 1. Temporal sequence of immunologic changes in primary nondisseminating coccidioidomycosis. Skin test, delayed response to coccidioidin; Precip., precipitins determined
by TP test; CF, complement-fixing antibodies. N.B.: Skin test results in the broader
contemporary clinical experience would likely not achieve the levels in groups noted by
Smith *et al.*[18,21] and C. E. Smith 1955 (*Ped. Clin. North Am.* 2:109–125), from which these
data were derived.

by spherule wall fragments.[38] The antigen reactive with CF antibody is
heat labile (60°C); that reactive in the precipitin test is heat stable.

5.2. Nature and Quantitative Change in the Immunoglobulin Response

A general increase in the "gamma 1" and "alpha 2" proteins was
noted with coccidioidal infection, the level of these proteins increasing
roughly proportional to the severity of infection.[39] Smith *et al.*[21] had
previously demonstrated that CF antibodies pass the placenta and could
be found in the cord blood. An increase in IgG, IgA, and IgM was
recorded for patients with coccidioidomycosis.[40] Precipitin-positive patients tend to have elevated IgM (and IgA), precipitin-positive, CF-
positive patients have increased IgG too, and CF-positive patients tend
to have increased IgG levels associated with increased CF titers. This
reflects crudely studies[41,42] that indicated the early precipitins are IgM,
and CF antibodies IgG. Sawaki *et al.*[42] also demonstrated an increase in
IgA, but its relationship to serologic tests and to patient response to
infection has not been established.

The CF titer is generally higher in the serum than in the CSF, joint, or pleural fluid, though this is not invariable. Precipitins are infrequently detected in the CSF,[21,43] but can be detected in the pleural fluid.

5.3. Influence of Skin Tests

The coccidioidin and spherulin skin tests do not influence coccidioidal serologic tests.[4,44,45] The coccidioidin skin test may induce the appearance of or a rise in histoplasmal antibody, but the extent and clinical significance of this is not yet established.[44]

5.4. Relationship of Serologic Findings and Clinical Status

5.4.1. Precipitins

Precipitins (as detected by tube precipitin, latex particle agglutination, or immunodiffusion using concentrated serum) are usually indicative of a recent primary coccidioidal infection. They usually appear before detectable CF antibodies and therefore may be the only detectable antibody in the early diagnosis of primary acute coccidioidomycosis. The precipitins are not quantitated, their detection alone being sufficient for diagnostic or prognostic conclusions. Precipitins generally do not persist, but they may be particularly persistent in some patients who undergo dissemination, and they may reappear (perhaps after persisting at very low levels) in patients with chronic pulmonary cavities that develop bronchopleural fistulae. (Precipitins can be detected by immunodiffusion in sera concentrated by evaporation from patients with chronic pulmonary cavities.) Precipitins may also reappear in patients with coccidioidal meningitis who reinfect themselves systemically by way of ventriculoatrial or ventriculoperitoneal shunts, and may provide an early clue to such systemic reinfection.

5.4.2. Complement Fixation

Complement fixation not only is of use in diagnosis but is particularly useful because of its quantitative aspects. The correlation of CF titer with the extent and severity of coccidioidal infection was established by Smith et al.[18,21] Using the Kolmer method with 2-hr binding of complement at 37°C, Smith concluded that over 80% of patients with extensive disseminated disease produced a CF titer of 1 : 16 or higher. With a single extrapulmonary site of dissemination, however, only 15% of patients were found to have a serum CF titer 1 : 16 or higher. It must be emphasized that potentially fatal coccidioidal meningitis may occur with serum CF titers less than 1 : 16 in 50% of patients. Fewer than 10% of primary nondisseminating coccidioidomycosis had titers greater than 1 : 16. Limited coccidioidal disease, e.g., a chronic pulmonary cavity or solitary pulmonary granuloma, is usually accompanied by serum CF titers less than 1 : 16. Sixty percent of the cases with cavitary coccidi- oidomycosis had diagnostic fixation of complement (at least 4+ at 1 : 2 dilution of serum), but with the solitary pulmonary granuloma more than 70% had titers of 1 : 2 or less.

It is important to note that the "critical" titer of 1 : 16 was obtained with one method of performance of the CF test; and with other techniques one may obtain other critical titers. The extensive correlation of titer and clinical status accomplished by Smith has not been carried out in a similar manner utilizing other techniques. One must therefore recognize the limitation of comparing titers obtained from different laboratories.

Sequential sera should be tested *simultaneously* to obtain valid comparison of changes in CF titer, owing to the multiple variables utilized in the CF test. Sequential sera should generally be tested at 3- to 4-week intervals to permit detectable changes in CF titer. A significant change in titer is represented by a fourfold ("two tube") change in titer, a rising titer being associated with extension or worsening of coccidioidal disease. The serum CF titer continues to rise until death in those with continuing extension of the disease, though with fulminating disease death can occur without a substantial rise in titer. A declining CF titer (fourfold) is regarded as a favorable change.

Other body fluids—CSF, pleural, ascitic, joint fluids—can be used for measurement of CF titer. Comparison of titers of sequential speci- mens must be made between specimens from the same anatomical source. Thus, lumbar fluid can be compared only with lumbar fluid, cisternal with cisternal fluid, etc.

Diagnostic fixation of complement by CSF (4+ fixation at a 1 : 2 or higher dilution) usually denotes presence of coccidioidal meningitis. (Undiluted CSF rather than the 1 : 2 dilution is the lowest dilution tested in some laboratories, though the lowest dilution utilized in the studies of C. E. Smith was the 1 : 2 dilution of CSF.) An extradural lesion, e.g., paralumbar or vertebral abscess, may yield diagnostic levels of CF antibody in the CSF. In the latter case, however, the CSF protein is elevated but cells and glucose are usually normal. Contamination of the CSF by blood of a patient with a high CF titer could possibly also yield a CF reaction in the absence of meningitis. A rising CF titer in the CSF means worsening of the meningeal infection, a falling titer indicates improvement. Persistent fixation of complement by CSF indicates persisting meningitis even if the glucose, protein, and cells have become normal. Ventricular fluid may be deceptively normal while the basilar meningitis flourishes (see Chapter 11, Section 5.1).

Generally the CF titer of other fluids is lower than that of serum obtained simultaneously. However, infrequently the CF titer detected in these fluids may exceed that in the serum. It is advisable to test both serum and the particular fluid for diagnosis and in following the course of infection, particularly sequential CSF specimens. As with serum, a declining CF titer in these fluids reflects improvement.

5.4.3. Serologic Negativity and Active Disease

Serologic negativity in patients with active coccidioidal disease generally has been infrequent; however, relatively more serologic failures have occurred among the small group of patients undergoing renal transplants and coccidioidal infection than in others.

5.5. Serologic Identification of Cultures

One additional use of serologic studies has been the identification of cultures suspected of being *C. immitis* by using immunodiffusion to detect specific cell-free antigens.[46] (See Chapter 3, Section 3.3.3.)

6. SUMMARY

The usual formation of two kinds of antibody in clinically apparent coccidioidomycosis provides diagnostic information and assistance in prognosis. Precipitins (IgM) detected by TP, by latex particle agglutination, or (under certain circumstances) by immunodiffusion are present early after onset of symptoms and are usually transient. Precipitins may be the only detectable antibody early in the course of coccidioidal infection, preceding detectable CF (IgG) antibody. CF antibody, detectable also by immunodiffusion, persists longer than precipitins, and may be present for years. The CF titer is generally proportional to severity. Depending on the method and antigen, a CF titer above 1 : 16 in the serum should lead to careful assessment of the patient for possible metapulmonary dissemination of infection. Presence of CF antibody in the CSF, usually but not always after its appearance in the serum, generally is diagnostic of coccidioidal meningitis. CF antibody, usually in low titer, may be detected in the serum of patients with old coccidioidal pulmonary residuals, e.g., a cavity or solitary pulmonary nodule, but absence of antibody does not exclude the coccidioidal etiology of such lesions. Despite the general sensitivity and specificity of coccidioidal serology, it should be supported where possible with histologic and/or cultural demonstration of *C. immitis* for diagnosis.

7. REFERENCES

1. J. V. Cooke, Immunity tests in coccidioidal granuloma, *Proc. Soc. Exp. Biol. Med.* **12:**35 (1914).
2. D. J. Davis, Coccidioidal granuloma with certain serologic and experimental observations, *Arch. Dermatol. Syphilol.* **9:**577–587 (1924).
3. C. E. Smith, Reminiscences of the Flying Chlamydospore and its allies, in: *Coccidioidomycosis* (L. Ajello, ed.), University of Arizona Press, Tucson (1967), pp. xiii–xxii.
4. C. E. Smith, E. G. Whiting, E. E. Baker, H. G. Rosenberger, R. R. Beard, and M. T. Saito, The use of coccidioidin, *Am. Rev. Tuberc.* **57:**330–360 (1948).
5. D. Pappagianis and G. S. Kobayashi, Production of extracellular polysaccharide in cultures of *Coccidioides immitis, Mycologia* **50:**229–238 (1958).
6. D. Pappagianis, C. E. Smith, M. T. Saito, and G. S. Kobayashi, Preparation and property of a complement-fixing antigen from mycelia of *Coccidioides immitis*, in: *Proceedings of the Symposium on Coccidioidomycosis, U.S. Public Health Serv. Publ. No. 575*, pp. 57–63 (1957).
7. D. Pappagianis, C. E. Smith, G. S. Kobayashi, and M. T. Saito, Studies of antigens from young mycelia of *Coccidioides immitis, J. Infect. Dis.* **108:**35–44 (1961).
8. D. Pappagianis and G. S. Kobayashi, Approaches to the physiology of *Coccidioides immitis, Ann. N.Y. Acad. Sci.* **89:**109–121 (1960).
9. M. Huppert and J. W. Bailey, The use of immunodiffusion tests in coccidioidomycosis. I. The accuracy and reproducibility of the immunodiffusion test which correlates with complement fixation, *Am. J. Clin. Pathol.* **44:**364–368 (1965*a*).
10. L. Ajello, K. Walls, J. C. Moore, and R. Falcone, Rapid production of complement fixation antigens for systemic mycotic diseases: I. Coccidioidin; influence of media and mechanical agitation in its development, *J. Bacteriol.* **77:**753–756 (1959).
11. K. Kaufman and M. J. Clark, Value of the concomitant use of complement fixation and immunodiffusion tests in the diagnosis of coccidioidomycosis, *Appl. Microbiol.* **28:**641–643 (1974).
12. J. L. Converse, Effect of surface active agents on endosporulation of *Coccidioides immitis* in a chemically defined medium, *J. Bacteriol.* **74:**106–107 (1957).
13. H. B. Levine, J. M. Cobb, and C. E. Smith, Immunity to coccidioidomycosis induced in mice by purified spherule, arthrospore and mycelial vaccines, *Trans. N.Y. Acad. Sci.* **22:**436–449 (1960).
14. M. Landay, R. W. Wheat, N. F. Conant, E. P. Lowe, and J. Converse, Serological comparison of the three morphological phases of *Coccidioides immitis, J. Bacteriol.* **93:**1–6 (1967).
15. G. M. Scalarone, H. B. Levine, D. Pappagianis, and S. Chaparas, Spherulin as a complement-fixing antigen in human coccidioidomycosis, *Am. Rev. Resp. Dis.* **110:**324–328 (1974).
16. F. G. Aguilar-Torres, L. J. Jackson, J. E. Ferstenfeld, D. Pappagianis, and M. W. Rytel, Counterimmunoelectrophoresis in the detection of antibodies against *Coccidioides immitis, Ann. Intern. Med.* **85:**740–744 (1976).

17. M. Huppert, I. Krasnow, K. R. Vukovich, S. H. Sun, E. H. Rice, and L. J. Kutner, Comparison of coccidioidin and spherulin in complement fixation tests for coccidioidomycosis, *J. Clin. Microbiol.* **6:**33–41 (1977).

18. C. E. Smith, M. T. Saito, R. R. Beard, R. Kepp, R. W. Clark, and B. U. Eddie, Serological tests in the diagnosis and prognosis of coccidioidomycosis, *Am. J. Hyg.* **52:**1–21 (1950).

19. C. E. Smith and C. C. Campbell, Question and answer period on the serology of coccidioidomycosis, in: *Proceedings of the Symposium on Coccidioidomycosis, U.S. Public Health Serv. Publ. No. 575,* pp. 53–56 (1957).

20. M. Huppert, Serology of coccidioidomycosis, *Mycopathol. Mycol. Appl.* **41:**107–113 (1970).

21. C. E. Smith, M. T. Saito, and S. A. Simons, Pattern of 39,500 serologic tests in coccidioidomycosis, *J. Am. Med. Assoc.* **160:**546–552, (1956).

22. C. Mulder, S. Kiddy, and K. Lou, A rapid latex slide test for coccidioidomycosis, *Bacteriol. Proc.,* p. 141 (1966).

23. M. Huppert, E. T. Peterson, S. H. Sun, P. A. Chitjian, and W. J. Derrevere, Evaluation of a latex particle agglutination test for coccidioidomycosis, *Am. J. Clin. Pathol.* **49:**96–102 (1968).

24. D. Pappagianis, I. Krasnow, and S. Beall, False-positive reactions of cerebrospinal fluid and diluted sera with the coccidioidal latex-agglutination test. *Am. J. Clin. Pathol.* **66:**916–921 (1976).

25. D. Pappagianis, M. T. Saito, and K. Van Hoosear, Antibody in cerebrospinal fluid in non-meningitic coccidioidomycosis, *Sabouraudia* **10:**173–179 (1972).

26. D. C. Heiner, Diagnosis of histoplasmosis using precipitin reactions in agar gel, *Pediatrics* **22:**616–627 (1958).

27. D. Pappagianis, E. W. Putman, and G. S. Kobayashi, Polysaccharide of *Coccidioides immitis, J. Bacteriol.* **82:**714–723 (1961).

28. M. Huppert and J. W. Bailey, The use of immunodiffusion tests in coccidioidomycosis. II. An immunodiffusion test as a substitute for the tube precipitin test, *Am. J. Clin. Pathol.* **44:**369–373 (1965*b*).

29. M. Huppert, J. W. Bailey, and P. Chitjian, Immunodiffusion as a substitute for complement fixation and tube precipitin tests in coccidioidomycosis, in: *Coccidioidomycosis* (L. Ajello, ed.), University of Arizona Press, Tucson (1967), pp. 221–225.

30. I. Krasnow and M. Huppert, An alternate to the complement fixation test in coccidioidomycosis, *Abstr. Annu. Meet. Am. Soc. Microbiol.,* p. 127 (1977).

31. J. G. Ray, Jr., The agar-gel precipitin-inhibition test used in the serum titration of human and animal coccidioidomycosis, in: *Coccidioidomycosis* (L. Ajello, ed.), University of Arizona Press, Tucson (1967), pp. 215–220.

32. W. Kaplan, Application of the fluorescent antibody technique to the diagnosis and study of coccidioidomycosis, in: *Coccidioidomycosis* (L. Ajello, ed.), University of Arizona Press, Tucson (1967), pp. 227–231.

33. C. C. Campbell and G. E. Binkley, Serologic diagnosis with respect to histoplasmosis, coccidioidomycosis, and blastomycosis and the problem of cross reactions, *J. Lab. Clin. Med.* **42:**896–906 (1953).

34. S. B. Salvin, M. L. Furcolow, and J. Nishio, Serologic studies on an outbreak of pulmonary disease at Camp Gruber, Oklahoma, *Arch. Intern. Med.* **93:**906–910 (1954).

35. J. E. Johnson, R. A. DeRemee, F. Kueppers, and G. D. Roberts, Prevalence of fungal complement-fixing antibodies in sarcoidosis, *Am. Rev. Resp. Dis.* **116:**145–147 (1977).

36. J. S. Chapman, Mycobacterial and mycotic antibodies in sera of patients with sarcoidosis, *Ann. Intern. Med.* **55:**918–924 (1961).

37. J. H. Schubert and C. R. Hampson, An appraisal of serologic tests for coccidioido-mycosis, *Am. J. Hyg.* **76**:144–148 (1962).
38. M. S. Collins, D. Pappagianis, and J. Yee, Enzymatic solubilization of precipitin and complement fixing antigen from endospores, spherules and spherule fraction of *Coccidioides immitis,* in: *Coccidioidomycosis: Current Clinical and Diagnostic Status* (L. Ajello, ed.), Symposia Specialists, Miami, (1977), pp. 429–444.
39. W. B. Reed, C. Heiskell, C. W. Holeman, and C. M. Carpenter, Serum protein profiles in coccidioidomycosis, *J. Invest. Dermatol.* **40**:147–158 (1963).
40. E. M. McKelvy and J. L. Fahey, Immunoglobulin changes in disease: Quantitation on the basis of heavy polypeptide chains, IgG (γG), IgA (γA), and IgM (γM), and of light polypeptide chains, Type K (I) and Type L (II), *J. Clin. Invest.* **44**:1778–1787 (1965).
41. D. Pappagianis, N. Lindsay, C. E. Smith, and M. T. Saito, Antibodies in human coccidioidomycosis: Immunoelectrophoretic properties, *Proc. Soc. Exp. Biol. Med.* **118**:118–122 (1965).
42. Y. Sawaki, M. Huppert, J. W. Bailey, and Y. Yagi, Patterns of human antibody reactions in coccidioidomycosis, *J. Bact.* **91**:422–427 (1966).
43. D. Pappagianis and R. Crane, Survival in coccidioidal meningitis since introduction of amphotericin B, in: *Coccidioidomycosis: Current Clinical and Diagnostic Status* (L. Ajello, ed.), Symposia Specialists, Miami (1977), pp. 223–237.
44. D. Pappagianis, C. E. Smith, and C. C. Campbell, Serologic status after positive coccidioidin skin reactions, *Am. Rev. Resp. Dis.* **96**:520–523 (1967).
45. S. C. Deresinski, H. B. Levine, P. C. Kelly, R. J. Creasman, and D. A. Stevens, Spherulin skin testing and histoplasmal and coccidioidal serology: lack of effect. *Am. Rev. Resp. Dis.* **116**:1116–1118 (1977).
46. P. G. Standard and L. Kaufman, Immunological procedure for the rapid and specific identification of *Coccidioides immitis* cultures, *J. Clin. Microbiol.* **5**:149–153 (1977).

7

Pathology of Coccidioidomycosis

Robert W. Huntington

1. SCOPE OF THIS CHAPTER

The pathologist continues to have an essential part in the study of coccidioidomycosis, for the clinician and the epidemiologist must press for diagnostic accuracy, and the most accurate diagnosis will often be that of the pathologist who reviews clinical and laboratory data in the light of anatomical findings.

The pathology of various manifestations of coccidioidomycosis, in various organ systems, is alluded to in the chapters to follow. Our aim here is to review some of the common elements of the pathological picture of the disease.

The diagnosis of the disease by examination of and by cultures of clinical specimens has been discussed in detail in Chapter 3. These methods are essential in the workup of specimens commonly received by the pathologist, including biopsy and autopsy material, as well as to specimens which may also be processed by the clinical microbiologist, cytologist, or pathologist, such as sputum, pus, or urine.

The principal aim of this chapter will be to offer suggestions, based on the writer's experience, on help which the pathologist may offer the clinician and the clinician may seek from the pathologist, in the recognition and differential diagnosis of coccidioidomycosis, and in the study of complications and sequelae of the infection and of its treatment.

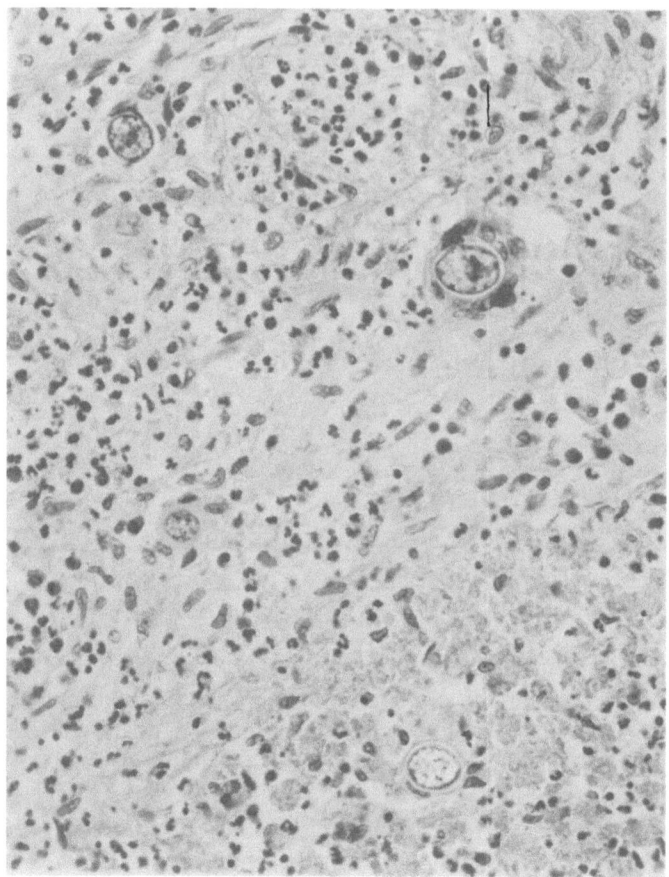

Figure 1. Pneumonic process, showing diffuse admixture of granulomatous and suppurative reaction patterns. Note the polymorphonuclear infiltrate, the fibrosis, the early caseation in the lower portion, and the giant cells, some of which contain spherules. The section is from case 9, reference 1. H & E stain, original magnification ×350.

2. MICROSCOPIC AND GROSS EXAMINATION

In our experience, it has not proved profitable to attempt wet mount studies in material which was not from the center of a lesion. Wet mounts are most apt to be helpful when the material is pus, though they are sometimes worthwhile with material which has to be crumbled. The material is emulsified in 10% KOH, and examined under reduced illumination.

In tissue, *C. immitis* is spherular (Fig. 1), save in some cases of pulmonary cavitation (in the interior margins),[1] and in at least one reported case of primary cutaneous infection[2] (Fig. 2). However, the writer's awareness of the variability of coccidioides as seen in tissue sections is largely based on material in which the morphology of the organisms might be regarded by eager taxonomists as atypical, but from which typical coccidioides has been readily cultured. In material from an actively infected patient in which the actual number of organisms may be small, culture may prove more informative than direct microscopic

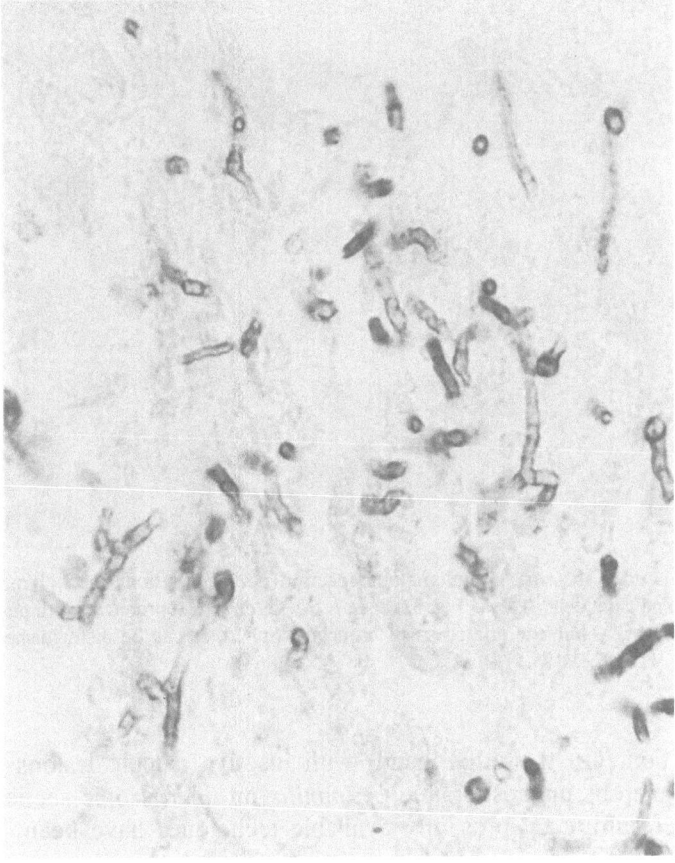

Figure 2. Mycelial phase coccidioides in the scalp of an agricultural worker. This was a primary lesion at the site of a grapevine scratch. This photograph has not been previously reproduced, but the case is number 1 of reference 2. Grocott–Gomori Methenamine Silver stain, ×800. Mycelial phase coccidioides occurs occasionally in the walls of pulmonary cavities.

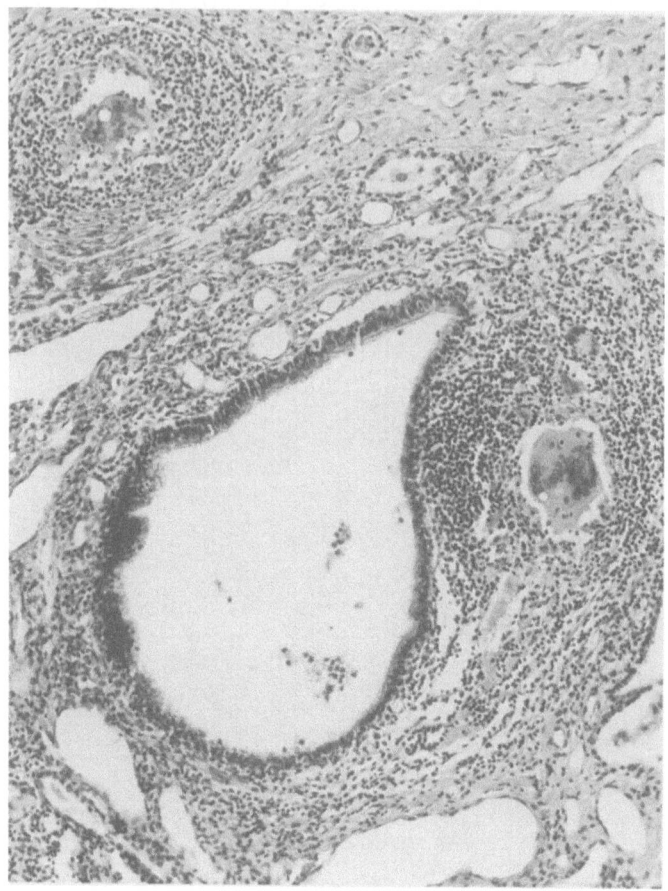

Figure 3. Lung, showing granulomatous reaction pattern, with fibrosis, lymphocytic infiltrate, and giant cells. This is Fig. 32, case 7, of reference 1, reproduced with permission of the publisher. Note the dilated small bronchus. Spherules can be distinguished in the giant cells. H & E, ×125.

examination. On the other hand, with inactive calcific lesions which show numerous unquestionable *C. immitis* on microscopic section, the results of culture by presently available techniques have been, in the writer's experience, consistently negative.

On gross examination, coccidioidal lesions may be miliary or massive; red, gray, or pale; nodular or diffuse; firm, hard, calcific, caseous, liquefactive, or cavitary. Some gross appearances in specific locations may alert the pathologist to the possibility of coccidioidomycosis. They can hardly do more than that. Coccidioidal involvement of the liver, spleen, and kidney is usually microscopic; the lesions may be either microabscesses or miliary granulomata.

Some of the characteristics of the lesions are shown in the illustrations. The pattern of tissue reaction may be granulomatous (Figs. 3 and 4) or suppurative (Figs. 5 and 6), or, perhaps most commonly and characteristically, mixed. Fibrosis may occur in older lesions. The granulomatous pattern may include lymphocytes, mononuclear and epithelioid cells, giant cells, fibrosis, caseation and calcification. Suppurative patterns will exhibit polymorphonuclear cells, and may go on to liquefaction or caseation. Quite often one may discern a "microabscess" in

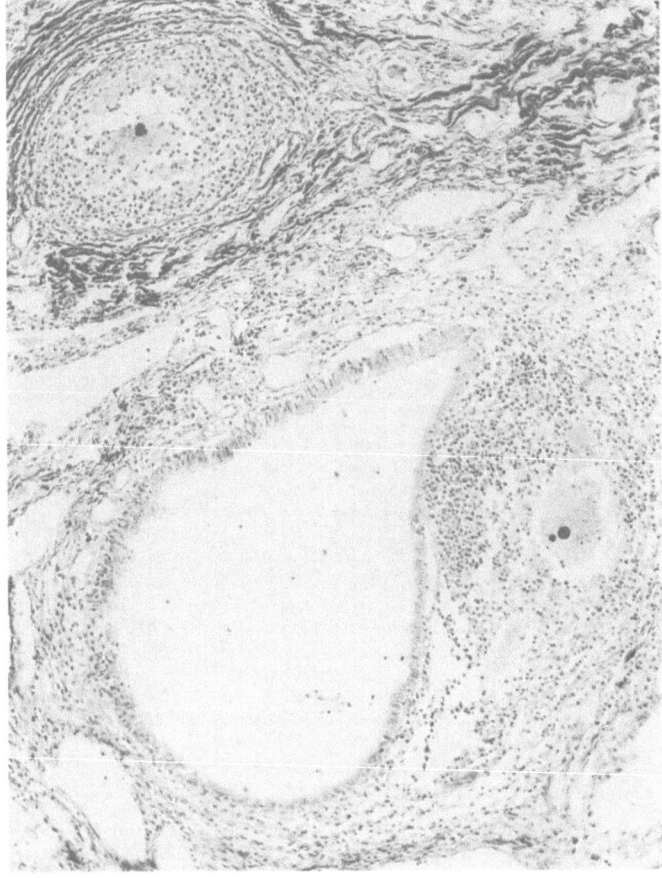

Figure 4. Same area and magnification, Grocott–Gomori stain. This is Fig. 33 of reference 1, reproduced by permission of the publisher. Note the deep staining of the spherules within the giant cells.

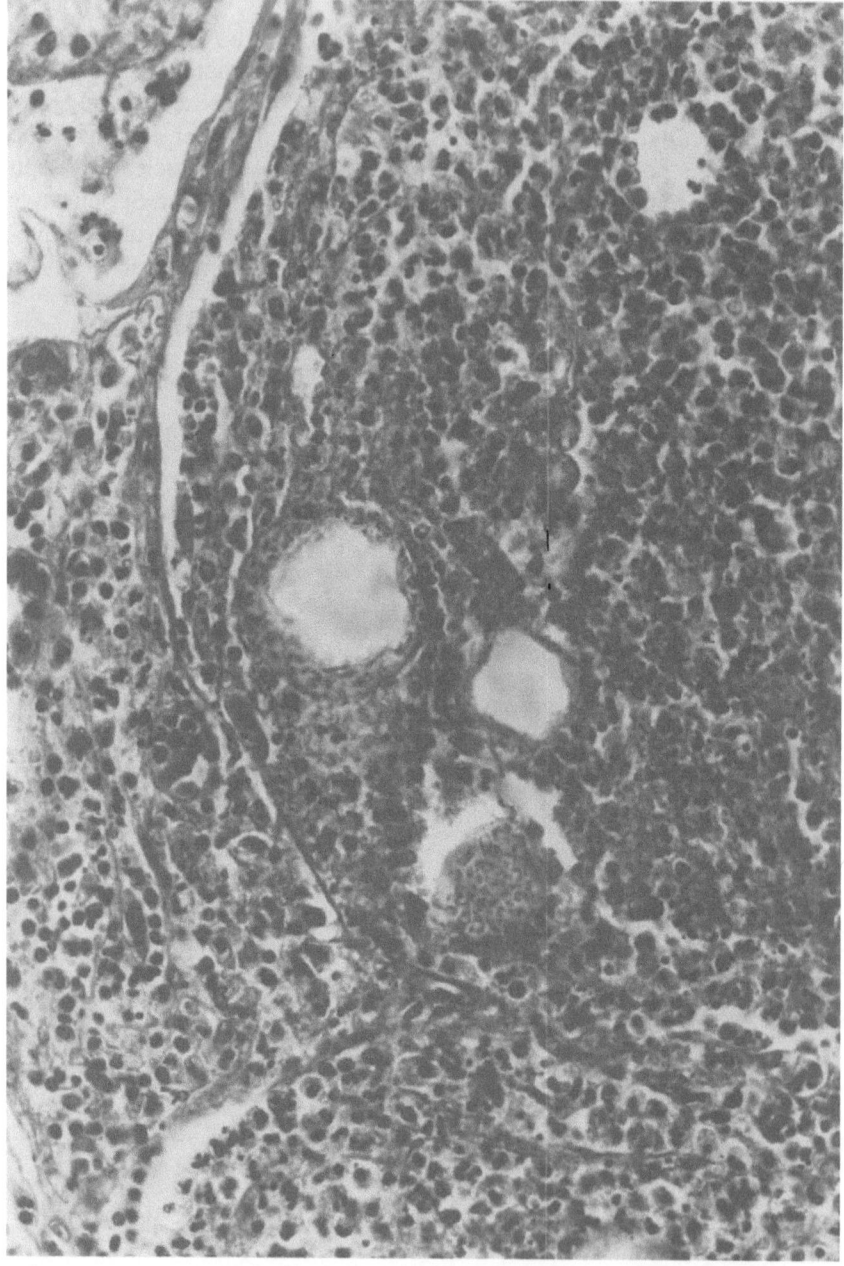

Figure 5. This is Fig. 16 of reference 1, reproduced with permission of the publisher. The section is from case D 2, reference 6. Suppurative pneumonia, showing several endosporulating sporangia. H & E, ×400.

the midst of an epithelioid "tubercle" (Fig. 7). The all-important part of histopathologic study of known or suspected coccidioidomycosis is the search for coccidioides organisms. The hunt for coccidioides may be quick and easy, or tedious and difficult. Sometimes organisms are readily found with hematoxylin and eosin (H & E) staining, but special stains are quite often necessary. Spherules are sometimes easy to spot within giant cells. Microabscesses are good places to look for them (Fig. 8). In the sort of field which is likely to be selected for didactic presentation,

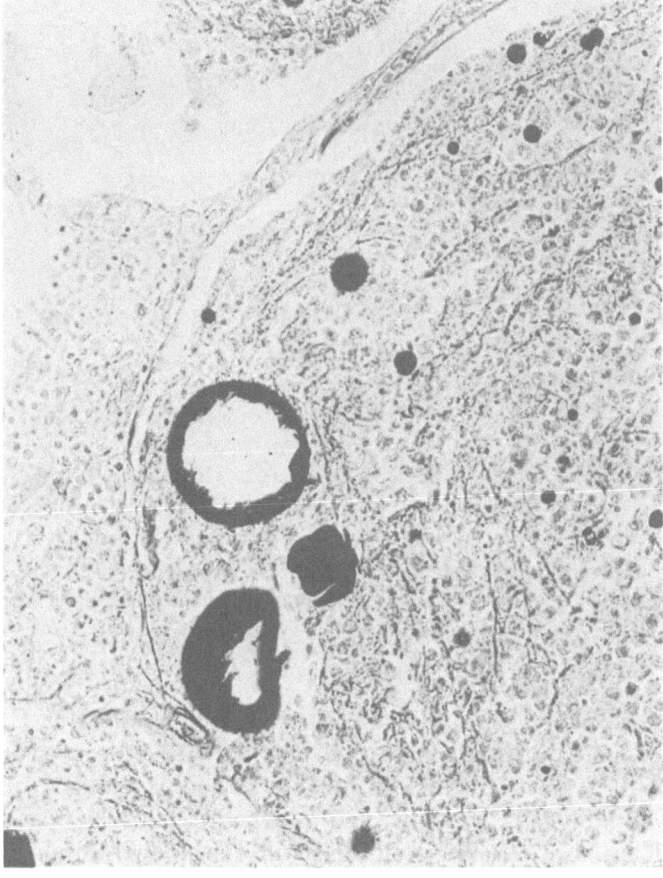

Figure 6. This is Fig. 17 of reference 1, reproduced with permission of the publisher. Area and magnification are those of Fig. 5, but stain is Grocott–Gomori. Note that several small spherules are discernible which were not clear in Fig. 5. However, the staining of the larger organisms is so deep and diffuse that endosporulation cannot be recognized here, though it was obvious in the previous figure.

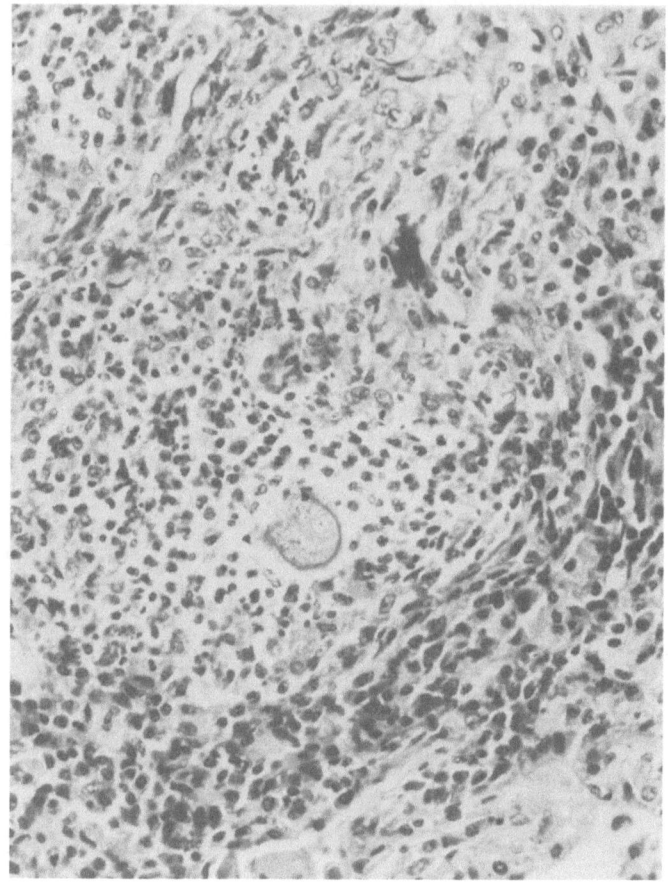

Figure 7. Lung, showing circumscribed microabscess within epithelioid "tubercle." This is a common combination. Note the rupturing sporangium in the center of the microabscess. H & E, ×300.

coccidioides spherules are so numerous and striking with H & E staining that one might be disposed to question the need for special stains. However, in caseous, calcific, or liquefactive foci, spherules will not be shown well with H & E stains, and in general, unless very numerous, they will be more readily found and will appear more abundant with special stains than with H & E. If coccidioidomycosis or other fungus infection is suspected, and fungi cannot be found on H & E, microscopic study will be inadequate without special stains.

Choice among the proposed "fungus stains" is a personal one. After an extensive trial with the Hotchkiss–McManus Periodic Acid–Schiff

(PAS) stain, and some experience with the Gridley,[3,4] the writer came to prefer the Grocott-Gomori Methenamine Silver.[5] The fungi stand out as black against a green background. Appropriate use and interpretation of any of these stains requires a degree of experience and sophistication. They are stains for oxidizable but insoluble polysaccharide, of which fungi usually contain a good deal. They are not "specific" for fungi even in the limited sense in which Ziehl–Nielsen stains may be said to be specific for mycobacteria. Among the tissue elements emphasized by "fungus stains" are mucus droplets, glycogen granules, corpora amylacea of the brain, cross-striations of voluntary muscle, and some fibrillar

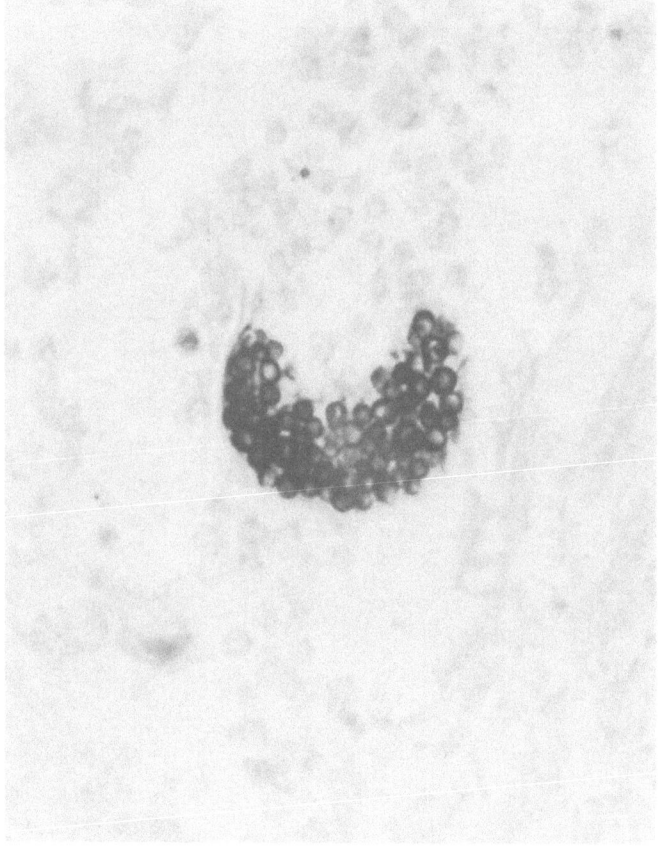

Figure 8. Pneumonic process, showing microabscess with rupturing sporangium. Grocott–Gomori, ×650. The section is from case 9, reference 1. Note that the walls of the endospores stain well, while the wall of the "old sporangium" stains very poorly.

components of connective tissue. Unstained anthracotic dust may look a good deal like silver-stained particulate polysaccharide.

Stains of adjoining sections from the same block with H & E and with methenamine silver are shown in Figs. 3, 4, 5, 6, 9, and 10. Clearly spherular coccidioides which could have been missed with H & E may be readily visible with methenamine silver (Figs. 5, 6, 9, and 10). Sometimes endosporulation is well brought out by the special stain. In other instances, however, the interior of a sporangium may be stained too deeply and diffusely to permit recognition of endosporulation (Fig. 6). Moreover, the outer wall of a ruptured sporangium will often, indeed rather regularly, stain poorly with methenamine silver (Fig. 8). Thus

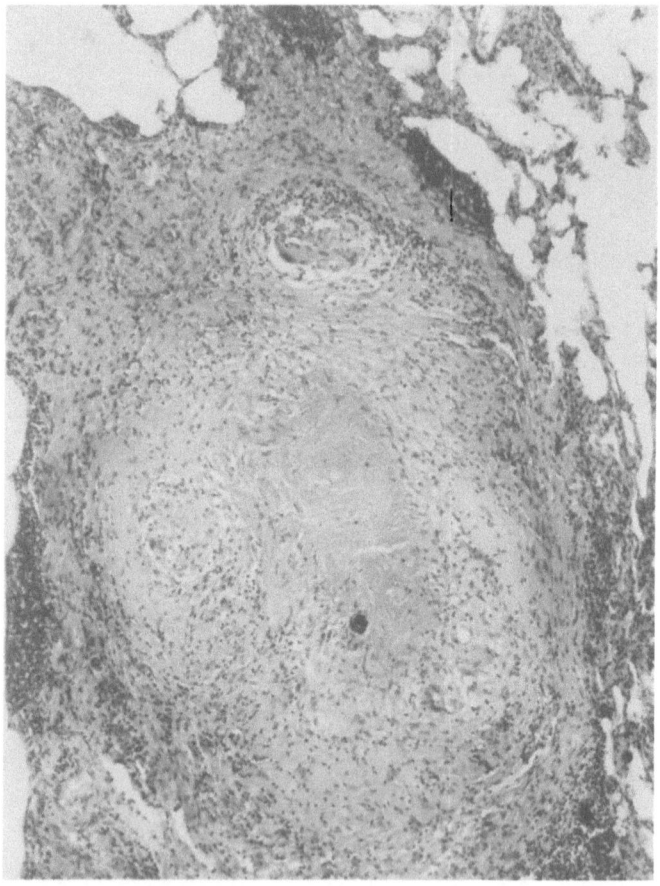

Figure 9. Lung, caseous miliary "tubercle." The section is from case B 5, reference 6. H & E, ×75.

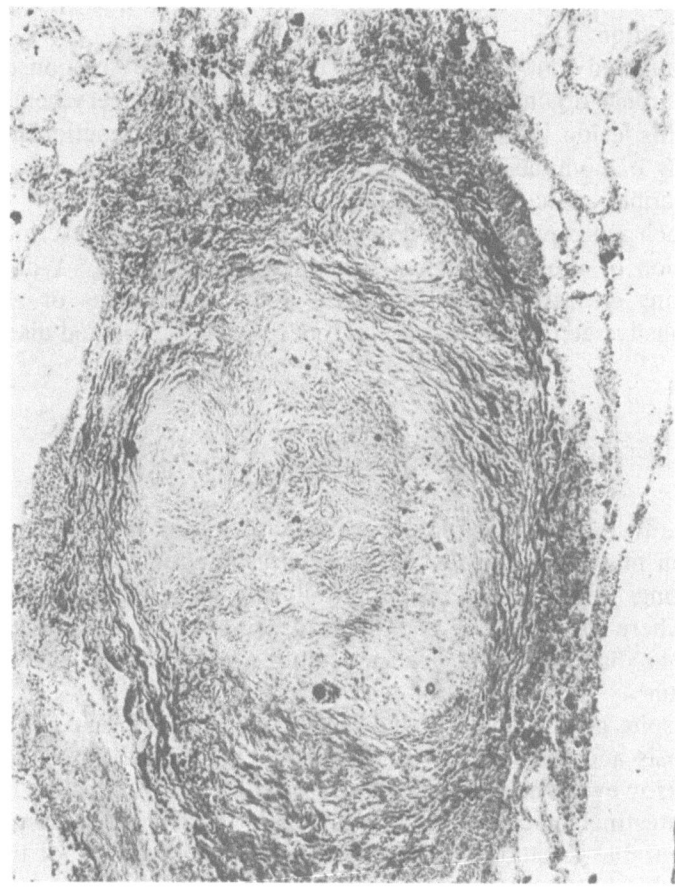

Figure 10. Same area and magnification as Fig. 9, Grocott–Gomori stain. The dark-staining spherules can be readily discerned even at this low magnification.

endosporulation is sometimes (not always) more readily discernable with H & E than with special stains (Figs. 5 and 6).

Newer techniques, such as identification of coccidioides in tissue sections with fluorescent-labeled antibody,[7,8] may be useful in sections with few organisms.

The sequence of host cell infiltration, and the relation of this to the metamorphosis of the fungus and its further replication in tissue, is discussed in Chapter 5.

Some patterns do not fit the pictures described above. Thus, in the spleens of subjects with "fungemia," the writer and his colleagues have encountered[6] considerable numbers of organisms with little or no tissue response. This phenomenon may be attributed to anergy and agonal dissemination.

In marked contrast to this pattern is the "allergic" response without demonstrable organisms, encountered in coccidioidal erythema nodosum.[9] This lesion is thought to represent an allergic reaction to soluble products or components of the organism. Histologically, it is a rather nondescript panniculitis and angiitis.

Much more puzzling in its pathogenesis is the nondescript cellular infiltration of the myocardium discussed by Reingold.[10] While this is something entirely distinct from the focal granulomas or abscesses occasionally seen in that tissue, both occur in disseminated disease.

3. DIFFERENTIAL DIAGNOSIS

The histopathologic picture of the suppurative type of coccidioidal infection may resemble that of a bacterial infection. Infections due to other fungi resemble histopathologically the granulomatous pattern. In cases where the organism is difficult to demonstrate, the travel history and other diagnostic aids such as cultures and serology become more important.

Despite great ecological and epidemiological differences, coccidioidomycosis and tuberculosis offer striking clinical and pathologic parallelism. However, the writer has yet to see coccidioidal infection involving gastrointestinal mucosa. While coccidioidal meningitis is common, he has been able to study but one case of "coccidioidoma" of the brain, comparable to tuberculomas.[11] Otherwise the parallelism has been fairly consistent. Polymorphonuclear or mixed patterns of cellular response, though perhaps less conspicuous in tuberculosis than in coccidioidomycosis, can hardly be classed as rare. Differential diagnosis, therefore, will usually require demonstration of one organism or the other. It must be remembered that patients who have had one infection can subsequently get the other. Thus the writer has studied several cases in which the subject, who unquestionably did have tuberculosis, has developed coccidioidomycosis while under sanitorium treatment for his tuberculosis.

In a praiseworthy attempt to discern differences between coccidioidal and tuberculous lung cavities, radiologist colleagues have emphasized a "thin-walled" appearance of some coccidioidal cavities. Yet, particularly since the advent of effective chemotherapy for tuberculosis, thin-walled tuberculous cavities are not uncommon. Moreover, some of the coccidioidal cavities which radiologists have described as thin-walled prior to resection have looked quite thick-walled when brought to the pathology laboratory. After considerable study of tuberculous and coccidioidal cavities, the writer has had to acknowledge that the only way he can differentiate them is by demonstration of the etiologic organism.

Coccidioidal infection, the "great imitator" pathologically as well as clinically, can also sometimes produce a histologic appearance easily confused with sarcoidosis.

4. MICROSCOPIC DISTINCTION FROM OTHER FUNGI

4.1. *Rhinosporidium seeberi*

R. seeberi, which may be an alga rather than a fungus, has apparently not been cultured *in vitro.* Its sporangia are characteristically so huge that confusion with those of *Coccidioides* would seem unlikely.[12] They also stain with mucicarmine, which spherules do not.

4.2. *Paracoccidioides brasiliensis*

The first students to observe *Paracoccidioides brasiliensis* did, in fact, confuse it with *C. immitis.*[13] One might guess that they had perhaps overlooked the multiple budding with everted buds now deemed characteristic and diagnostic, and may have concentrated on what looks like inward budding. Whether the latter pattern is an artifact due to plane of section does not concern us, nor does any other explanation, for that pattern is indeed readily confused with that of endosporulation. In paracoccidioidal material given to me, the everted budding pattern was not difficult to find.

4.3. *Histoplasma capsulatum*

Ordinarily the yeast form of *H. capsulatum* is much smaller and more uniform that the average-sized spherule of *C. immitis.* "Huge forms" of *H. capsulatum,* as illustrated in Schwartz's Fig. 6 in reference 14 could readily be mistaken for coccidioides. An aggregate of normal-sized *H. capsulatum* might be mistaken for an aggregate of just released coccidioidal endospores, and it is unsafe, therefore, to acclaim an aggregate of small round fungi as "newborn" coccidioides without finding a bit of remaining wall of a parent sporangium (Fig. 11).

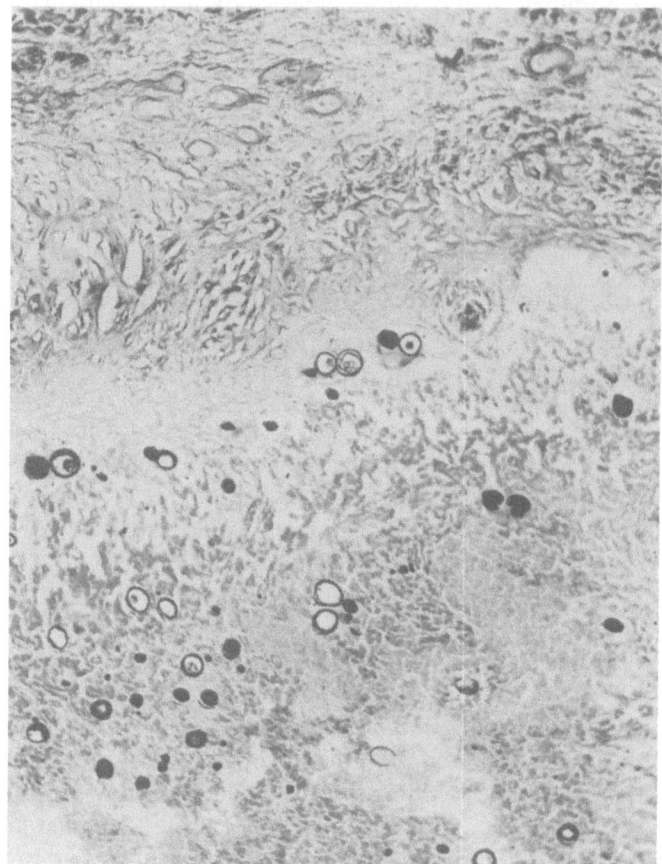

Figure 11. This, like Fig. 12, is from the meninges of case 2, reference 1. The stain is Grocott–Gomori and the magnification ×125. Note that spherules are numerous, but none of them are large, and endosporulation is not discernible.

4.4. Histoplasma duboisii

From African histoplasmosis material graciously given to me, I recognize that I might have real difficulty in distinguishing *H. duboisii* from nonendosporulating *C. immitis* in tissue sections.[15]

4.5. Cryptococcus neofomans

If typical cryptococcus cells of *C. neofomans* with large capsules are present, they should be readily distinguishable from *C. immitis*.[16]

4.6. *Blastomyces dermatitidis*

In the North American blastomycosis material which I have had the opportunity to study, budding of the fungus has been consistently obvious.[17] While pairs of *C. immitis* are not rare, in the blastomycosis material, the budding has been unmistakable and omnipresent. With the Grocott–Gomori stain, *B. dermatitidis* has stained much less vividly than coccidioides, and its organisms have tended to be smaller.

5. POSTMORTEM EXAMINATION

Wet mounts at the autopsy table are often helpful, and cultures should be taken freely. Positive culture cannot be expected from tissue fixed in 10% formalin, but tissue concentrations of formaldehyde obtained on ordinary intravascular embalming are not necessarily lethal to coccidioides, for I have quite often obtained positive cultures from embalmed bodies. It may be appropriate to warn undertakers of the risk they incur in handling bodies of victims of disseminated coccidioidomycosis.[18] The problem is not that of ordinary contagion, but of inoculation from a puncture wound. While no organ or tissue should be neglected, attention is often appropriately centered on the lungs and meninges.

In chronic disseminated coccidioidomycosis, one may find little or nothing in the lungs. Even the primary lesion may have disappeared. On the other hand, there may be miliary disseminated disease in the lungs, and confluent coccidioidal penumonia may occur early or late. One should be particularly concerned not to miss cases of pneumonic coccidioidomycosis with early rapid fatality. Massive pneumonic reaction with excavation (cavity formation) may occur.

From study of various stages and patterns of coccidioidal pneumonia, the writer is convinced that this process can and sometimes does lead to bronchiectasis (Figs. 3 and 4), and that in endemic areas some cases of bronchiectasis which show no trace of their ultimate etiology may well have been due to coccidioidomycosis.

Since the signs and symptoms of coccidioidal meningitis are often vague and ambiguous, exploration and examination of the cranial cavity and removal of a sizeable portion of spinal cord should, whenever possible, be made routine in autopsies on subjects with known or suspected coccidioidomycosis. Of course, in some cases limitation of extent of autopsy is necessary to obtain consent for any autopsy at all. However, when unconditional consent for autopsy has been obtained, opening the skull should not be omitted on account of fatigue, inertia, or belief that the case has already been adequately clarified.

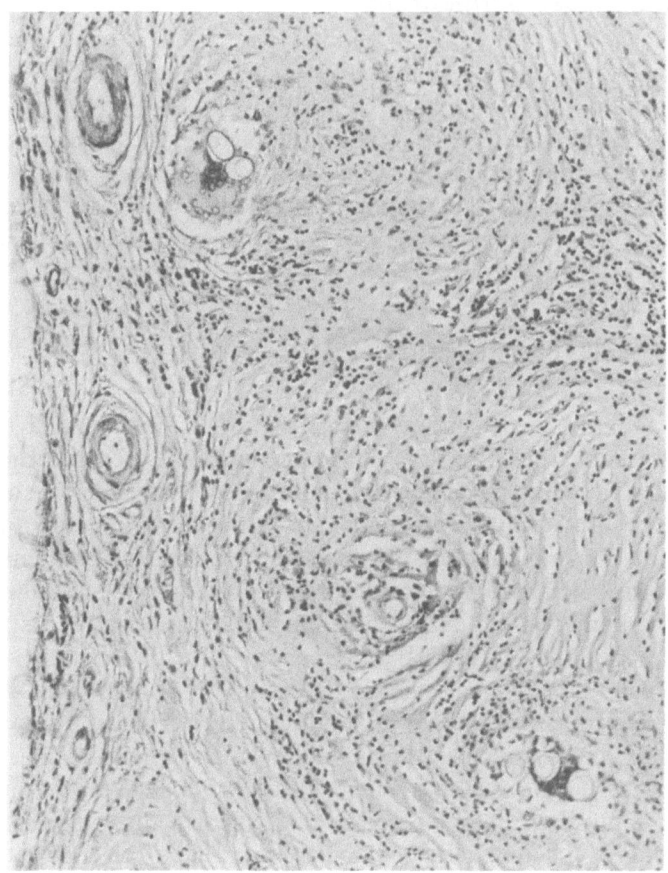

Figure 12. Chronic meningitis with hyaline fibrosis, and giant cells containing spherules. The section is from case 2, reference 1. H & E, ×125.

Coccidioidal meningitis is seldom impressive on gross examination. It tends to involve depths of sulci rather than peaks of gyri and, especially when chronic, to be basilar rather than supracortical. The leptomeninges of the spinal cord merit careful microscopic examination. Cultures may be helpful, especially if the case has not been adequately studied *intra vitam*. Numerous blocks should be taken for microscopic study.

Particularly upon prolonged amphotericin treatment, coccidioidal meningitis can become very indolent and fibrotic, and death in such cases may be due to sequelae (Fig. 12). Such chronic meningitis frequently results in interference with spinal fluid circulation and reabsorption; this in turn results in ventricular dilation with cortical thinning, i.e., in hydrocephalus.

Since granulomatous cerebral arteritis is sometimes conspicuous in coccidioidal meningitis, and the process when chronic and basilar may concentrate upon the vicinity of the Circle of Willis, the frequent occurrence of multifocal ischemic cortical encephalomalacia in chronic coccidioidal meningitis is hardly surprising. Cortical lesions in coccidioidal meningitis have usually proved to be of this character. Further discussion of the sequelae of central nervous system infection can be found in Chapter 11.

Secondary infections of the lungs, or of the central nervous system (consequent to repeated spinal fluid punctures or neurosurgical procedures), may be a source of confusion at postmortem examination.

Sequelae of amphotericin treatment should be carefully distinguished

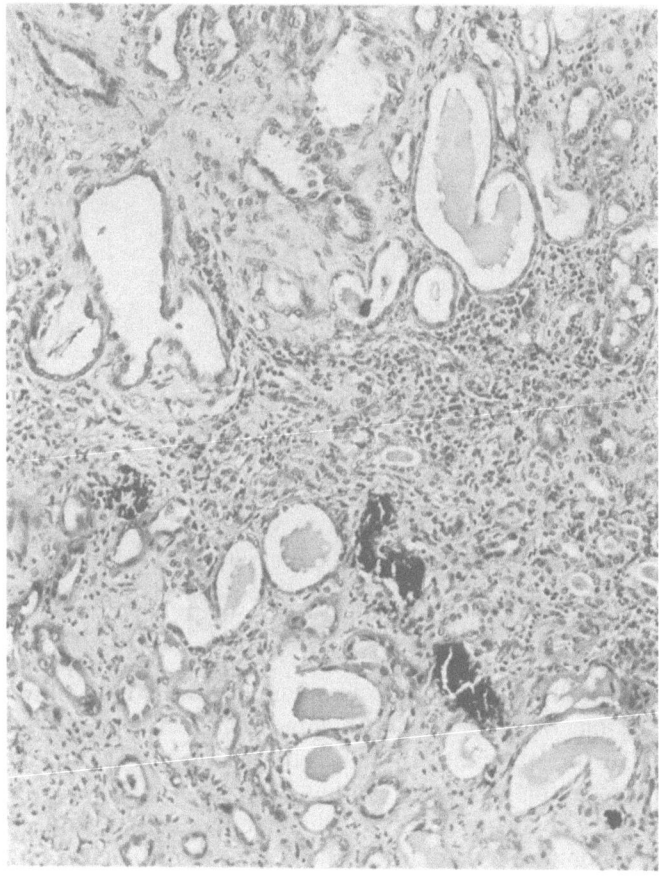

Figure 13. End-stage nephropathy due to amphotericin. H & E, ×125. Note atrophy and distortion of tubules, interstitial fibrosis and calcification, and patchy round cell infiltrate.

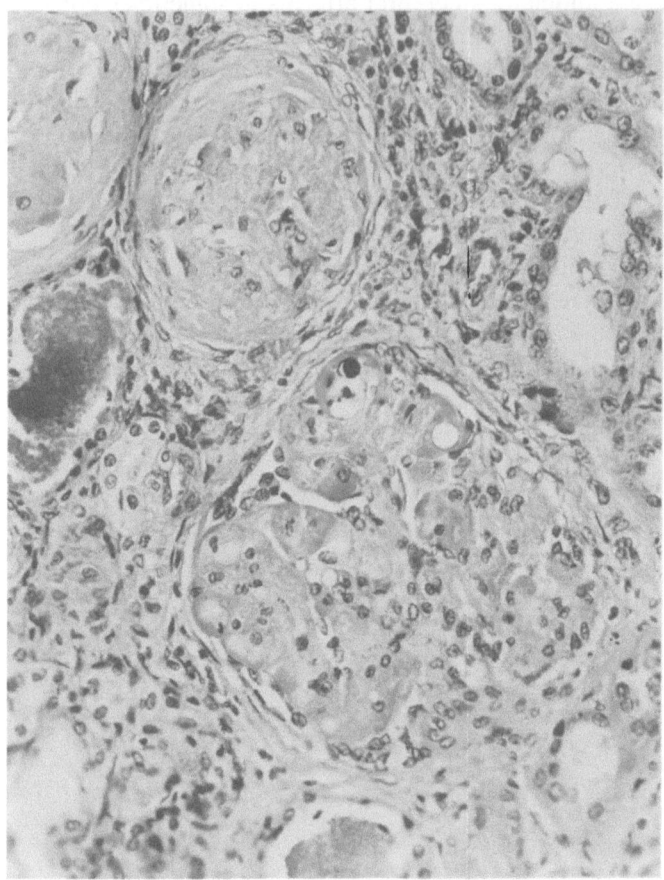

Figure 14. Glomerulopathy in end-stage amphotericin nephropathy. H & E, ×250.

from direct results of the infection. With reiterated injection of amphotericin into the spinal fluid, there will sometimes be meningeal accumulation of extraneous material. It is uncertain whether this is amphotericin, or a component of the vehicle.

In cases of disseminated coccidioidomycosis involving an extremity intraarterial injection has been attempted, with result disastrous to the circulation in the extremity. In a recent case, constriction of a spinal artery with resulting myelomalacia has been noted following intrathecal amphotericin.[19] This is evidently a phenomenon distinct from the multifocal encephalomalacia mentioned as a sequel to meningitis.

With massive and prolonged amphotericin treatment, at autopsy one may encounter the "end stage" kidney, with extensive tubular, interstitial, and glomerular alteration (Figs. 13 and 14). Early lesions are predominantly tubular and are reversible, later glomerular lesions become conspicuous. It appears the nephropathy can progress during life[20,21] after the last dose of amphotericin, consistent with that drug's persistence in the body.

In previous studies by the writer, meningitis was found in the majority of coccidioidal fatalities[1,6] and, when found, was assumed to be the cause of death. In cases of chronic meningitis, this assumption seems safe enough. In many such cases, extrameningeal lesions have been sparse or undetectable. However, in quite a number of cases the meningitis, fairly recent, has been associated with massive coccidioidal pneumonia, and one may question which of the two lesions has the major responsibility for the fatality.

ACKNOWLEDGMENTS.   Permission to reproduce some of the figures from a preceding article[6] was granted by the University of Arizona Press.

6. REFERENCES

1. R. W. Huntington, Coccidioidomycosis, in: *Human Infection with Fungi: Actinomycetes and Algae,* (R. Baker, ed.), Chapter VI, Springer-Verlag, Berlin (1971).
2. N. Levan and R. W. Huntington, Primary cutaneous coccidioidomycosis of agricultural workers, *Arch. Derm.* **92**:215–220 (1965).
3. A. Kligman, H. Mescon, and E. Delameter, The Hotchkiss-McManus Stain for the histopathologic diagnosis of fungus diseases, *Am. J. Clin. Pathol.* **21**:86–91 (1951).
4. M. Gridley, A stain for fungi in tissue sections, *Am. J. Clin. Pathol.* **23**:303–307, 1953.
5. R. Grocott, A stain for fungi in tissue sections and smears, using Gomori's methenamine silver nitrate technique, *Am. J. Clin. Pathol.* **25**:975–979, 1955.
6. R. W. Huntington, W. J. Waldmann, J. A. Sargent, H. O'Connell, R. Wybel, and D. Croll, Pathologic and clinical observations on 142 cases of fatal coccidioidomycosis with necropsy, in: *Coccidioidomycosis* (L. Ajello, ed.), University of Arizona Press, Tucson (1967), pp. 143–167.
7. W. Kaplan, Application of the fluorescent antibody technique to the diagnosis and study of coccidioidomycosis, in: *Coccidioidomycosis* (L. Ajello, ed.), University of Arizona Press, Tucson (1967), pp. 227–232.
8. W. Kaplan and D. Kraft, Demonstration of pathogenic fungi in formalin-fixed tissues by immunofluorescence, *Am. J. Clin. Pathol.* **52**:420–432 (1969).
9. A. Allen, *The Skin. A Clinicopathological Treatise,* 2nd ed., Grune and Stratton, New York (1967), p. 517.
10. I. Reingold, Myocardial lesions in disseminated coccidioidomycosis, *Am. J. Clin. Pathol.* **20**:1044–1049 (1950).
11. A. Rhoden, Coccidioidal brain abscess, *Bull. Los Angeles Neurol. Soc.* **11**:80–85 (1946).
12. L. N. Mohapatra, Rhinosporidiosis, in: *Human Infection with Fungi, Actinomycetes and Algae* (R. Baker, ed.), Chapter XIV, Springer-Verlag, Berlin (1971).

13. A. Angulo O. and L. Pollak, Paracoccidioidomycosis, in: *Human Infection with Fungi, Actinomycetes and Algae* (R. Baker, ed.), Chapter X, Springer-Verlag, Berlin (1971).

14. J. Schwarz, Histoplasmosis, in: *Human Infection with Fungi, Actinomycetes and Algae* (R. Baker, ed.), Chapter IV, Springer-Verlag, Berlin (1971).

15. J. Schwarz, African Histoplasmosis, in: *Human Infection with Fungi, Actinomycetes and Algae* (R. Baker, ed.), Chapter V, Springer-Verlag, Berlin (1971).

16. K. Salfelder, Cryptococcosis, in: *Human Infection with Fungi, Actinomycetes and Algae* (R. Baker, ed.), Chapter VII, Springer-Verlag, Berlin (1971).

17. E. W. Chick, North American Blastomycosis, in: *Human Infection with Fungi, Actinomycetes and Algae* (R. Baker, ed.), Chapter IX, Springer-Verlag, Berlin (1971).

18. J. Wilson, C. Smith, and O. Plunkett, Primary cutaneous coccidioidomycosis. The criteria for diagnosis and report of a case, *Calif. Med.* **79**:233–239 (1953).

19. N. T. Carnevale, J. N. Galgiani, J. W. Langston, and D. A. Stevens, Myelopathy due to intrathecal amphotericin B, in: *Coccidioidomycosis: Current Clinical and Diagnostic Status* (L. Ajello, ed.), Symposia Specialists, Miami (1977), pp. 259–260.

20. E. Reynolds, Z. Tomkiewics, and G. Dammin, The renal lesion related to amphotericin B treatment for coccidioidomycosis, *Med. Clin. North Am.* **47**:1149–1154 (1963).

21. F. Takacs, Z. Tomkiewics, and J. Merrill, Amphotericin B nephrotoxicity with irreversible renal failure, *Ann. Intern. Med.* **59**:716–724 (1963).

8

Classification of Coccidioidomycosis

David Salkin

1. INTRODUCTION

As in other diseases, the classification of coccidioidomycosis is a method of describing the disease by grouping its various manifestations into special categories and patterns to give as complete a picture as possible of the history of the disease and its state in any patient at any time. It may be used to compare different series of cases, in research programs, and for statistical and record-keeping purposes. However, it must be dynamic and subject to change as new developments occur in pathogenesis, immunology and other host-organism relationships, treatments, and the use of vaccines which may alter the relative importance of established categories. As an infectious disease, it has a number of features in common with other granulomatous diseases.

The broad relationships between the organism and the host are:

1. No infection.
2. Infection without disease.
3. Infection with disease.
4. Prophylactic vaccination and chemotherapy.

The description of these relationships follows:

1. No infection—no exposure to the endemic area or its products, no symptoms, negative skin test and other immunological tests, negative mycologic studies, and no roentgen findings.
2. Infection without disease—positive skin test, possibly a low complement fixation titer, no specific symptoms, negative mycologic studies, no compatible active X-ray findings.

3. Infection with disease—to be described.

4. Prophylactic—must be considered as present and future research with vaccines and chemotherapeutic agents are developed and utilized.

2. THE DISEASE: COCCIDIOIDOMYCOSIS

2.1. Pathogenesis

Primary disease: May be asymptomatic or symptomatic and usually produces a high degree of immunity.

Recurrent disease:

1. Endogenous—extension or reactivation even years after apparent quiescence or healing (postprimary progression).

2. Exogenous—a new exogenous infection occurring rarely, in a previously healing or healed or even a still active lesion (superinfection).

Dissemination: Usually occurs as a complication of the primary disease, but some cases become manifest after a year or more (may have no history of a symptomatic primary), may occur with chronic lesions, or in states of immune debility may reactivate previously quiescent primary disease and disseminate.

2.2. Clinical Types

Asymptomatic disease: No clinical symptoms but shows a recent conversion of the skin test, positive precipitin or complement fixation tests, densities on the X-ray film, or positive sputum cultures (may be induced). One or more of these features may be present.

Acute pulmonary disease: May be very mild to very severe and show no X-ray changes or an extensive pneumonia. Although it occurs usually as a primary disease process, it may be an acute reaction representing a reactivation. Clinical activity classification always "Active."

Subacute disease: A relatively small number of cases; a phase between a prolonged acute and chronic disease. Because of the small numbers, this category may be omitted and classified with chronic disease.

Chronic pulmonary disease: includes cavitary, nodular, and fibrosing disease, chronic pneumonitis, or mixtures of these which may be "residual" from the acute disease or develop after years of apparent healing. The lesions may be progressive, regressive, stable, or unstable. See Chapter 10.

Dissemination: May be pulmonary and extrapulmonary.

2.3. Clinical Activity

The three main stages are active, quiescent, and inactive, and are judged by the symptoms and signs, roentgenograms, mycologic studies, immunology, and duration (should be stated).

Active: Symptoms and signs usually present (absent if heading toward inactive status); the X-ray may show progression, regression, or even stable disease; mycologic studies usually positive; serology and skin tests usually positive; pathology if available shows an active process.

Quiescent: Shows a healing or stable process and no symptoms, but the complement fixation titer is high ($>1 : 16^*$), mycologic studies variable.

Inactive: Shows no symptoms, X-ray lesion stable if present, negative mycologic studies, a negative or positive skin test, no precipitins, and a low complement fixation titer ($<1 : 16^*$); these conditions are to have existed for more than 6 months.

2.4. Location

The *primary* disease is usually pulmonary but also involves the regional nodes in the hilum and mediastinum, and may involve the pleura and resulting effusions. The pericardium may also be involved. A generalized rash (several types) may be present without pulmonary disease.

When dissemination occurs, it may also involve the lung secondarily. Usually, the dissemination is extrapleural and must be listed. Almost every tissue in the body may be involved. Dissemination may be general (miliary), or it may involve one or more systems. They include:

---

* Titers refer to procedure of Smith *et al.;* see Chapter 6.

1. *Lymphatic system*—if cervical nodes are involved in the primary phase, it should be considered dissemination unless proven otherwise. More distant lymph nodes mean dissemination.

2. *Bones and joints.*

3. *Skin and subcutaneous tissue.*

4. *Central nervous system.*

5. *Abdominal viscera*—spleen and liver.

6. *Serous cavities*—pleura, pericardium, and peritoneum.

7. *Genitourinary*—kidneys, ureter, bladder; prostate, epididymis; uterus, tubes and ovaries.

8. *Endocrine*—pancreas, adrenals, and thyroid.

9. *Other*—skeletal muscle, eyes, middle ear, myocardium, and pericardium.

2.5. X-ray Findings

The *pulmonary* findings should be described with regard to the side involved, the lobes, and the nature of the lesions, which can be pneumonic, nodular, cavitary, fibrous, or calcified; the patterns are often mixed. The lung findings should include the hilar and mediastinal lymph nodes, the pleural and pericardial reactions.

The *extrapulmonary* lesions should have roentgen examinations (sometimes radionuclide scans) when feasible, especially the bones and joints, and the extent of sinus tracts and fistulas defined by sinograms.

2.6. Extent of Disease

The extent of the pulmonary lesions may be added to those described with the X-ray findings, and may be described as localized or extensive, lateralization, lung fields involved, and should include the size of cavities and their locations. The latter are especially important in surgical cases.

Disseminated lesions require detailed descriptions depending upon radiologic and nuclear methods as well as physical and laboratory examinations.

2.7. Therapeutic Status

The classification of therapy is described as follows:

1. None (or symptomatic).

2. Chemotherapy—drug used, total dosage.
3. Surgical—pulmonary, extrapulmonary.

2.8. Mycology

Coccidioides immitis should be sought in every case, and if there is no sputum where pulmonary infection is possible, sputum should be induced. Gastric lavage has low yield but may be tried. The findings should be described as positive (by smear, by culture or by animal), negative, pending or not done. Number of cultures may be of interest in serial observations.

2.9. Immunology

The three tests of importance include the specific skin test, the serological precipitin test, and the complement fixation test.

The skin test preferred is the intradermal, and coccidioidin and/or spherulin may be used. One should note the dilution used and whether the test was positive (record induration in mm, longest axis of reaction), negative, doubtful, or not done.

The precipitin test is read as positive or negative. If done by the test tube method, it should be noted, if positive, in what dilution.

The complement fixation test may be done by immunodiffusion test, or by the dilution method (highest positive dilution noted).

2.10. Racial Susceptibility

There is a marked difference in the racial reaction to the disease (see Chapter 4). Ancestry should be recorded.

2.11. Sex Differences

Sex differences are discussed in Chapters 4, 9, and 17. Sex should be noted.

2.12. Age Differences.

See Chapter 18. Age should be noted.

2.13. Concomitant Diseases and Therapy

Concomitant diseases and therapy should be listed as pulmonary and nonpulmonary diseases which may influence the coccidioidal disease and, in turn, be affected.

The pulmonary diseases to be noted particularly are tuberculosis, chronic bronchitis, sarcoidosis, other granulomata, important infections, and tumors.

The nonpulmonary diseases of particular significance include diabetes, alcoholism, malignant tumors, and states of debility and low immunity.

Use of immunosuppressive agents such as corticosteroids, radiotherapy, and cytotoxic drugs should be noted (see Chapter 19).

3. EXAMPLE OF CLASSIFICATION OF COCCIDIOIDOMYCOSIS

The various categories described may be divided into those that are *basic* and those that are *supplementary*. Although all categories may be important, the basic ones, as a rule, include the pathogenesis, clinical type, clinical activity, and the location of the lesions. The others are to be added as their importance indicates in the particular patient described.

3.1. Case: Male, White, Age 30 Years

Admission diagnosis—Coccidioidomycosis: pulmonary, active primary disease, acute, positive skin test (7-mm induration to spherulin, Usual Test Strength) and complement fixation test in 1 : 256 dilution, positive precipitins, small bilateral pneumonic pulmonary densities (lower lobes), and adenopathy, duration 3 months. To start chemotherapy. Sputum cultures (two of three) positive for *C. immitis*. Juvenile onset diabetes mellitus.

Final diagnosis—Coccidioidomycosis: pulmonary, primary, inactive, asymptomatic, skin test positive (8-mm induration to spherulin, Usual Test Strength), no precipitins, complement fixation test is 1 : 8 dilution, complete X-ray clearing. Chemotherapy (amphotericin B) completed (675 mg total dose over 6 weeks). Sputum cultures negative (zero of three) for *C. immitis*. Juvenile onset diabetes mellitus.

9

Primary Coccidioidomycosis

Antonino Catanzaro and David J. Drutz

1. INTRODUCTION

That approximately 60% of coccidioidal infections are asymptomatic has been discussed in Chapter 4. Forty percent of patients are symptomatic with a disease spectrum ranging from mild influenzalike complaints to frank pneumonia. Ordinarily the symptoms are sufficiently vague that no specific diagnosis is suggested. Thus, the epidemiologic history is of major value.

The most common symptoms of primary coccidioidomycosis are cough, fever, and chest pain. Cough is often not productive of sputum. Chest pain is often pleuritic. Fever is more commonly accompanied by chilly sensations than by frank shaking chills; night sweats are not unusual.

Other symptoms include headache, malaise, sore throat, myalgias, and anorexia. It should be noted that headache may be a nonspecific symptom, and does not necessarily indicate that the patient is experiencing concurrent dissemination of infection to the meninges. Nevertheless, if there is any doubt, lumbar puncture should always be carried out for two reasons: (1) Dissemination of coccidioidomycosis characteristically occurs early in the course of infection; therefore, early meningeal dissemination is not necessarily unusual. (2) The prognosis for recovery from meningitis is limited, but there may be some advantage to early therapeutic intervention, as will be discussed in Chapter 10.

Three aspects of primary coccidioidomycosis are somewhat more helpful diagnostically, and deserve special comment.

2. TOXIC ERYTHEMA

Since the very earliest observations of primary pulmonary coccidi-oidomycosis by Dickson, it has been appreciated that a nonspecific rash may accompany acquisition of the infection.[1-4] This is not to be confused with erythema nodosum or erythema multiforme. Toxic erythema generally occurs in the first few days of illness, before coccidioidin sensitivity is established, and tends to disappear before the patient seeks medical advice.[5] The rash is generally fine, diffuse, erythematous, and macular, and it may cover the trunk and extremities[6-9]; there may be an associated oral enanthem.[10,11] The rash generally occurs in about 10% of patients,[12] but appears to be more common in children.[11] Fully one-half of the archeology students in Werner's series manifested "toxic erythema"; several of these students were treated for allergic or contact dermatitis with systemic steroids.[7,9] This rash has also be confused with measles,[1,3] scarlet fever,[3] heat rash,[2] and urticaria.[9,12] The etiology of "toxic erythema" is unknown. We have been unable to find studies in the literature in which immunopathologic analysis of the skin eruption has been undertaken. The occurrence of the rash seems to have no bearing on the outcome of coccidioidomycosis. Excellent color photographs of "toxic erythema," erythema multiforme, and erythema nodosum may be found in an article by Harvey and Greendyke.[8]

3. "VALLEY FEVER" (ERYTHEMA NODOSUM, ERYTHEMA MULTIFORME; ARTHRALGIAS, ARTHRITIS)

Erythema nodosum and erythema multiforme constitute the principal manifestations of the "valley fever" complex, which also includes arthralgias ("desert rheumatism") and a mild nonspecific conjunctivitis sometimes accompanied by episcleritis or keratitis.[1,2,4,5,8,12-18]

In contrast to "toxic erythema," erythema nodosum and erythema multiforme have been referred to as the "specific erythemas" of coccid-ioidomycosis.[8,12] Erythema nodosum is the most common accompaniment of primary coccidioidomycosis in most series.[4,16,17] There are exceptions, however.[8] Erythema nodosum tends to occur at about the time that the coccidioidin skin-test reaction becomes positive and is considered to reflect the development of "hypersensitivity" to *Coccidioides immitis*.[1,19] This impression is supported by the characteristic violence of the coccidioidin skin test in this setting.[2,13,14,16,20] Although it is generally assumed that erythema multiforme has the same relationship to coccidioidin sensitivity,[8,12] the situation is less clear. At least two papers suggest that erythema multiforme may antedate erythema nodosum.[8,11] In one, erythema multiforme accompanied the toxic erythema and preceded coccidioidin reactivity.[11] Whether these two "specific" eruptions have the same clinical significance is not clear; what we do know about valley fever is largely based on observations of erythema nodosum.

Erythema nodosum and erythema multiforme may occur in patients who have been otherwise asymptomatic, or in whom influenzalike symptoms have waned. Often, the frightening appearance and the pain of erythema nodosum cause a patient to seek medical advice when other symptoms might have been ignored.[1,13,14]

Erythema nodosum and erythema multiforme are described in Chapter 13. Recurrences are extremely rare.[1,12]

Erythema nodosum has several characteristic associations: As indicated in two classic studies,[1,14] erythema nodosum is more common in women with coccidioidomycosis. In a retrospective study of 432 residents of the San Joaquin Valley who had experienced valley fever, there were only 4 men for every 10 women with erythema nodosum.[1] This figure contrasts starkly with the figures for dissemination, as discussed in Chapter 4. The female predisposition to erythema nodosum does not obtain before puberty; boys and girls have the same susceptibility to erythema nodosum.[1]

In prospective studies conducted among airmen stationed at San Joaquin Valley airbases during World War II, erythema nodosum occurred in 5% of patients whose coccidioidin skin-test reaction became positive.[19] Expressed in terms of the symptomatic (rather than the total) skin-test converters, 20% of men experienced erythema nodosum. Studies in women were limited, but 10/41 members of the Women's Army Corps (25%) in this same series experienced erythema nodosum in association with coccidiodin skin-test conversion. Of the women who had symptomatic infection, 50% had erythema nodosum.

Erythema nodosum is far more common in whites than in persons of other races. Of the 432 persons noted above, 428 were white, despite the fact that considerable numbers of persons of Filipino and black ancestry did live in the area.[1] None of the 94 black soldiers stationed in the San Joaquin Valley in Smith's study experienced erythema nodosum or erythema multiforme.[19]

Erythema nodosum is widely regarded as predictive of a good prognosis with regard to dissemination of coccidioidomycosis. For example, as indicated, white women, who have a greater propensity to develop erythema nodosum, are also less susceptible to dissemination.

The protective value of erythema nodosum is far from complete; the literature is filled with case reports of patients who have disseminated disease despite previous valley fever. As a result, a physician is not justified in assuming that erythema nodosum confers guaranteed safety from dissemination of the disease.

Approximately one-third of patients with erythema nodosum or erythema multiforme experience simultaneous articular symptoms.[5,12,15–18,21] On rare occasions the joints are involved in the absence of a skin rash.[5] Joints are not red, but are tender to pressure, painful on motion, and may be slightly edematous.[4,5,17] Symptoms may be worse than objective clinical findings.[17] Radiographs of joints have been normal.[16] There are no published data concerning analysis of synovial fluid in these patients, probably because a significant degree of joint effusion is not common.[5,8,16]

Although the arthritis is not migratory, the simultaneous occurrence of skin rash and joint manifestations may raise the possibilities of acute rheumatic fever[15] or the preicteric immune complex phenomena of viral hepatitis[22] in the differential diagnosis.

Careful immunopathologic studies of the synovium and skin have not been carried out in patients with valley fever. Hence, the immunologic explanation for the syndrome remains unclear.

Eosinophilia is a common accompaniment of primary coccidioidomycosis.[5,12,15–17,23] In one large series, 66 of 75 patients (88%) with acute symptomatic pulmonary coccidioidomycosis had eosinophil counts ranging from 3 to 26% of the total peripheral white blood cell count.[16] In most instances, the proportion of eosinophils ranges between 3 and 10%.[15] However, at least one patient has been reported with 89% eosinophils in his peripheral blood.[24]

Peak eosinophilia tends to occur between the 2nd and 3rd weeks of illness.[16] There is no apparent relationship between the occurrence of erythema nodosum or erythema multiforme and eosinophilia.[16] Persistent eosinophilia may be encountered in patients who experience coccidioidal dissemination.[12]

4. PRIMARY PULMONARY COCCIDIOIDOMYCOSIS

The majority of patients with primary pulmonary coccidioidomycosis report chest pain and a cough which is productive of sputum and occasional streaks of blood. When the airways are visualized through an endoscope, granulomatous inflammation is commonly seen.[25] Radiographic changes are frequent, being noted in about 80% of infections severe enough to require hospitalization,[12] and may be quite varied. Infiltrates, the most common X-ray abnormality, may be single or multiple and often have a segmental or lobar distribution. Characteristically, they are soft and hazy, but homogeneous.[26] Coalescence of many patchy infiltrates with varying amounts of atelectasis is common. Hilar adenopathy is present in 20% of cases, almost always on the same side as the infiltrate. However, hilar adenopathy (unilateral or bilateral) may also occur in the absence of pulmonary infiltrative disease.[12,27] Bilateral hilar adenopathy may suggest the diagnosis of sarcoidosis and thus be confusing. The presence of mediastinal or paratracheal adenopathy should raise the possibility of dissemination, because such nodes represent the second line of defense which must be breached if dissemination is to occur.[26] Supraclavicular nodes as well as these nodes may be culture positive, however, in cases of primary infection which do not go on to dissemination.

Involvement of the pleura is common in primary infection, but the exact frequency depends on the definition employed. If the definition is pleuritic chest pain, the frequency is 70%. If the definition is blunting of the costophrenic angle on chest X-ray, the frequency is 20%.[28] If the definition is a more generous amount of pleural fluid, the frequency varies between 2 and 6%.[25,29]

A recent study of 28 cases of acute coccidioidal pleural effusion demonstrated that fever and chest pain were universal findings and that fully 48% of patients had erythema nodosum or erythema multiforme.[30] A small amount of fluid was usually noted early during the period of observation, but there was an increase with time, sometimes to the point of complete opacification of the hemithorax. Half the cases were associated with an ipsilateral pulmonary infiltrate which extended to the edge of the lung. Unlike the situation in tuberculous pleurisy, removal of pleural fluid at thoracentesis often discloses an obvious parenchymal lesion.[26] Thus, it is possible that coccidioidal effusion occurs by direct contiguous spread across the pleural space.

The characteristics of the pleural fluid in the 28 cases were not diagnostic: mean WBC 4600/mm^3 with 66% mononuclear cells; protein 4.7 ± 0.8 g/dl; glucose 89.2 ± 17 mg/dl. C. immitis was identified in the pleural fluid in only 3 of 15 patients studied. However, the parietal pleura contained C. immitis in all 8 patients biopsied. Peripheral eosinophilia ($> 5\%$) was present in half the patients, but pleural fluid eosinophilia was only seen in 1. Complement fixation (CF) titers were positive in serum in all cases; the coccidioidin skin test (1 : 100) was positive in 85% of the patients. Eight patients had CF titers $\geq 1 : 64$. Two patients developed systemic dissemination (one with a CF of 1 : 32; another with a CF $\geq 1 : 64$); both were from racially susceptible groups.

The frequent occurrence of erythema nodosum and erythema multiforme as well as skin-test reactivity to coccidioidin and a relatively high titer of CF antibody suggest that the immune response in patients with pleural effusion due to C. immitis is quite vigorous. The pleural fluid resolved spontaneously in 25 patients; therapeutic thoracentesis was rarely required. Apparently coccidioidal pleural effusion is a largely self-limited process.

In general, patients with uncomplicated primary pulmonary coccidioidomycosis require no antifungal chemotherapy. Chemotherapy may be useful in preventing extrapulmonary spread in those predisposed to dissemination by virtue of race, sex, or immunosuppression (see Chapter 4).

ACKNOWLEDGMENTS   Dr. Catanzaro is the recipient of Research Corporation/Brown Hazen Grant No. BH-986R. We thank the *American Review of Respiratory Diseases* for permission to publish parts of this chapter that appeared initially in an article by us in that journal [*Am. Rev. Resp. Dis.* 117:559–585, 727–771 (1978)].

REFERENCES

1. C. E. Smith, Epidemiology of acute coccidioidomycosis with erythema nodosum ("San Joaquin" or "Valley Fever"), *Am. J. Public Health* 30:600–611 (1940).
2. E. C. Dickson, "Valley Fever" of the San Joaquin Valley and fungus coccidioides, *Calif. West. Med.* 47:151–155 (1937).
3. C. E. Smith, Diagnosis of pulmonary coccidioidal infections, *Calif. Med.* 75:385–391 (1951).
4. H. K. Faber, C. E. Smith, and E. C. Dickson, Acute coccidioidomycosis with erythema nodosum in children, *J. Pediat.* 15:163–171 (1939).
5. C. E. Smith, Coccidioidomycosis, *Med. Clin. North Am.* 27:790–807 (1943).
6. S. B. Werner and D. Pappagianis, Coccidioidomycosis in northern California. An outbreak among archeology students near Red Bluff, *Calif. Med.* 119:16–20 (1973).
7. S. B. Werner, D. Pappagianis, I. Heindl, and A. Mickel, An epidemic of coccidioidomycosis among archeology students in northern California, *N. Engl. J. Med.* 286:507–512 (1972).
8. W. C. Harvey and W. H. Greendyke, Skin lesions in acute coccidioidomycosis, *Am. Fam. Physician.* 2:81–85 (1970).
9. S. B. Werner, Coccidioidomycosis misdiagnosed as contact dermatitis. *Calif. Med.* 117:59–61 (1972).
10. D. G. Ramras, H. A. Walch, J. P. Murray, and B. H. Davidson, An epidemic of coccidioidomycosis in the Pacific Beach area of San Diego, *Am. Rev. Resp. Dis.* 101:975–978 (1970).
11. H. B. Richardson, Jr., J. A. Anderson, and B. M. McKay, Acute pulmonary coccidioidomycosis in children, *J. Pediatr.* 70:376–382 (1967).
12. M. J. Fiese, *Coccidioidomycosis*, Charles C. Thomas, Springfield, Ill. (1958).
13. E. C. Dickson, Coccidioidomycosis—The preliminary acute infection with fungus coccidioides, *J. Am. Med. Assoc.* 111:1362–1365 (1938).
14. E. C. Dickson and M. A. Gifford, Coccodioides infection (coccidioidomycosis). II. The primary type of infection, *Arch. Intern. Med.* 62:853–871 (1938).
15. C. E. Smith, Coccidioidomycosis. *Pediatr. Clin. North Am.* 2:109–125 (1955).

16. D. M. Goldstein and S. Louie, Primary pulmonary coccidioidomycosis—Report of an epidemic of seventy-five cases, *War Med.* **4**:299–317 (1943).
17. F. M. Willett and A. Weiss, Coccidioidomycosis in southern California: Report of a new endemic area with a review of 100 cases, *Ann. Intern. Med.* **23**:349–375 (1945).
18. R. A. Carter, Infectious granulomas of bones and joints, with special reference to coccidioidal granuloma, *Radiology* **23**:1–16 (1934).
19. C. E. Smith, R. R. Beard, E. G. Whiting, and H. G. Rosenberger, Varieties of coccidioidal infection in relation to the epidemiology and control of the diseases, *Am. J. Public Health* **36**:1394–1402 (1946).
20. C. E. Smith, E. G. Whiting, E. E. Baker, H. G. Rosenberger, R. R. Beard, and M. T. Saito, The use of coccidioidin, *Am. Rev. Tuberc.* **57**:330–360 (1948).
21. E. F. Rosenberg, M. B. Dockerty, and H. W. Meyerding, Coccidioidal arthritis. Report of a case in which the ankles were involved and the condition was unaffected by sulfanilamide and roentgen therapy, *Arch. Intern. Med.* **69**:238–250 (1942).
22. E. Alpert, K. J. Isselbacher, and P. H. Schur, The pathogenesis of arthritis associated with viral hepatitis. Complement-component studies, *N. Engl. J. Med.* **285**:185–189 (1971).
23. E. C. Dickson, Primary coccidioidomycosis—The initial acute infection which results in coccidioidal granuloma, *Am. Rev. Tuberc.* **38**:722–729 (1938).
24. F. M. Willett, and E. Opperheim, Pulmonary infiltration with associated eosinophilia, *Am. J. Med. Sci.* **212**:606–612 (1946).
25. J. W. Birsner, The roentgen aspects of five hundred cases of pulmonary coccidioidomycosis, *Am. J. Roentgenol. Radium. Ther. Nucl. Med.* **72**:556–573 (1954).
26. W. H. Greendyke, D. I. Resnick, and W. C. Harvey, The varied roentgen manifestations of primary coccidioidomycosis, *Am J. Roentgenol. Radium. Ther. Nucl. Med.* **109**:491–499 (1970).
27. H. E. Einstein, Bilateral hilar adenopathy, *Ann. Int. Med.* **78**:787 (1973).
28. H. W. Jamison, A roentgen study of chronic pulmonary coccidioidomycosis, *Am. J. Roentgenol.* **55**:396–412 (1946).
29. C. F. Sweigert, J. W. Turner, and J. B. Gillespie, Clinical and roentgenologic aspects of coccidioidomycosis, *Am. J. Med. Sci.* **212**:652–673 (1946).
30. S. A. Lonky, A. Catanzaro, K. M. Moser, and H. Einstein, Acute coccidioidal pleural effusion, *Am. Rev. Resp. Dis.* **114**:681–688 (1976).

10

Pulmonary Coccidioidomycosis

Antonino Catanzaro and David J. Drutz

The most common manifestation of respiratory infection due to *Coccidioides immitis* occurs during the primary infection. This facet is dealt with in Chapter 9.

1. PERSISTENT PULMONARY COCCIDIOIDOMYCOSIS

Persistent pulmonary infection is the most common form of coccidioidal disease with which clinicians must deal. Symptoms of primary pulmonary coccidioidomycosis generally clear within 2 to 3 weeks of the initial infection. Patients whose symptoms or radiographic abnormalities persist beyond 6 to 8 weeks may be considered to have persistent coccidioidomycosis. Manifestations of persistent infection include pneumonia, chronic progressive pneumonia, miliary disease, pulmonary nodules, and pulmonary cavitation. Healing of these processes may result in fibrosis, bronchiectasis and calcification.

1.1. Persistent Coccidioidal Pneumonia

These patients are often, but need not be, very ill. Typical symptoms include persistent fever, prostration, chest pain, productive cough, and occasionally hemoptysis. If untreated, their symptoms may persist for months.[1] Infiltrates may be quite variable in extent, in some cases occupying more than one-third of the lung field. Areas of dense infiltration clear very slowly—8 months in one series.[1]

In Rowland's analysis of host factors in fatal coccidioidal pneumonia,[2] there were two striking observations: (1) 84% of fatal cases occurred in immunocompromised hosts; (2) 50% died of pulmonary coccidioidomycosis without evidence of dissemination. Fatal coccidioidal pneumonia is certainly not confined to the immunocompromised host. Huntington described 45 autopsied cases of fatal coccidioidal pneumonia.[3] In this group, collected from the San Joaquin Valley, only 1 case might be classified as immunocompromised.

1.2. Chronic Progressive Coccidioidal Pneumonia

Chronic progressive coccidioidal pneumonia accounts for a small fraction of coccidioidal pulmonary disease.[4] Two features are characteristic of this group: (1) prolonged symptoms (in one series, 7 to 162 months, average 40 months) including cough, weight loss, fever, hemoptysis, chest pain, and dyspnea; (2) biapical fibronodular lesions and multiple cavities with retraction, very similar in appearance to chronic tuberculosis or chronic histoplasmosis (Fig. 1). In a recent study of 20 patients with this form of coccidioidomycosis, the complement-fixation (CF) antibody test was positive in 14 of 15 patients tested, with a mean titer of 1 : 64. The height of the titer was not related to the extent of disease, nor did patients with high titers show apparent evidence of dissemination. Of interest, skin test reactions to coccidioidin 1 : 100 were positive in only 4 of 17 patients tested; no additional reactors were identified using coccidioidin 1 : 10. Half of the group reacted to PPD (5 or 250 tuberculin units). Sputa were positive for *C. immitis* in all but one case (none of the patients had positive sputum cultures for *M. tuberculosis*).

2. MILIARY COCCIDIOIDOMYCOSIS

Approximately 4% of hospitalized patients with coccidioidomycosis have miliary pulmonary lesions. Miliary spread usually occurs early in the disease but may also be a late complication of chronic pulmonary or extrapulmonary disease (Fig. 2, A, B). Occasionally the clinical picture is that of mild chronic symptoms which are less than one would expect in view of the radiographic picture. Before the advent of amphotericin B, mortality in miliary coccidioidomycosis was extremely high, particularly in cases where extrapulmonary lesions developed within the 1st month of the illness.[1] In one series, symptoms of meningitis were not apparent in two-thirds of cases until the chest lesions cleared.[5] Therefore,

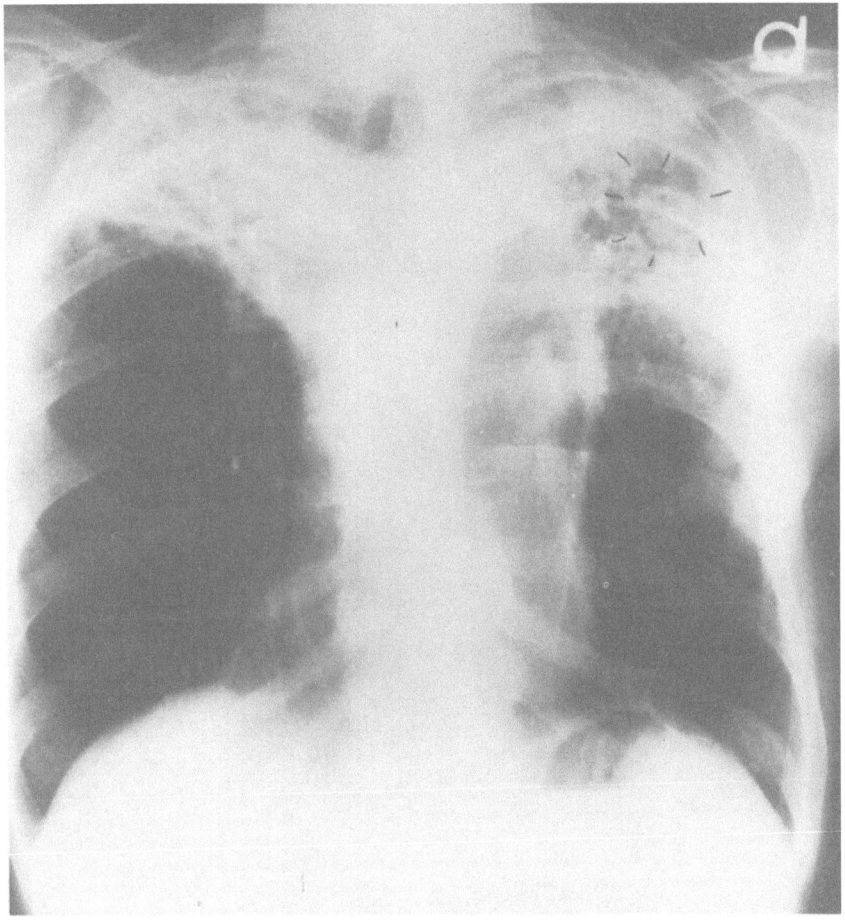

Figure 1. Bilateral apical fibrocavitary coccidioidomycosis. Note multilocular cavity in left upper lobe.

we recommend examination of cerebrospinal fluid in all cases of miliary coccidioidomycosis.

Miliary coccidioidomycosis can also present as rapidly progressive pulmonary disease with respiratory failure, particularly in immunocompromised hosts. In a recent report of six such cases, the mean A-aO$_2$ gradient was 72 mm without hypercarbia.[6] Fungemia may be present in fulminating miliary disease.[7] Serologic tests are usually positive, but, like the blood cultures, may not be available in time to be helpful diagnostically.[6,7]

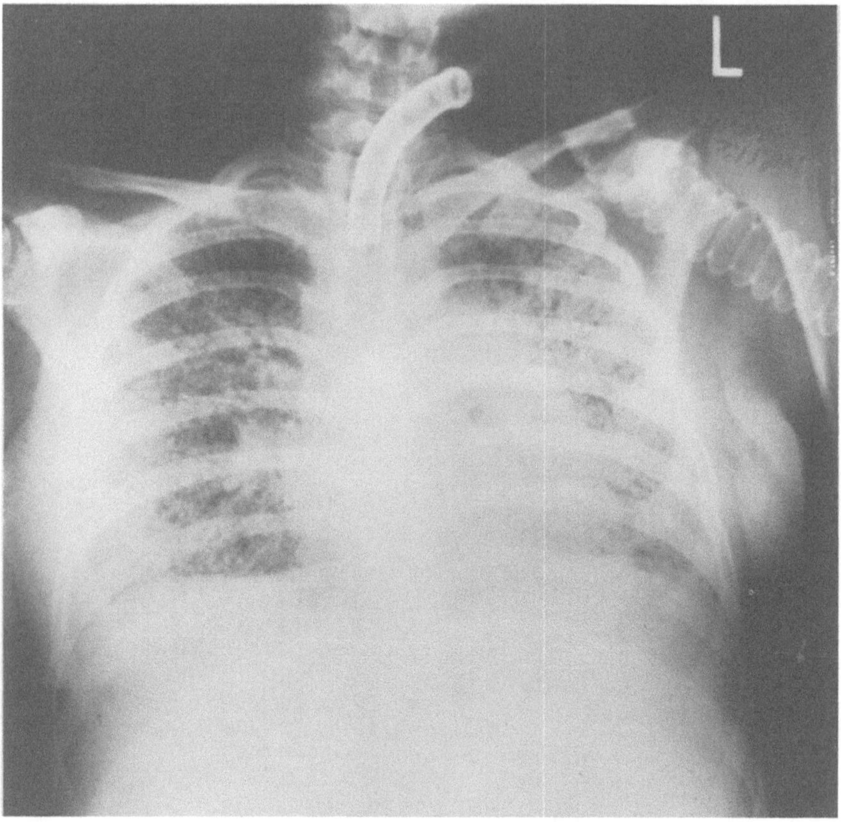

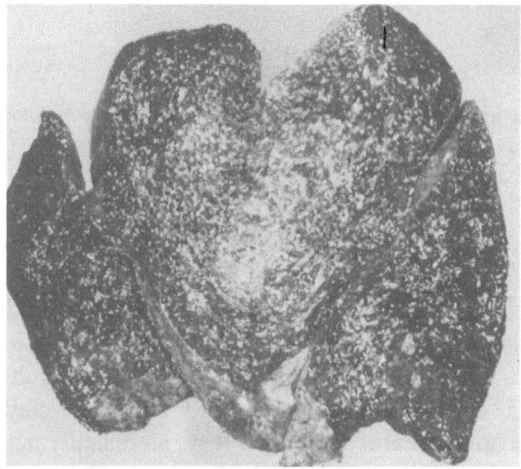

Figure 2. (a) Miliary pulmonary coccidioidomycosis; (b) miliary coccidioidomycosis of lung at autopsy. Note multiple white miliary nodules.

3. COCCIDIOIDAL NODULES

Many cases of coccidioidal pneumonia undergo a characteristic evolution from the typical soft infiltrate to a spherical, dense nodule (coccidioidoma) without surrounding infiltration. Clinical symptoms do not distinguish these patients from others. The evolution may occur in 10 days to 3 months.[1] Nodules tend to occur in the midlung field, within 5 cm of the hilum. Most are single and range in size from 1 to 4 cm. However, multiple nodules may also occur.[1,8,9] Nodules are not simply static residua of past events. When removed, nearly all have a semiliquid or gelatinous center in which *C. immitis* is usually identifiable. In one study of 35 nodular lesions, spherules were seen in tissue section in 24; and *C. immitis* was cultured from tissue in 11.[10] One case report described viable organisms present 15 years after infection.[11]

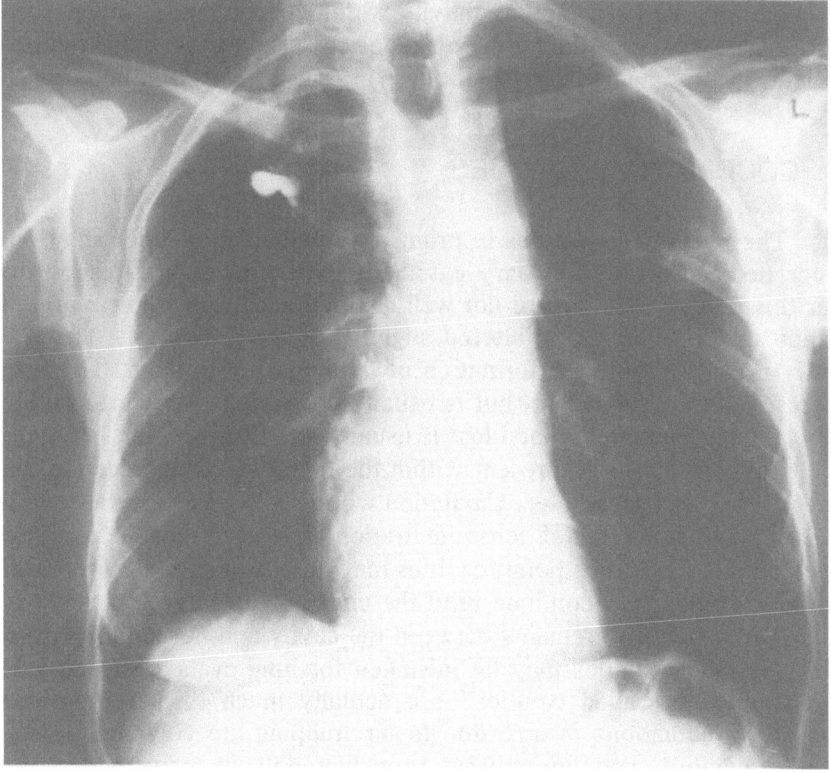

Figure 3. Bilateral cavitary pulmonary coccidioidomycosis. Right apical thin-walled cavity, with lower margin extending from radio-opaque intracavitary dye to mediastinum. Multilocular thicker-walled cavity in left mid-upper lung field near pleural margin.

C. immitis may be recovered from sputum in 14% of patients with coccidioidal nodules, and a draining bronchus can often be identified at pathologic examination.[10] It would appear that coccidioidal nodules often represent undrained or poorly draining lung abscesses. Clues to their central cavitation may be detected by careful radiographic study, particularly with special views including tomography.[12] Perhaps computerized tomography scanning may be able to identify such liquid centers.

Salkin and Huppert[13] studied sequential chest X-rays in 300 cases of coccidioidal nodules drawn from a highly selected group of cases followed at military hospitals, including the VA. The follow-up period was 10 years in most cases. Thirty-three of the nodules drained or "shelled out," leaving behind a cavity which in some was thin-walled, in others, thick-walled (Fig. 3). Occasionally the cavity refilled and regained its original appearance of a nodule. The nodules that retained their solid appearance sometimes underwent a change in size over the years. Eighteen decreased slowly in size, a few disappearing entirely; 14 increased in size.

Despite the frequency of activity within coccidioidal nodules, calcification may occur.[10] Sargent *et al.* reported two cases in which multiple calcifications ranging from 0.3 to 1 cm in size developed in both lungs.[9]

4. COCCIDIOIDAL CAVITIES

The pneumonic process in primary coccidioidal infection may produce necrosis with pulmonary cavitation. The host factors responsible for this type of reaction are not well characterized. The clinical presentation in this subgroup is altered slightly in that hemoptysis occurs in 70% of cases during the formation of pulmonary cavitation. The hemoptysis may be significant, but is usually not serious enough to be life-threatening (volume of blood lost is usually less than 100 ml).

Cavitation may be present within the first 10 days of infection, but more typically occurs later. Cavitation will usually be evident as central clearing within an area of dense infiltration or within a nodule, if X-rays are taken early. At this point, cavities may have a thick, "shaggy" wall. "Shelling out" may continue until the entire involved area is removed and only a thin wall remains between the cavity and normal lung tissue (Fig. 3). Such cavities may be mistaken for lung cysts. However, the walls of "thin-walled cavities" are actually much thicker than they appear. Fluctuations in size due to air trapping are common in thin-walled cavities, and intermittent bronchial potency may lead to the collection of fluid.

Once a coccidioidal cavity has formed, it can persist for some time.

Since the formation of the cavity may have been subclinical (in the manner of most cases of primary coccidioidomycosis), it is not surprising that many patients are first recognized when a chest radiograph is taken for some other reason.

The symptoms reportedly exhibited by patients who first come to medical attention after cavity formation has already occurred are more highly dependent upon authors and their case selection processes than on intrinsic clinical or radiologic aspects of the illness. For example, in military populations where patients are X-rayed on a routine basis, the finding is most often made on a routine film, and symptoms are absent. When patients are symptomatic, the most common complaint is hemoptysis (25 to 50% of cases).

From a radiographic point of view, 90% of coccidioidal cavities are single, 70% are in the upper lung fields, and 5% cross fissures. The cavities are less than 2 cm in diameter in 25%, 2 to 4 cm in 58%, 4 to 6 cm in 10%, and greater than 6 cm (up to 14 cm) in 7% of cases.[14]

Both Winn[14] and Smith et al.[15] in their early series, which included long-term follow-up of nearly 400 patients with cavitary disease, stressed the benign nature of coccidioidal cavities. Specifically, they pointed out that even though sputum from these cases was usually positive for C. immitis, neither airway spread nor extrapulmonary spread occurred. The subsequent literature does record occasional cases of dissemination from previously stable cavities, however.

Hyde specifically addressed the issue of spontaneous cavity closure in a study of 211 coccidioidal cavities. Spontaneous closure occurred in 50% of the "control" group, which received neither surgery nor amphotericin B. The mean period for cavity closure was 2 years.[16] Likewise, Winn reported that 27% of 200 cases of coccidioidal cavities closed spontaneously and "permanently." All closures occurred within 4 years of observation.[17]

There are three major potential complications of coccidioidal cavities.

1. *Infection.* Obviously, clearance mechanisms in coccidioidal cavities are not ideal. Intermittent obstruction may produce a ball valve effect with rapid changes in the size of the cavity. Impaired mechanisms for the removal of contaminating particles and microorganisms set the stage for secondary infection. Cavities may become infected with pyogenic microorganisms and fill with the byproduct of such infection. Fungal contamination may result in the formation of a mycetoma or fungal ball. *Aspergillus* fungus balls have been reported to form in cavities of any etiology. Several cases of fungus ball due to mycelial elements of *C. immitis* have also been reported.[18,19] The presentation in these cases is not unlike those with aspergillus mycetoma, except that

precipitins to aspergillus are not found. Furthermore, sputum cultures are usually positive for *C. immitis*.

2. *Pyopneumothorax*. Coccidioidal cavities which are large or sub-pleural in location are considered by some to be in danger of rupture.[19a,20,21] The fact is that whereas coccidioidal cavities are common, pyopneumothorax is rare.[22] Two large series reporting long-term obser-vations of more than 500 cases of pulmonary coccidioidomycosis do not include any cases of pyopneumothorax.[1,5] Smith's analysis of 274 patients with coccidioidal cavities included 7 (2.6%) who developed pyopneu-mothorax.[15] In 6 additional cases, pyopneumothorax developed in the absence of antecedent cavitation; 2 of these occurred during primary infection. Rivkin *et al.* reported 4 cases of pyopneumothorax. Only 1 patient was known to have an antecedent cavity; it was neither large nor subpleural;[10] 1.4% of Winn's 300 cases and 3% of Hyde's 211 cases of coccidioidal cavities developed pyopneumothorax.[14,16]

Cases of pyopneumothorax present usually as bronchopleural fistu-las. Cultures of both sputum and pleural fluid are generally positive for *C. immitis*. Surgical treatment with resection of the bronchopleural fistula is usually recommended in these cases.[12]

3. *Pulmonary hemorrhage*. Hemoptysis may occur in 25 to 50% of patients with coccidioidal cavities during the period of observation. Although this generally consists of "occasional blood-streaked sputum," several cases have been described in which hemorrhage is "frighteningly brisk." These cases stand out as rare exceptions among the more than 1000 cases of coccidioidal cavities reported in the literature.[1,14,15,23,24]

5. COMPLICATING FACTORS

Clinical manifestations of pulmonary coccidioidomycosis as well as dissemination are influenced by a number of factors. Age, race, and sex are discussed in Chapters 4 and 18. Immunosuppression, whether sec-ondary to a disease which effects the immune system such as Hodgkin's disease, or due to drugs, has a profound effect on the pulmonary disease seen in coccidioidomycosis (see Chapter 19). Pregnancy also has a significant effect (discussed in Chapter 17).

The effects of diabetes mellitus or tuberculosis also appear impor-tant. Diabetics appear more likely to develop pulmonary cavitation, and diabetics are overrepresented in series of patients reported with cavitary disease. The likelihood of recavitation, either at the same site or a new site, is much greater. For this reason, surgical resection of cavities in diabetics should only be done for the most pressing indications.

Coexisting pulmonary tuberculosis and pulmonary coccidioidomycosis has been reported several times, including mixed infection in the same focus and separate infections in multiple foci. The response of the tuberculosis to antituberculous therapy is generally unchanged, though the coccidioidal disease appears more refractory to treatment.

Bronchiectasis may be a sequela of chronic or severe acute pulmonary coccidioidomycosis.

6. GUIDELINES FOR THERAPY—CHEMOTHERAPY

The therapeutic alternatives in treatment of coccidioidal disease are limited. Amphotericin B is the standard for chemotherapy, since over 20 years' experience has been accumulated with it in pulmonary coccidioidomycosis. Since the toxicity of amphotericin B is significant, its indications must be carefully weighed against its toxicities. If a clearly more effective, less toxic antifungal agent were available, the indications for therapy could alter quickly.

Fortunately, coccidioidal infection usually progresses slowly. There is adequate opportunity to weigh the pertinent risk factors (race, sex, pregnancy, concomitant disease). More important, one has an adequate opportunity to assess the host response to this particular infection, e.g., toxicity, weight loss, spread of disease, CF titer, and skin test response to coccidioidal antigens.

Those patients with persistent pneumonia,[2] chronic progressive pneumonia,[4] bronchopleural fistula and empyema, or those with thick-walled cavities and prominent symptoms should be treated to limit symptoms or extent of disease. With amphotericin B, the dose recommended is arbitrary, generally ranging from 500 to 2500 mg, depending upon the severity of the disease process. Available evidence suggests that amphotericin B is not sufficient to eradicate *C. immitis* from the lung when significant structural changes have occurred.[25] However, persistent pneumonia (6 weeks), particularly in a symptomatic patient, is a clear indication for treatment. If a bronchopleural fistula with empyema has developed, surgical closure of the fistula is necessary. Often this is most easily performed in conjunction with resection of the diseased pulmonary tissue. Amphotericin is often given to such patients but is probably not essential to a good response.

Chronic progressive coccidioidal pneumonia (also called fibrocavitary) is another indication for treatment. Without treatment these patients remain infected with *C. immitis* for many years. They usually undergo very slow destruction of pulmonary parenchyma. Short courses of amphotericin (0.5 to 1 g) usually result in mild improvement in symptoms. In addition, following treatment sputum will be rendered free of *C.*

immitis for several months, perhaps longer. It is difficult to be certain whether this has an effect on the course of the disease. It has been suggested that longer courses (>30 mg/kg total dose) correlate best with successful outcome in chronic disease.[4]

A thick-walled or expanding cavity, particularly in a symptomatic patient, may be taken as an indication for a brief course of chemotherapy (e.g., amphotericin, 0.5 to 1 g). Again, one can expect to clear *C. immitis* from the sputum and improve the symptoms. There is no predictable effect on cavity closure. One cannot predict the period of time before symptoms of chronic infection or bleeding may return.

Miliary infection is so commonly lethal that it demands aggressive treatment. Coccidioidal nodules, even when manipulated at bronchoscopy or surgery, rarely require drug therapy.

The ultimate goal of treatment is marked clinical improvement, healing of all apparent lesions, and a reduction of CF antibody titers to the lowest possible level. As a practical point, a fourfold reduction of CF antibody titer, especially if maintained, is considered to indicate a favorable therapeutic response.[26]

Relapses may occur, and close followup of treated patients is crucial so that therapy may be reintroduced as needed.[25]

The decision of when to discontinue amphotericin B is perhaps the most difficult of all. some authors regard the patient to be at risk of relapse for as long as the coccidioidin skin test is negative, and would recommend continuation of therapy until the state of anergy is corrected.[27] In patients with proven propensity to relapse, one might consider therapy two to three times weekly on an outpatient basis until skin test reactivity returns. However, this may be an elusive goal; some patients may never regain cutaneous reactivity to *C. immitis*. As a practical matter, amphotericin is so toxic that most physicians are not willing to push therapy beyond the point of apparent return to good health in an attempt to correct an underlying immune defect.[28] In most cases this should not exceed a total dose of 3 g. Long-term suppressive therapy is likely to become a realistic goal only when an orally absorbable, nontoxic drug becomes available.

Nebulization of amphotericin B has been utilized in therapy[29] and could be a potential modality in all forms of pulmonary coccidioidomycosis, possibly free of the systemic side effects of the drug. Absorption would presumably be small, making it logical only for endobronchial or cavitary disease. Further data with this approach is needed.

A new synthetic imidazole, miconazole, has been reported to produce responses in two-thirds of a series of patients with chronic pulmonary coccidioidomycosis, almost all of whom had failed amphotericin therapy.[30] One-third of the responders, however, subsequently relapsed during follow-up. Determination of the place of this drug relative to amphotericin for therapy of pulmonary coccidioidomycosis awaits appropriate comparative trials. Ketoeonazole is an imidazole which is absorbed following oral ingestion.[30a] Preliminary studies with the drug are encouraging; this could be the drug which would dramatically alter the therapeutic approach to pulmonary coccidioidomycosis.

7. PULMONARY RESECTIONAL SURGERY

As the full spectrum of pulmonary coccidioidomycosis began to unfold, many students of the disease noted its apparent similarity to tuberculosis. It is not surprising that attempts were made to apply lessons learned in tuberculosis to patients with pulmonary coccidioidomycosis. Even though earlier investigators were aware of the benign nature of coccidioidal cavities, various attempts to facilitate closure were tried. Bed rest, sandbags applied to the chest, pneumothorax, pneumoperitoneum, thoracoplasty, phrenic nerve crush, and other procedures were used and were credited with some role in cavity closure. Of course, any treatment would have resulted in closure of 50% of cavities in the time frame Hyde demonstrated.[16]

Complications of surgical procedures, especially bronchopleural fistulas, were a matter of great concern.[22,24] With the development of techniques, and greater familiarity of surgeons with the disease, resectional surgery was introduced. Melick reported the results of such surgery in 400 patients operated upon by 66 surgeons between 1950 and 1953. The complication rate was 13%, consisting mostly of postoperative bronchopleural fistulas or pulmonary recavitation.[24] Cotton et al. reported the results of surgery in 100 patients.[20] Here, the surgery tended to be more extensive, with 17 pneumonectomies, 41 lobectomies, and 35 subsegmental lobectomies. Complications were held to a minimum, with only 1 case of recavitation due to coccidioidomycosis, 1 due to tuberculosis, and 1 death due to myocardial disease.

Unfortunately, other workers have not matched these results. Aronstam and Hopeman reported an overall complication rate of 20% following lobectomy, and 40% following segmental resection.[19a] Many of the complications, however, were not serious. Rivkin and his colleagues reported complications due to C. immitis in 15% of surgical cases.[10] Grant and Melick reported a complication rate of 8.7%, with only 5.7% "significant" complications.[21] Hyde reported on 108 patients who underwent resection of a coccidioidal cavity. Thirty percent developed a bronchopleural fistula, and 18% developed a new coccidioidal cavity in the area of the resection.[16] The explanation for local coccidioidal cavitary recurrences may be appreciated by microscopic examination of pathologic material. Whereas the typical coccidioidal cavity seen on chest radiograph is thin-walled, and apparently free of surrounding infiltration, histopathologic examination often shows a small number of coccidioidal abscesses in the surrounding tissue.[31] Both the debilitating effect of surgery and the mechanical stretching of the tissue after resection are considered to favor recavitation.

To reduce the incidence of postoperative coccidioidal complications, Grant and Melick introduced the concept of using amphotericin B as a "therapeutic umbrella."[21] In 1960, they began the practice of administering 400 to 600 mg of the drug during the preoperative period. Depending upon the operative findings, another gram might be administered postoperatively. The reported reduction in complications was marked, from 20% "preumbrella" to 4.2% "postumbrella." A number of other variables may have influenced these results. Because of the high incidence of complications with segmental and wedge resections, lobectomy had become the procedure of choice during the course of this study. Further, all patients without amphotericin B coverage had surgery prior to 1960, whereas all patients operated upon subsequent to 1960 were treated with amphotericin B. The influence of the evolving techniques and surgical experience on these results cannot be ignored. The mix of active and nonactive cavitary disease in the two populations is also an important variable.

Other reports regarding the use of the "amphotericin B umbrella" have been unimpressive, and no properly controlled trials have been performed. Fosburg et al. administered amphotericin B to 14 patients judged to be at increased risk of coccidioidal dissemination in the postoperative period.[32] High-risk factors were identified as a cavity greater than 5 cm in diameter, a cavity which appeared to involve more than one lobe ("fissure-jumper") and patients whose sputum was positive for C. immitis. The incidence of complications in the umbrella group was the same as that in a group which was perceived to be at low risk, and therefore received no amphotericin B. In view of the selection process, the results cannot be properly evaluated. Preoperative amphotericin B has not been studied any further, since it has not gained notable support or usage. However, use of amphotericin B coverage may be advisable in surgical procedures involving extensive manipulation of infected tissue.

At the present time, the least controversial indication for pulmonary surgery in coccidioidal disease is to establish the diagnosis. This problem arises most commonly in the evaluation of a pulmonary nodule. Cutaneous reactivity to coccidioidin or spherulin and detection of a CF antibody titer does not prove that a nodule is coccidioidal in origin. Even when C. immitis is demonstrated in the sputum, one cannot be certain that the fungi are coming from the nodule, or that there is no possibility of concomitant malignancy. When the evolution from primary coccidioidal infection to a pulmonary nodule has been observed, surgery can be avoided. Brushing and biopsying a lesion via the fiberoptic bronchoscope is difficult, but is occasionally rewarding in proving coccidioidal etiology of a pulmonary nodule. Even though more than 75% of coccidioidomas contain identifiable *C. immitis,* neither pulmonary nor disseminated spread has been reported following such diagnostic manipulations. Similarly, limited surgical resection of a coccidioidal nodule results in few complications.[10,32]

Surgery in cavitary pulmonary coccidioidomycosis is a matter of controversy. The literature is replete with lists of stated indications for resectional surgery.[10,12,20,22,25,33] The basis for formulating these indications is not given in most reports. As has been pointed out, the behavior of coccidioidal cavities is almost uniformly benign, in the absence of manipulation. Neither intrapulmonary nor extrapulmonary spread is common. Secondary infection, either with pyogenic bacteria or mycetoma-forming fungi, is uncommon. Cavitary rupture with pyopneumothorax occurs in no more than 3% of cases[5,14,15,16] and is reported as frequently in patients without known antecedent pulmonary cavitary disease.[15]

Although symptoms are common in patients with cavitary disease, most are generally mild. Hemoptysis is frequent, unpredictable and frightening. Nevertheless, hemoptysis which is recurrent or severe is unusual.[14-16] Only a few cases of fatal pulmonary hemorrhage from a cavity have been mentioned in the literature.[20,34]

In comparison with the natural history of unresected coccidioidal cavities, resectional surgery is often followed by a significant rate of complication, as has been noted above. Hyde has provided one of the few comparative studies of surgical and nonsurgical treatment of cavitary pulmonary coccidioidomycosis.[16] Cavity closure was accomplished in 82% of the surgical group and 50% of the nonsurgical group. New cavities developed in 18% of the surgically managed patients, but in only 1% of those managed without surgery. Bronchopleural fistula developed in 30% of the surgical group but in only 3% of the nonsurgical group.

Clearly, surgical treatment is not indicated for the majority of patients with coccidioidal cavities. On the other hand, as pointed out by Cotton *et al.,* the overall benign nature of the disease has little meaning to the patient who is suffering from one of the more alarming complications of chronic pulmonary coccidioidomycosis.[20,33] In our opinion, the clearest indications for surgery in cavitary pulmonary coccidioidomycosis are as follows: (1) rapidly expanding cavity with apparent imminent risk of rupture, (2) bronchopleural fistula, (3) symptomatic mycetoma, and (4) serious or persistent hemorrhage. Surgery must sometimes be considered in patients because they find it impossible to obtain insurance with a cavitary lesion present. Surgery may be needed to deal with the consequence of a ruptured cavity, or when lung expansion is restricted by residua of coccidioidal disease.

ACKNOWLEDGMENTS. Dr. Catanzaro is the recipient of Research Corporation/Brown Hazen Grant No. BH-986R. We thank the *American Review of Respiratory Diseases* for permission to publish parts of this chapter which appeared initially in an article by us in that journal [*Am. Rev. Resp. Dis.* 117:559–585, 727–771 (1978)].

REFERENCES

1. H. W. Jamison, A roentgen study of chronic pulmonary coccidioidomycosis, *Am. J. Roentgenol.* **55**:396–412 (1946).
2. V. S. Rowland, R. E. Westfall, and W. A. Hinchcliffe, Fatal coccidioidomycosis: Analysis of host factors, in: *Coccidioidomycosis: Current Clinical and Diagnostic Status* (L. Ajello, ed.), Symposia Specialists, Miami (1977), pp. 91–106.
3. R. W. Huntington, Acute fatal coccidioidal pneumonia, in: *Coccidioidomycosis: Current Clinical and Diagnostic Status* (L. Ajello, ed.), Symposia Specialists, Miami (1977), pp. 127–138.
4. G. A. Sarosi, J. D. Parker, I. L. Doto, and F. E. Tosh, Chronic pulmonary coccidioidomycosis *N. Engl. J. Med.* **283**:325–329 (1970).
5. J. W. Birsner, The roentgen aspects of five hundred cases of pulmonary coccidioidomycosis, *Am. J. Roentgenol. Radium Ther. Nucl. Med.* **72**:556–573 (1954).
6. V. S. Rowland, R. E. Westfall, W. A. Hinchcliffe, and P. B. Jarrett, Acute respiratory failure in miliary coccidioidomycosis, in: *Coccidioidomycosis: Current Clinical and Diagnostic Status* (L. Ajello, ed.), Symposia Specialists, Miami (1977), pp. 139–155.
7. W. R. Winn, S. M. Finegold, and R. W. Huntington, Jr., Coccidioidomycosis with fungemia, in: *Coccidioidomycosis* (L. Ajello, ed.), University of Arizona Press, Tucson (1967), pp. 93–109.
8. W. H. Greendyke, D. L. Resnick, and W. C. Harvey, The varied roentgen manifestations of primary coccidioidomycosis, *Am. J. Roentgenol. Radium Ther. Nucl. Med.* **109**:491–499 (1970)
9. E. N. Sargent, E. Balchum, A. L. Freed, and G. Jacobson, Multiple pulmonary calcifications due to coccidioidomycosis, *Am. J. Roentgenol. Radium Ther. Nucl. Med.* **109**:500–504 (1970).
10. L. M. Rivkin, D. F. Winn, and J. M. Salyer, The surgical treatment of pulmonary coccidioidomycosis, *J. Thorac. Cardiovasc. Surg.* **42**:401–412 (1961).
11. A. J. Cox and C. E. Smith, Arrested pulmonary coccidioidomycosis granuloma, *Arch. Pathol.* **27**:717–734 (1939).
12. A. R. Nelson, The surgical treatment of pulmonary coccidioidomycosis, *Curr. Probl. Surg.* 1974 (entire October issue).
13. D. Salkin and M. Huppert, Review of 706 cases in the VA-AF Cooperative Study, in: *Proc. 23rd Ann. Coccidioidomycosis Study Group Meeting*, abstract no. 12.
14. W. A. Winn, A long term study of 300 patients with cavitary-abscess lesions of the lung of coccidioidal origin. An analytical study with special reference to treatment, *Dis. Chest.* **1**:12–16 (1968).

15. C. E. Smith, R. R. Beard, and M. T. Saito, Pathogenesis of coccidioidomycosis with special reference to pulmonary cavitation, *Ann. Intern. Med.* **29:**623–655 (1948).
16. L. Hyde, Coccidioidal pulmonary cavitation, *Dis. Chest.* **54**(Suppl.):273–277 (1968).
17. W. A. Winn, A working classification of coccidioidomycosis and its application to therapy, in: *Coccidioidomycosis* (L. Ajello, ed.), University of Arizona Press, Tucson (1967), pp. 3–9.
18. R. Belgrad, Fungus ball—an unusual manifestation of coccidioidomycosis. A case report, *Radiology* **101:**289–290 (1971).
19. H. Thadepalli, F. A. Salem, A. K. Mandal, K. Rambhatla, and H. E. Einstein, Pulmonary mycetoma due to Coccidioides immitis. *Chest.* **71:**429–430 (1977).
19a. E. M. Aronstam and A. R. Hopeman, Surgical experiences with pulmonary coccidioidomycosis, a survey of 112 operative cases, *J. Thorac. Cardiovasc. Surg.* **42:**200–205 (1961).
20. B. H. Cotton, G. A. Paulsen, and J. W. Birsner, Surgical considerations in pulmonary coccidioidomycosis, report of 100 cases, *Am. J. Surg.* **90:**101–106 (1955).
21. A. R. Grant, and D. W. Melick, The surgical treatment of cavitary pulmonary coccidioidomycosis, *Arch. Surg.* **94:**559–566 (1967).
22. L. Hyde and D. C. Holman, Coccidioidal spontaneous pneumothorax, *Ann. Intern. Med.* **47:**1234–1242 (1957).
23. A. R. Grant, N. G. Steinhoff, and D. W. Melick, Resectional surgery in pulmonary coccidioidomycosis, a review of 263 cases, in: *Coccidioidomycosis: Current Clinical and Diagnostic Status (L. Ajello, ed.), Symposia Specialists, Miami (1977), pp. 209–221.*
24. D. W. Melick, The surgical treatment of pulmonary coccidioidomycosis with a comprehensive summary of the complications following this type of therapy, *Am. Rev. Tuberc.* **77:**17–21 (1958).
25. G. Hildick-Smith, H. Blank, and I. Sarkany (eds.), Coccidioidomycosis, in: *Fungus Diseases and Their Treatment,* Little, Brown, Boston (1964), p. 241.
26. C. E. Smith, Coccidioidomycosis, in: *Immunological Diseases* (M. Samter and H. L. Alexander, eds.), Little, Brown, Boston (1965), p. 439.
27. H. W. Buchsbaum, Clinical management of coccidioidal meningitis, in: *Coccidioidomycosis: Current Clinical and Diagnostic Status* (L. Ajello, ed.), Symposia Specialists, Miami (1977), pp. 191–199.
28. W. G. Sanford, J. R. Rasch, and R. B. Stonehill, A therapeutic dilemma. The treatment of disseminated coccidioidomycosis with amphotericin B, *Ann. Intern. Med.* **56:**553–563 (1962).
29. R. S. Eisenberg and W. H. Oatway, Nebulization of amphotericin B, *Am. Rev. Resp. Dis.* **103:**289–292 (1971).
30. D. A. Stevens, Miconazole in the treatment of systemic fungal infections, *Am. Rev. Resp. Dis.* **116:**801–806 (1977).
30a. D. Borelli, J. L. Bran, J. Fuentes, R. Legendre, E. Leiderman, H. B. Levine, A. Restrepo-M., and D. A. Stevens, Ketoconazole, an oral antifungal: Laboratory and clinical assessment of imidazole drugs, *Postgrad. Med. J.* **55:**657–661 (1979).
31. W. D. Forbus and A. M. Bestebreurtje, Coccidioidomycosis: A study of 95 cases of the disseminated type with special reference to the pathogenesis of the disease. *Mil. Surg.* **99:**653–719 (1946).
32. R. G. Fosburg, B. F. Baisch, and M. J. Trummer, Limited pulmonary resection for coccidioidomycosis, *Ann. Thorac. Surg.* **7:**420–427 (1969).
33. B. H. Cotton and J. W. Birsner, Surgical treatment in pulmonary coccidioidomycosis. Preliminary report of thirty cases, *J. Thorac. Surg.* **20:**429–442 (1950).
34. M. J. Fiese, *Coccidioidomycosis,* Charles C. Thomas, Springfield, Ill. (1958).

11

Coccidioidal Meningitis

Peter C. Kelly

Coccidioidal meningitis (CM) is a lethal, chronic granulomatous disease of the leptomeninges caused by *Coccidioides immitis*. Untreated CM is uniformly fatal and accounts for the majority of the deaths caused by coccidioidomycosis.[1,2,3] However, aggressive treatment with amphotericin B (AMB) reduces mortality and prolongs survival. This chapter will review our current concepts of CM, its diagnosis, and its treatment.

1. PATHOGENESIS

The leptomeninges become infected by hematogenous spread of organisms originating in a primary pulmonary focus. Evidence supporting the concept of the pulmonary origin of CM is the high frequency of pulmonary coccidioidal lesions among cases of CM[4-6] and epidemiologic studies[7,8] which show that pulmonary infection precedes disseminated disease. The frequency of overt pulmonary disease in clinical series of CM is 33–67%, while in autopsy series the frequency is 67–95%.[3] A clinically occult pulmonary focus may be the source of a fungemia which causes meningitis.[9] Pulmonary disease may be concomitant with meningitis or precede it by several weeks to months.[6] Of interest, there are cases where antecedent pulmonary lesions are resolving at the time meningitis becomes manifest.[9]

Rarely, central nervous system coccidioidomycosis results from direct extension of a parameningeal or juxtadural focus, such as skull or vertebral osteomyelitis.[10-14] Abbott and Cutler included two cases of skull bone osteomyelitis associated with CM; in both of these, epidural abscesses were observed.[10] Cervical[11] or thoracic[12-14] vertebral osteomyelitis may extend to the dura and spinal meninges, and when this occurs the clinical findings mimic a spinal cord tumor.

2. PATHOLOGY

The basic pathologic lesion of fatal CM is an exudative inflammatory process with areas of both suppuration and granuloma formation.[9,10,15] The process is widely but unevenly distributed over the leptomeninges, with the basilar portions being most severely affected in 71–86% of cases,[1,3,9,10,15,16] and sulci preferentially involved. Light microscopy reveals granulomas similar to tuberculous meningitis with mononuclear, epithelioid, and giant cell infiltration.[15] Suppurative areas show collections of polymorphonuclear leukocytes and fibrinous exudate.[9,10] Spherules of *C. immitis* (which are plentiful in some cases and scarce in others) may be seen in both granulomatous and suppurative areas.[15] The end result of this process is a thick, opaque, plastic membrane containing plasma cells and fibrous tissue which may obliterate the subarachnoid, space in some areas.[3,9,10] In the basilar region the thickened meninges frequently cause obstruction to the flow of CSF, which results in moderate to severe ventricular dilation.[9,10] The resulting hydrocephalus is an important cause of death.

Brain pathology is much less common than meningeal involvement in CM. The reported frequency of cerebral lesions is 1.2, 10.5, 20, and 29% in four series.[3,10,15,16] When present, the lesions are usually small nodules.[15,16] Any area of the brain may be involved. Rarely, a nodule may enlarge and present as a mass lesion.[17] Granulomatous cerebral arteritis may accompany CM.

Autopsied cases of CM can be divided into two categories regarding non-CNS coccidioidal pathology. First, cases where the meninges are the sole site of dissemination, and second, cases where the meninges are but one of multiple organs infected. The relative frequency of these groups in three series is shown in Table 1. Among the 48 cases of meningitis as the only site of dissemination (Table 1) the frequency of detectable pulmonary lesions was 31 of 46 cases (67%). (In two cases[16] insufficient data are available to exclude a pulmonary focus.) In Huntington's series,[3] among the 12 cases where no pulmonary lesion was found, 8 received AMB treatment which may have eradicated a lung infection. Fifty-three of 61 cases of multiple-organ dissemination (Table 1) included information about lung pathology, and in 50 of these 53 cases (94.3%) a pulmonary infection was present.

The pathology of coccidioidal involvement of the CNS is also discussed in Chapter 7.

TABLE 1
The Frequency of Solitary Meningitis and Multiple Organ Disease in Autopsy Series of
Coccidioidal Meningitis

Reference	Total number of cases	Meningitis alone		Meningitis and other organs	
		Number	%	Number	%
Abbott and Cutler[10]	14	7	50	7	50
Schlumberger[16]	13	5	38	8	62
Huntington et al.[3]	82	36	44	46	56
	TOTAL: 109	TOTAL: 48	MEDIAN: 44	TOTAL: 61	MEDIAN: 56

3. DEMOGRAPHY

There are no reliable, contemporary measurements of either the prevalence of CM or the proportion of meningitis among all cases of coccidioidomycosis. The older literature estimates the frequency of dissemination by counting the number of patients who develop coccidioidal granuloma (an older term for disseminated coccidioidomycosis) following an episode of primary pulmonary infection.[7] In 1936–37 physicians in the San Joaquin Valley reported 354 cases of "valley fever" with one case of coccidioidal granuloma,[7] and Goldstein and McDonald[18] reported 1 case of coccidioidal granuloma among 85 cases of primary infection. Schlumberger[16] stated that CM occurred in 25% of disseminated coccidioidomycosis but presented no evidence to support his estimate.

During World War II, C. E. Smith and co-workers[19] conducted extensive studies of coccidioidomycosis among Army personnel stationed in the San Joaquin Valley. Their data provide a basis for estimating the frequency of dissemination and CM. They reported that 1% of clinically manifest primary infections disseminated in white males and 12% in black males.[19] In a subsequent analysis of serologic tests for coccidioidomycosis, they found that 68 of 419 (16.2%) cases of disseminated coccidioidomycosis had meningeal disease.[20] The data of Smith et al.[19,20] lead to a calculated frequency of CM of 1 case per 625 primary pulmonary infections among whites, and of nearly 2 cases per 100 among blacks!

CM occurs in all age groups and races and in both sexes (Table 2). White males are the largest single group afflicted, but black males are disproportionally represented. Thus, in a large collection of cases 16% were black males, who represent only 3–5% of the general population.[5] This is also discussed in Chapter 4.

TABLE 2
Demographic Data from Selected Series of Coccidioidal Meningitis

Reference	Number of cases	Sex (%)		Age (yr)		Race (%)					Comment
		Male	Female	Mean	Range	White	Black	Oriental[a]	M-A[b]	Other	
Huntington et al.[3]	82	79	21	37.5	2 mo–86	35	38	16	10	1	Autopsy series, California
Winn[23]	31	77	23	34	7–61	74	13	—	13	—	Clinical series, California
Pappagianis and Crane[5]	265	82	18	—	2–80	53	19	6	10	12	Reference lab. series, 8.7% of race unknown and included with Other
Kelly et al.[21]	22	45	55	36	3–80	45	—	—	—	55	Arizona series. Race divided into white and nonwhite

[a] Includes Filipinos.
[b] Mexican-American.

4. CLINICAL MANIFESTATIONS AND COURSE OF CM

4.1. Signs and Symptoms

CM is usually an illness of insidious onset and progressive course. There are two reliable but nonspecific early symptoms—headache and behavioral changes.[4,21] The typical headache involves the whole head and is of moderate severity and stubborn persistence. Aspirin provides only temporary relief. The early behavioral changes are often subtle and include emotional lability, job dissatisfaction, and domestic difficulties. The patient may not recognize these symptoms, but family members are usually aware of changes in behavior. Later in the course more obvious changes are observed such as increased somnolence, disorientation, and stupor.

A geographic history is especially relevant when evaluating a patient who presents outside the endemic zone.[4,22] In nearly all instances the patient will either reside in or have visited the endemic zone. The length of time spent in the zone is of little significance. Even a brief visit to an endemic area is sufficient to acquire the disease. Rosen and Belber[22] report a case of CM occurring after an overnight visit to Bakersfield, California! Diagnosis may be further obscured by the fact that patients need not visit the endemic zone to acquire the disease. Fomite-acquired and laboratory-acquired coccidioidomycosis are discussed in Chapter 4.

Physical examination reveals signs of chronic meningitis. Fever of variable degree is usually present.[1] Neck stiffness is an inconstant finding, with one series[1] reporting it as "common" and another[21] as occurring in 40% of 22 cases. The degree of nuchal rigidity varies from mild to severe. Focal neurologic findings are unusual but can occur in those rare instances where CNS coccidioidomycosis presents as a mass lesion or produces occlusion of the spinal canal (Table 3). Careful examination of the skin and lymph nodes may reveal abnormalities which upon biopsy prove to be coccidioidal.

As mentioned, nonmeningeal coccidioidomycosis may antedate meningeal disease. In Winn's[23] series of 31 cases of CM the interval between onset of disease and onset of meningitis ranged from 1 month to 84 months, with over 50% of the meningitides evident within a month of the onset of disease (Fig. 1). Kelly et al.[21] reported antecedent coccidioidomycosis in 7 of 22 (33%) cases of CM with an interval between onset and meningitis of 1 week to 14 months. In 6 of these 7 cases the preceding infection was pulmonary only, and in 1 case disseminated. Pappagianis and Crane[5] reported that 31 of 51 (61%) cases of CM had antecedent respiratory or febrile illness within weeks or months of the onset of CM.

TABLE 3
Unusual Cases of CNS Coccidioidomycosis

Reference	Number of cases	Presentation —clinical	Clinical impression	Pathological finding	With CM	Outcome
Reeves and Baisinger[24]	1	(L) Ataxia (L)Babinski (R) Jacksonian seizure	(R) Frontal abscess	*C. immitis* infection in brain stem and cerebrum. No true abscess or mass.	Yes	Died
Rhoden[17]	1	Mild headache and nystagmus.	Diabetes mellitus and viral encephalitis.	*C. immitis* abscess of (L) cerebellar hemisphere.	No	Died
Ingham[12]	1	Paraplegia of (L) extremity and paraparesis of upper extremity with associated sensory defect. C-spine erosion on X-ray.	Epidural abscess	*C. immitis* infection of lungs, cervical vertebrae, and spinal cord.	Not recorded	Died

Reference	No.	Clinical features	Preoperative diagnosis	Operative/pathologic findings		Outcome
Rand[13]	2	a. Spastic paraplegia-associated sensory defect.	a. Spinal cord tumor at T9	a. *C. immitis* extradural mass, which extended into the thoracic cavity.	No	Recovered
		b. Ataxia and nuchal rigidity early. Flaccid quadriplegia later.	b. Spinal cord tumor	b. *C. immitis* granuloma of cervical spinal cord. Granulomatous tissue encircled the cord.	Yes	Died
Gottlieb[14]	1	Upper extremity weakness. Sensory level at T2–T4.	Not recorded	*C. immitis* granuloma encircling spinal cord, and thickened leptomeninges of cord and base of brain.	Yes	Died
Jackson *et al.*[11]	1	Quadriplegia with associated sensory defect. C-spine erosions on X-rays.	Epidural abscess due to *C. immitis*	*C. immitis* osteomyelitis of cervical vertebrae.	Yes	Recovered

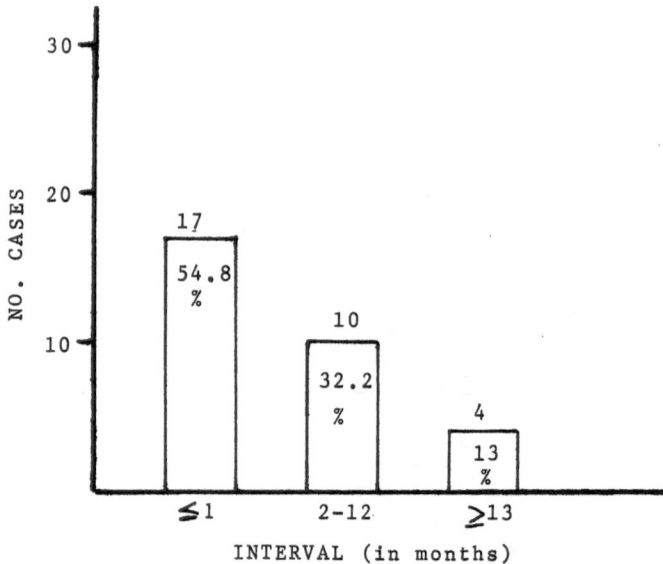

Figure 1. Interval between onset of coccidioidomycosis and onset of coccidioidal meningitis. Data computed from Winn.[23]

Of interest, 2 of Winn's 31 cases received intravenous AMB for their preceding coccidioidal infections, and yet meningitis subsequently developed.[23]

In recent years the therapeutic use of immunosuppressive drugs, and the prolonged survival of some patients with advanced Hodgkins disease and other forms of lymphoma have led to a group of patients predisposed to opportunistic infection. Fungal disease has emerged as a significant cause of mortality and morbidity among these patients. Although *C. immitis* is not ordinarily considered an opportunist, several referral centers located within or adjacent to the endemic zone have reported cases of coccidioidomycosis developing in patients with defects in cell-mediated immunity, and posing all the clinical problems associated with opportunistic infections caused by other fungi.[25-27] Deresinski and Stevens[25] reported 2 fatal cases of CM among 13 cases of coccidioidomycosis in compromised hosts diagnosed at Stanford University between 1961 and 1975. Smithline *et al.*[26] reported 2 cases of CNS coccidioidomycosis among 7 cases of coccidioidomycosis occurring in renal transplantation immunosuppressed patients at the University of Arizona. Rowland *et al.*[27] reviewed 21 fatal cases of coccidioidomycosis in immunocompromised patients and found that 3 patients had CM (see also Chapter 19).

4.2. Course of CM

In the absence of appropriate chemotherapy, coccidioidal meningitis follows a course of progressive deterioration which ends in death. Buss et al.[1] reported on 53 cases of coccidioidal meningitis diagnosed between 1936 and 1950. Fifty of the patients died, and 3 survived. Among the fatal cases, 15 died within 3 months of onset, 23 within 12 months, 7 survived for more than 1 year, and 2 lived almost 2 years. In the 3 remaining fatal cases the duration of illness was not known. Einstein and co-workers[28] briefly mention 31 cases diagnosed between 1947 and 1951; 29 died within a year, and the remaining 2 patients died within 2 years.

In contrast to this gloomy picture, several authors[29-32] have reported individual cases of prolonged survival without AMB (Table 4). One of the striking features of these cases is that the patients had long intervals where they were asymptomatic and able to work. These intervals would be followed by exacerbations and further neurologic deterioration. There is no information suggesting which host defense mechanism successfully prolonged life in these exceptional cases.

Aggressive AMB treatment has significantly improved the outlook for coccidioidal meningitis. With treatment the overall mortality is lower and prolonged survival is now common (see Section 7). The prognosis depends on several factors in addition to AMB therapy. Patients who start antifungal therapy shortly after the diagnosis of CM is established

TABLE 4
Prolonged Survival in Coccidioidal Meningitis without AMB

Reference	Number of cases	Diagnosis confirmed	Evidence whole course due to CM	Length of survival	Outcome
Rosen and Belber[22]	1	Yes by Clt.,[a] Srl., and PM	Clin.	4 yr, 8 mo	Died
Jenkins and Postlewaite[31]	2	Yes by Srl.	Clin. and Srl.	3 yr	Survived
		Yes by Srl. and PM	Clin. and Srl.	5 yr, 6 mo	Died
Norman and Miller[29]	1	Yes by Srl. and Clt.	Clin., Srl., and Clt.	10 yr, 2 mo	Survived
Sweigert and Turner[30]	1	Yes by Clt. and Srl.	Clin., Srl., and Clt.	4 yr	Died
Unterharnscheidt et al.[32]	1	Yes by PM	Clin.	7½ yr	Died

[a] Abbreviations: Clt., culture; Srl., serology; Clin., clinical; PM, postmortem.

fare better than patients whose treatment is delayed.[33,34] Patients with serious underlying diseases, particularly immunocompromised hosts, do worse than patients without complicating illnesses.[25–27] Communicating hydrocephalus is an ominous complication of CM and carries a mortality of 50–70%.[35] In one recent series 75% of the CM mortality occurred in patients with hydrocephalus.[21] Fortunately, modern techniques such as CAT scans and ventriculoperitoneal shunts permit early detection of hydrocephalus and allow for safe decompression.

5. LABORATORY MANIFESTATIONS OF CM

5.1. Essential Laboratory Tests

Thorough examination of the cerebrospinal fluid (CSF) is the key to prompt, accurate diagnosis of CM. Indeed, CSF examination is the only method which establishes the diagnosis short of biopsy of the leptomeninges or autopsy. The CSF is abnormal in *all* patients with CM and the composite abnormalities (especially the complement-fixing activity) are characteristic of the disease. The cellular and biochemical features of the CSF are those of granulomatous meningitis and are summarized in Table 5. The frequency of abnormal cellular and biochemical tests at the onset of the disease is reported by Pappagianis and Crane.[5] They found the cell count increased in 43 of 46 patients (93%), and of the 3 remaining patients, 2 showed an increase later. Similarly, the protein content was elevated in 40 of 44 patients (91%) initially and in all 44 later. Glucose was low in 41 of 43 patients (95%) at onset and later in all 43. The

TABLE 5
Pretreatment CSF Data in 22 Patients with Proven
Coccidioidal Meningitis[a]

	Mean	Range
Total cell count (cell/mm³)	371	25–1510
% Polymorphonuclear leukocytes	24	—
% Lymphocytes	76	—
Protein (mg/dl)	215	44–760
Glucose (mg/dl)	42	9–143
Ratio to serum glucose	0.35	0.15–0.60
Complement fixation titer	1 : 8	1 : 2–1 : 256
C. immitis isolates[b]	5/12	—

[a] Adapted from Kelly *et al.*[21]
[b] Data reported as number of patients with positive culture/number of patients cultured.

differential cell count typically shows predominence of lymphocytes, but early in the course polymorphonuclear leukocytes may predominate.

The pathognomonic abnormality of the CSF in CM is the fixation of complement in the presence of coccidioidin. The technique is described in Chapter 6. The complement-fixing activity in CM is due to IgG antibody produced by cells within the CNS.[36-39] Using the complement fixation technique Smith et al.[40] reported in 1956 that 70 of 92 patients (76%) with CM had complement-fixing activity in their spinal fluid. A generation later Pappagianis and Crane[5] reported that 44 of 47 patients (93%) with CM had CSF complement fixation, and that in a total of 265 patients with CM only 14 (5%) had CSF which failed to fix complement. The improvement in sensitivity is probably due to overnight cold incubation.[5] The titer of complement-fixing antibody in the CSF may vary over a wide range (Table 5) and is of no diagnostic significance, but titers are useful in following regression of the illness with AMB treatment.

The complement fixation test on CSF detects antibody formed within the CNS. In no instance does serum complement-fixing antibody diffuse into the CSF in a sufficient concentration to give a positive test.[20,40,41] However, recent experiments by Pappagianis et al.[41] demonstrate the presence of immunodiffusing antibody in concentrated CSF specimens of some patients known to have nonmeningeal coccidioidomycosis. This antibody forms a line of identity with serum complement-fixing antibody in gel diffusion plates. Hence, in some patients small amounts of serum complement-fixing antibody may enter the CSF. The presence of this antibody (i.e., detectable by immunodiffusion but not by complement fixation) in an otherwise normal CSF is not adequate evidence for CM. Smith[20,40] and Pappagianis[41] emphasize the importance of a complete examination of CSF for establishing a diagnosis of CM. Patients with CM will have abnormal CSF cell counts, protein, and glucose concentrations in addition to complement-fixing antibody.[5,18] There is no disease other than CM or juxtadural coccidioidomycosis which is associated with a positive complement fixation test in the CSF. Precipitins, an early-appearing IgM antibody to coccidioidin, are rarely found in the CSF of patients with CM.[5,40]

Culture of CSF infrequently yields C. immitis in cases of CM. Kelly et al.[21] report that only 5 of 12 cultured pretreatment CSF specimens grew C. immitis. The yield might be improved by submitting large volumes (~10-15 cc) of CSF or by centrifugation techniques, as discussed in Chapter 3, but a negative CSF culture is of no value in excluding CM. However, a positive culture is diagnostic of CM.

It should be noted that in a few cases of CM the initial CSF specimen may not show all the typical findings. Hence repeated examinations are indicated if CM is genuinely suspected.

5.2. Adjunctive Laboratory Tests

Laboratory tests aimed at detecting *C. immitis* in nonmeningeal body sites or at detecting a systemic immunologic response to the organism can be helpful in evaluating patients with granulomatous meningitis. The results of adjunctive tests may provide support for the diagnosis of CM but can never provide proof.

Serum complement-fixing antibody is present in virtually all cases of CM. Smith and co-workers[40] reported that 100% of 92 cases had serum complement-fixing antibody and that in 70% the titer was 1 : 16 or greater. Kelly *et al.*[21] reported that 100% of 22 patients had antibody in serum with a median titer of 1 : 32 and a range of 1 : 4 to 1 : 512. Serum precipitins are variably present in CM.[20,21,40]

Coccidioidin skin tests may be either positive or negative and are of no diagnostic value in CM. Kelly *et al.*[21] reported that 3 of 16 patients tested had a positive test with 1 : 100 coccidioidin and that 1 of 11 tested was positive with 1 : 10 coccidioidin. Buss *et al.*[1] reported positive skin tests in only 3 of 53 patients. Pappagianis and Crane[5] found positive skin tests in 25 of 47 (53%) cases.

Isolates of *C. immitis* from a nonmeningeal body site may be helpful in suggesting the etiology of an otherwise cryptic granulomatous meningitis. In a series of 22 patients with CM, 5 patients had isolates from the respiratory tract and 1 from lymph nodes and skin biopsy.[21] Coccidioidouria was found in 5 patients with CM reported by Petersen *et al.*[42]

Roengentography is occasionally helpful in evaluating suspected cases of CM. Pappagianis and Crane[5] reported that 24 of 35 cases of CM had pulmonary disease at the time of meningitis. Among these 24 cases, 13 had pulmonary infiltrates, 4 hilar adenopathy, 4 cavity formation, 2 granuloma, and 1 miliary disease. Other authors[43] have also reported that cavitary pulmonary coccidioidomycosis may be associated with meningitis. In those unusual cases where meningitis results from direct extension of vertebral or skull osteomyelitis, X-rays may demonstrate erosion of vertebral bodies[11,12] or "punched out" lesions of the skull[15] (see also figure in Chapter 12).

6. THE DIAGNOSIS OF CM

The differential diagnosis of granulomatous meningitis includes mycobacterial, fungal, parasitic, neoplastic, and noninfectious granulomatous disease. A detailed discussion of these is beyond the scope of this chapter and is available elsewhere.[44] The two principal diseases that might be confused with CM are tuberculous and cryptococcal meningitis.* Both can usually be excluded by detecting complement-fixing activity against coccidioidin in the patient's spinal fluid.

In a patient with clinical and CSF findings of granulomatous meningitis a diagnosis of CM may be proven by any of the following findings:

1. Detection of complement-fixing antibody in the CSF. This is the most expeditious method to establish the diagnosis. There are no "false positive" tests. In rare instances where complement fixation occurs in a CSF without the cellular and biochemical changes of meningitis, two alternatives should be considered. First, the patient in fact has CM but cellular and biochemical changes have not yet occurred.

Second, the patient has a juxtadural focus of coccidioidal disease such as vertebral osteomyelitis or a paravertebral abscess. The characteristic CSF findings of juxtadural coccidioidomycosis are an elevated protein concentration with normal cell count and glucose content.[41] The diagnosis may be facilitated by clinical findings such as local pain or focal neurologic defects, and by X-rays of suspect bones. It is important to distinguish juxtadural disease from true meningitis because surgical resection may be indicated in the former. For example, Jackson et al.[11] completely reversed quadriplegia in a 22-year-old man with surgical debridement of C4 and C5 coccidioidal osteomyelitis.

2. Growth of C. immitis from a culture of CSF. As mentioned above, isolation of the organism is inconstant and should not be relied upon. However, when C. immitis grows the diagnosis is certain.

3. Microscopic examination of the leptomeninges or brain shows spherules of C. immitis. These procedures are most often used in cases diagnosed at autopsy. Meningeal biopsy is not an established technique for diagnosis of CM in a living patient.

A diagnosis of probable CM can be made in the absence of CSF complement fixation when (1) clinical and CSF findings suggest a granulomatous process; and (2) coccidioidal infection is found at another site by culture, microscopy, or serum serology. As noted above, in the 1950s Smith et al.[40] noted that in as many as 25% of CM cases the CSF failed to fix complement. Winn[23] reported that 6 of 31 cases (19%) had no complement-fixing activity in the CSF. In more recent times using overnight incubation of CSF at 4°C, Pappagianis and Crane[5] reported that initial CSF fixed complement in 34 of 49 patients (71%) but that later specimens demonstrated fixation in 44 of 47 patients (94%). Thus, repeat

---

*Buss et al.[1] reported a patient with simultaneous tuberculous and coccidioidal meningitis! Fortunately, cases of that ilk are rare. After all, one granulomatous meningitis is enough for anybody!

examinations of the CSF will increase diagnostic accuracy, and only a small group (approximately 5–6%) of patients will be labeled as "probable" CM.

Physicians living outside the endemic zone often lack familiarity with the vagaries of coccidioidomycosis.[4] Consequently, the diagnosis may be delayed or missed entirely. This situation can be avoided by obtaining a geographic history on each patient with granulomatous meningitis. If the patient has been in the endemic zone —however briefly, however far in the past—CSF and serum should be tested for complement-fixing antibody.

7. TREATMENT OF CM

7.1. Amphotericin B

7.1.1. Introduction

The principal antimicrobial agent for treating CM is AMB. Since its introduction in the late 1950s, the mortality rate of the disease has decreased and the length of survival increased. The current concepts of treatment which evolved from the work of Winn[6,23,33,45] and Einstein and co-workers[28] recognize two important features of the drug. First, AMB is fungistatic only, and the minimal inhibitory concentration for most strains of *C. immitis* approaches the peak serum levels attained with conventional doses.[46,47] AMB may arrest *C. immitis* infection, but eradication is difficult. In this regard Winn[33] points out that the inhibitory action of AMB provides time for development of adequate immunity by the host that will sustain the arrest of infection when treatment is discontinued. Second, intravenous AMB penetrates poorly into the CSF, and intrathecal dosing is necessary to achieve fungistatic concentrations within the spinal fluid.[6,47]

7.1.2. Treatment Strategy

William Winn[6,23,33,45] pioneered the use of AMB in the treatment of CM. His treatment plan consisted of combined intravenous and intrathecal AMB administered over an extended interval and discontinued only when either the CSF was normal or toxicity prohibited further treatment. The original treatment schedule,[6] which was published in 1959, called for intravenous AMB 6 days a week (at doses of 1 mg/kg for adults and 1.25

to 1.50 mg/kg for children), and lumbar intrathecal AMB every 48 hr (at doses no greater than 0.7 mg per injection).

By 1964 the treatment schedule was modified in several important ways.[33] Initial intensive treatment consisted of alternating lumbar and cisternal intrathecal doses of AMB, providing four treatment days each week; and intravenous AMB at 1 mg/kg per dose every 48 hr with a total dose no greater than 5 g. Winn[33] emphasized that the cisternal route is preferred because of its "direct approach to the usual site of coccidioidal infection at the base of the brain" and because it "eliminates the danger of arachnoiditis which frequently follows continued injections . . . into the lumbar sac." Intensive treatment was continued until the CSF cell count, glucose, protein, and complement-fixing activity had improved. Then sustained suppressive therapy was instituted immediately. It consisted of outpatient injections of intracisternal AMB at intervals of 3 to 7 days until the CSF failed to fix complement. Treatment was suspended several months after the CSF complement fixation was negative.

Nearly 20 years have passed since Winn[6] and Einstein et al.[28] advocated combined intravenous and intrathecal AMB for treatment of CM. During that time many patients with CM have been treated by these methods, and while conclusive proof of efficacy is lacking, combined AMB therapy is the current treatment of choice for CM.

See also Section 7.1.4.2 on duration of treatment.

7.1.3. Outcome of Treatment

Winn's methods are followed by other physicians, and the impact of combined intravenous and intrathecal AMB treatment on the outcome of CM can be judged by reviewing several published series (Table 6). The mortality rate of CM in published series ranges from 19 to 49% and would depend on the duration of follow-up, with a mean survival time among fatalities from 9.2 months to 50.3 months. While none of the published series included concurrent untreated controls, Einstein[28] did include 78 untreated patients collected retrospectively. Among these cases the 1-year mortality was 85.9% and the 2-year mortality 100%. Thus AMB reduces mortality, and prolongs life among ultimately fatal cases.

Fifty-nine to 69.3% of the published cases are nonfatal, with mean survival times at time of reporting from 19.2 to 162 months (Table 6). Among the 50 reported survivors, 27 remained on AMB treatment, while 23 did not require therapy. The majority of survivors are ambulatory and have returned to useful life. Prolonged survival is reported by Pappagianis and Crane[5] and Holeman and Johnson.[48] The former authors document

TABLE 6

Effect of Amphotericin B on the Outcome of Coccidioidal Meningitis

Reference	Number of cases	Fatalities					Survivors			
		Total	CM mortality	Survival time[a]	Number off Rx[b]	Survival time	Number on Rx	Survival time	Total	Survival time
Einstein et al.[28]	11	4/11 36.3%	4/11 36.3%	18.9 4.5–34	0	—	7/11 63.6%	19.2 7–37	7/11 63.6%	19.2 7–37
Winn[33]	31	10/31 32%	6/31 19%	50.3 22–99	13/31 41.9%	53 16–95	8/31 25.8%	25.2 4–59	21/31 67.8%	42.4 4–95
Pappagianis and Crane[5]	265	130/265 49%	N.R.[c]	N.R.	N.R.	N.R.	N.R.	N.R.	N.R.	N.R.
Kelly et al.[21]	22	9/22 40.9%	8/22 36.4%	9.2 0.5–47.3	6/22 27.2%	38.3 16–75	7/22 31.8%	26 2–56	13/22 59%	31.5 2–75
Holeman and Johnson[48]	13	4/13 30.7%	4/13 30.7%	36.5 4–72	4/13 30.7%	162 120–216	5/13 38.4%	— <24–156	9/13 69.3%	— <24–216

a Survival time is mean number of months and range in months from time of diagnosis or first treatment.
b Rx refers to AMB treatment.
c N.R. = not recorded.
d Includes three patients with active disease who dropped out of treatment.

survival for up to 19 years with no deaths among patients surviving 8 years or longer. Holeman and Johnson report three 13-year and one 18-year survivor, off therapy for 24–45 months.

Cures of CM are infrequent despite aggressive, apparently adequate AMB treatment, because of the long-term threat of a relapse. In Winn's series of 31 cases, 7 relapses occurred in 6 patients (Fig. 2 and Table 7).[23] Four of the relapses occurred after an interval of approximately 2 years without overt disease! Therefore, survivorship is not synonymous with cure. Three of 6 relapsed patients ultimately died.

The morbidity of CM is substantial both in frequency and in impact on the lives of survivors. Among the 50 survivors listed in Table 6, 27 (54%) required continuing suppressive AMB. These treatments are protracted, painful, expensive interruptions of normal living, and they are only partially effective. Irreversible physical defects occur in some survivors. For example, among 7 survivors on suppressive AMB, 3 had moderate impairment of mental status, 2 had abnormal gait, 2 had urinary incontinence, and 1 was blind.[21] Only 2 of the 7 returned to their premeningitis life style.[21]

Communicating hydrocephalus probably makes a major contribution to CM morbidity. Kelly et al. reported hydrocephalus in 11 of 22 cases, with 10 patients requiring a ventriculoperitoneal shunt.[21] In Winn's series of 31 cases of CM, 5 patients required a ventriculoatrial shunt, and among these 5, 3 died and 2 remained on treatment with restricted physical activity.[23]

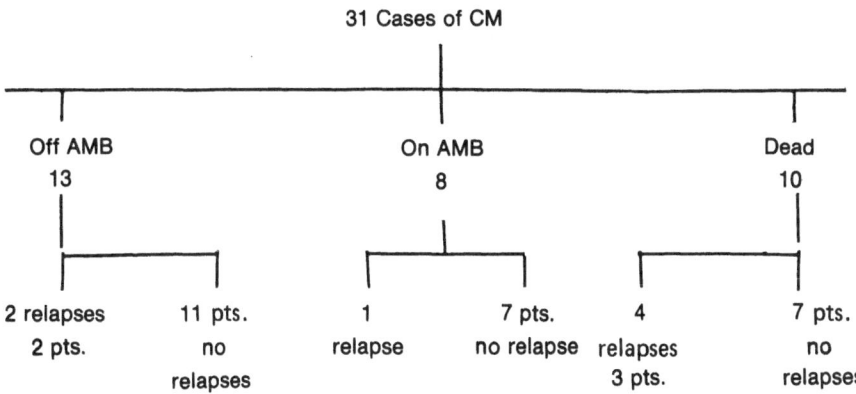

Figure 2. Frequency of relapses among 31 cases of coccidioidal meningitis. Data adapted from Winn.[23]

TABLE 7
Data on Relapsed Cases of Coccidioidal Meningitis[a]

Case No.		Interval[b]	Outcome of relapse
9		22	Patient well, CSF negative, off AMB 15 months
10		5	Patient well, CSF negative, off AMB 5 months
15		19	Patient working, on suppressive AMB
22	Relapse 1:	23	Patient relapsed a second time 3 months off AMB
	Relapse 2:	23	Death
24		27	Death
27		9	Death

[a] Data adapted from Winn.[23]
[b] Interval is the time in months from a negative CSF to onset of relapse. Patients did not receive AMB during this interval.

7.1.4. Practical Considerations

The pharmacokinetics of AMB are understood poorly and investigated incompletely. Empiric consideration such as clinical improvement, drug toxicity, and the recorded experience of skilled clinicians[5,6,21,23,28,45,48–50] are used to determine route of administration, dose, and duration of treatment.

7.1.4.1. Route of Administration and Dose. Intravenous AMB: Conventional intravenous doses of AMB (i.e., about 50 mg IV QOD) do not produce measurable concentrations of drug in CSF.[6,47] Despite this fact its use in CM is recommended by knowledgeable physicians[6,21,23,28,49] and is *de rigueur* in treatment regimens. There is one recorded case of cure of CM with only intravenous AMB.[5,51]

The total dose and duration of intravenous AMB for CM reported in the literature varies widely. Kelly *et al.*[22] administered a mean total intravenous dose of 1.6 g over a mean of 19 weeks among 14 surviving patients. Winn[23,33] used larger doses delivered over a longer interval and suggested that the total dose not exceed 5 g. Einstein[49] recommends a dose of 1 g. In contemporary practice the trend is toward a total intravenous dose of 2 g or less given early in the course of treatment.

Intrathecal AMB: Intrathecal AMB is administered by entering the subarachnoid space at one or more of several possible sites. The commonly used sites are the lumbar sac and the cisterna magna; less frequently used sites are the subarachnoid space at C1-C2 (lateral cervical puncture) and the lateral cerebral ventricle (via a reservoir). Therapy by any of these routes may be frustrated by obstruction to flow due to inflammation.

Lumbar sac injections are used to initiate intrathecal therapy.[33] The advantages of this route are safety and widespread physician familiarity with lumbar puncture. Two important disadvantages limit the long-term utility of lumbar punctures. First, repeated installation of AMB in the sac usually results in symptomatic arachnoiditis, which precludes further injections.[23,33] Second, the lumbar sac is remote from the infected basal meninges, and the flow of AMB to the base of the brain is sluggish and incomplete.[33]

Alazraki and co-workers[52,53] modified the lumbar technique to promote gravity-dependent flow of AMB to the cisterna magna. They mixed AMB with 10% glucose in water and placed the subjects in 25% Trendelenberg position (hyperbaric glucose AMB). In monkey experiments[52] they showed that AMB appeared in cisternal fluid more rapidly in hyperbaric glucose-AMB treated animals than in controls. In a human case of CM[53] they demonstrated that hyperbaric glucose-AMB facilitated the flow of a radiolabeled albumin marker from the lumbar sac to the basal cisterns. The patient was treated for 2 years with this technique and made an excellent recovery. Twenty-three patients treated with the hyperbaric technique were reported by Pappagianis and Crane.[5] Seventeen of these either improved or did not progress, but in 6 cases no effect on the meningitis was evident. Side effects occurred in 12 patients, and 7 expired. The side effects were arachnoiditis, possible induction of a spinal canal block (1 case), and transverse myelitis (2 cases). Thus, the addition of hyperbaric glucose to lumbar AMB has improved distribution of the drug but has not alleviated the problem of arachnoiditis.

Repeated injections of AMB into the lumbar sac results in symptomatic arachnoiditis in most cases of CM (see below). But several authors[4,5,23,54] report effective treatment without associated arachnoiditis using lumbar injections as the only intrathecal route of administration. Therefore, if lumbar treatment is successfully controlling the disease and if arachnoiditis does not supervene, long-term use of lumbar sac injections is acceptable.

Injection of AMB directly into the cisterna magna is common practice in the management of CM. Several experienced clinicians state that cisternal injections are the preferred intrathecal route of administration because of the proximity of the cistern to the site of infection and the lack of arachnoiditis. Winn[23,33] recommends starting cisternal treatments early in therapy and continuing them throughout the suppressive phase. Einstein[49] uses cisternal injections as a "primary form of treatment." Holeman and Johnson[48] and Buchsbaum[50] rely on the cisternal route for intrathecal treatment.

The hazards of repeated cisternal punctures are real but occur infrequently. Winn[23] performed "hundreds" of punctures without any "serious results." Holeman and Johnson[48] had no mortality associated with 1600 cisternal punctures. Other physicians have reported individual patients with complications. Buchsbaum[50] had three serious complications (one unilateral deafness, one posterior fossa hematoma, and one permanent T4 paraparesis) among 26 patients with CM managed with repeated cisternal injections. Sung and Grendahl[55] reported an intracisternal hemorrhage due to trauma during a cisternal puncture. Keane[56] reported two serious complications (one fatal subarachnoid hemorrhage, and one nonfatal brain stem trauma) in patients with CM and reviewed the literature on the hazards of cisternal puncture. The serious complications are subarachnoid hemorrhage and needle trauma of brain tissue, either of which may be fatal.[56] Death from subarachnoid hemorrhage is caused by the mass effect of blood accumulating in the cisterna magna and compressing the brain stem. Surgical decompression of the posterior fossa is indicated in these cases. Brain stem trauma is less frequent and less likely to be fatal than subarachnoid hemorrhage.[56] In view of the fatal course of CM and the established benefits of intrathecal AMB, the prudent use of cisternal puncture seems a justifiable risk. Cisternal puncture adverse effects are also mentioned in Section 7.1.5.

Lateral cervical puncture enters the subarachnoid space between the spinous processes of C1 and C2 by percutaneous insertion of a spinal needle 1 cm inferior and 5 cm posterior to the tip of the mastoid process.[57] This route is used extensively for myelography,[58] but its use in fungal meningitis is recent. Underman[57] used the technique over 300 times without any morbidity in eight patients with fungal meningitis (7 CM, one cryptococcal). He feels the technique is safe and allows injection of AMB 1.5–2.0 cm below the cisterna magna in an area adjacent to the disease process.

Ventriculostomy with an Ommaya reservoir is used in a minority of CM patients[5,23]; it provides access to infected ventricles for administration of AMB. (Indications for placement are discussed in Section 7.3). Unfortunately, Ommaya reservoirs have a high incidence of bacterial superinfection and/or mechanical problems.[5,35,59,60] Pappagianis and Crane[5] include 51 patients with Ommaya intraventricular catheters in their report on treatment of CM. Among these cases 14 (28%) died, with 4 deaths caused by "secondary bacterial sepsis." Twenty-one patients (38%) developed bacterial infection of the Ommaya device, and 11 (22%) experienced obstruction, or breakage of the catheter. CSF leakage, hemorrhage, and wound infection have also been reported. Thus, ventriculostomy with an Ommaya reservoir should be reserved for selected patients with coccidioidal ventriculitis.

The dose of intrathecal AMB (both individual injection and total cumulative dose) used to treat CM is determined wholly on an empiric basis. The determinants of dose are the patient's response to treatment and his tolerance of treatment. There is no predetermined total amount of intrathecal AMB that will supress all cases of CM, nor is there any universally well-tolerated single injection dose. The treating physician must adjust the dose so that treatment is timely, regular, and well tolerated. This requires forbearance, persistence, and patient rapport.

Lumbar or cisternal therapy begins with a small amount (0.05–0.1 mg) of AMB mixed with 25 mg of hydrocortisone (or a comparable amount of other corticosteroids). The drug is injected slowly with the barbotage technique. Injections are performed three to four times a week on an alternate-day schedule in the early stages of treatment. The dose is *gradually* increased as patient tolerance permits. Most patients will tolerate doses of 0.25–0.5 mg per injection; an occasional patient can tolerate 0.75–1 mg. Volumes used for cisternal treatment are advised to be ≤1.5 ml. Toxic reactions to intrathecal AMB are frequent but usually can be managed with preinjection sedation and postinjection analgesia. If reactions unduly distress the patient, it is best to decrease the dose to a previously well-tolerated level and/or increase the interval between injections. Wise physicians realize that patient-to-patient tolerance of AMB is variable and adjust the treatment schedule accordingly.

Once a satisfactory regimen is established, intensive treatment continues until the patient improves as judged by clinical condition and the return of CSF parameters toward normal. Then suppressive treatment commences, and the interval between doses usually can be increased. Holeman and Johnson[48] used CSF cell counts to vary intrathecal dosing intervals. If the cell count was 10/mm³ or less, the interval between doses was gradually increased up to but no less frequently than every 6 weeks for a substantial period. If the cell count increased to greater than 10/mm³, intensive therapy was reinstituted.

The pharmacokinetics of intrathecal AMB were studied by Bindschadler and co-workers[47,61] in three patients with cryptococcal meningitis who received intraventricular AMB via an Ommaya reservoir. Peak concentrations of AMB in ventricular CSF were 0.5–0.8 µg/ml after doses of 0.1–0.3 mg. The CSF concentrations 24 hr after 0.2- to 0.3-mg doses were 0.19–0.29 µg/ml, and 48 hr after 0.3 mg, the concentration was 0.14 µg/ml. The investigators[61] have proposed a two-compartment model for CNS handling of AMB. One compartment is the measurable amount of CSF and approximates a volume of 140 ml. The drug is removed from this compartment via bulk flow and is diluted by addition of new CSF from the choroid plexus. The second compartment, which is thought to be the extracellular space of the brain, has a volume of approximately

680 ml and serves as a reservoir of AMB within the CNS. Drug in the second compartment diffuses back into the CSF and thereby maintains AMB within the CSF between injections. The validity of this model is not yet established.

7.1.4.2. Duration of Treatment. (See also Section 7.1.2.) The duration of intrathecal therapy is determined by the patient's response to treatment, which is estimated by clinical improvement and repeated examinations of the CSF. In fully treated cases the CSF cell count, protein concentration, and glucose concentration are normal or nearly so, and complement-fixing antibody is absent.[23,33] The latter test is considered by Winn[23,33] to be the single most important tool for estimating response to treatment. He recommends stopping intrathecal therapy when CSF complement fixation is absent for 3 months.[23,33]

In actual practice CM patients are treated for many months or years. For example, among Winn's 13 patients who were well and off all treatment, the mean duration of cisternal therapy was 12.4 months with a range of 1–35 months.[23] Einstein[49] states that cisternal treatments continue "usually for a period of years" and that "some never have . . . cessation of therapy." Holeman[48] discontinues therapy only after at least 1 year of normal CSF on treatment schedule of once every 6 weeks. CSF examinations are then continued for 1–2 years. CSF pleocytosis or chemical abnormalities generally precede CSF antibody in relapses.

The collection site of CSF is an important variable when judging response to treatment. Ventricular fluid collected via an Ommaya reservoir was diagnostically misleading in three cases studied by Goldstein *et al.*[62] When compared with lumbar fluid, the ventricular fluid consistently underestimated cell counts, protein concentration, and complement fixation titer and overestimated glucose concentration, thereby falsely indicating a favorable response. Hence, only lumbar or cisternal fluid should be used to evaluate progress of treatment.[33,62]

7.1.5. Adverse Effects

Intrathecal AMB treatment is always associated with undesirable local side effects, and the drug preparation itself produces an inflammatory response within the CNS.[33] The commercial preparation of AMB contains sodium deoxycholate and buffers in addition to the active drug.[63] When doses appropriate for treating CM (i.e., 0.025–1 mg) are injected into the lumbar sac of a normal human, a pleocytosis of several hundred cells and a mild increase in CSF protein often occurs.[33] Thus, the treating physician should expect side effects and plan for their management.

The adverse effects of intrathecal AMB are local in distribution and putatively inflammatory in nature. Their clinical manifestations range from mild to severe and from transient to prolonged or even permanent. The most common side effect is headache or back pain which may be accompanied by nausea and vomiting, and occurs shortly after an intrathecal injection. This reaction is usually transient and of mild to moderate severity. It is managed by adequate premedication and by postinjection analgesics.[23,33] Usually this side effect diminishes in frequency and severity as therapy progresses but tends to recur as the dose of AMB is increased.

Repeated lumbar intrathecal AMB injections commonly lead to a syndrome referred to as "arachnoiditis,"[5,23,33] which is manifested by prolonged back, leg or saddle pain, paresthesias and/or weakness in the lower extremities, bladder dysfunction, impotence, and large amounts of protein in the CSF. All symptoms are not seen in each patient and when present may fluctuate in severity, often exacerbating after an injection. If this syndrome is recognized early and treatment discontinued, symptoms dissipate; but if lumbar injections continue, the condition will worsen and symptoms may be prolonged or even permanent. Onset of the symptoms mentioned is an indication to stop lumbar sac injections.

The prevalence of this syndrome is not reported in the published series, but it is the consensus of most experienced clinicians that the effect is common[5,23,33,49] (if not inevitable) with prolonged lumbar therapy. The syndrome may be either more frequent or more severe in patients treated with the hyperbaric glucose technique.[5] Hydrocortisone (25 mg) is usually added to intrathecal AMB in an attempt to prevent or ameliorate "arachnoiditis" by reducing the local inflammatory response of the meninges.

It is customary to attribute the lower extremity and bladder symptoms described above to inflammatory arachnoiditis,[5,23,33] but two recently reported cases demonstrate spinal cord myelopathy associated with intrathecal AMB.[64,65] One patient developed a flaccid paralysis with a T4 sensory level and the other a partial Brown–Sequard syndrome at T8. Myelography did not suggest arachnoiditis in either case, and autopsy of the patient with the Brown–Sequard syndrome showed necrosis of the left half of the spinal cord at T8. These cases indicate that intrathecal AMB has a potential for direct damage to CNS tissue. The prevalence of "AMB myelopathy" and its distinction from arachnoiditis are not clear at this time.

Cisternal AMB injections may be complicated by acute headache as mentioned above (see also Section 7.1.4.1), cranial nerve palsies which are usually transient, arterial hypertension and bradycardia, other arrhythmias, nausea and vomiting, and gait disturbances.[48] The mechanism of these adverse effects is obscure, but in the past they were ascribed to arachnoiditis. Because of reports of spinal cord myelopathy,[64,65] a direct neurotoxic mechanism should also be considered. Some of the complications may be dose related, and in clinical practice the amount of drug administered is adjusted to produce only minimal headache.[48]

7.2. Miconazole

Until recently, AMB was the only antimicrobial agent available for treating *C. immitis* infections. In the early years of this decade, a synthetic imidazole derivative, miconazole (MCZ), was found to be fungistatic for *C. immitis in vitro* and effective in treating experimental murine coccidioidomycosis.[66] Human trials were performed in patients with coccidioidomycosis and other deep fungal infections, and the results of these trials reported.[34,55,67,68] Our concern here is with the use of MCZ in CM (see also Chapter 20).

The relevant *in vitro* and pharmacologic data for evaluating MCZ in CM are summarized in Table 8. It is noteworthy that intravenous MCZ penetrates into the CSF to some extent.[67,68] However, the degree of penetration is unpredictable, and there is no apparent correlation between CSF levels of MCZ after intravenous administration and the degree of CNS inflammation (as measured by CSF pleocytosis and CSF protein concentration), nor is there any correlation between intravenous dose and subsequent CSF concentration.[68] MCZ can be safely administered intrathecally into the lumbar sac, cisterna magna, and lateral cerebral ventricle in doses of up to 20 mg.[68] Twenty-four hours after a 20-mg intrathecal injection, the mean CSF concentration of MCZ is above the minimal inhibitory concentration of most strains of *C. immitis*.

Only a few patients with CM have received MCZ therapy.[34,55,67,68] The results of treatment in most of these cases were collected by Deresinski *et al.*[34] and presented at the Third International Coccidioidomycosis Symposium. They reported on 17 courses of MCZ in 13 cases of CM. Twelve of the 13 patients had already been treated with intravenous and intrathecal AMB, and 5 were moribund when MCZ was begun. All 5 moribund patients died despite intravenous and intrathecal MCZ. Five of the remaining 8 patients responded to MCZ. Four of the 5 responders had CM of less than 6 months' duration and received only intravenous MCZ. The total intravenous dose in responders ranged

TABLE 8
In Vitro and Pharmocologic Data for Miconazole[a]

Minimal inhibitory concentration	14 strains, mycelial phase mean 0.87 $\mu g/ml$, range 0.32 –1.7 $\mu g/ml$. Endospore phase is 33% to 79% lower than corresponding mycelial phase.
Plasma half life	Early phase 30 min. Late phase 20 hr.
Peak serum concentration @ dose of 9 mg/kg	71% of tests show > 1 $\mu g/ml$ with maximum of 7.5 $\mu g/ml$.
CSF concentration shortly after intravenous dose	32 tests in 9 patients. 45% of values < 0.1 $\mu g/ml$. Among values > 0.1 $\mu g/ml$ the range was 0.77 –0.1 $\mu g/ml$ with a mean of 22% of simultaneous serum concentration.
CSF concentration after 20 mg MCZ intrathecally	24 hr postinjection, mean 1.1 $\mu g/ml$, range 0.29 –1.6 $\mu g/ml$. 48 hr postinjection, mean 0.25, range 0.13 –0.34 $\mu g/ml$. 72 hr postinjection, range < 0.1 –0.17 $\mu g/ml$

[a] Data from Deresinski et al.[34]

between 41.4 and 113.8 g (median, 55.2 g) delivered over 17–49 days (median, 23 days). One responder who was treated within a week of diagnosis was alive and free of meningitis 18 months after discontinuing MCZ. Two of the responders relapsed 3 and 9 weeks after MCZ was stopped. Three nonmoribund patients ultimately died (one ruptured esophageal varices, one obstructive hydrocephalus, one ventricular catheter complication).

Seven of 12 patients who had post MCZ CSF examinations showed a 40% or greater decrease in protein concentration. Among 5 patients with pretreatment CSF pleocytosis, 3 showed a significant decrease after treatment. Only 1 patient had a fall in CSF complement fixation titer.

The numbers of MCZ-treated CM patients reported was expanded in a subsequent editorial,[69] and the earlier results were confirmed.

It is difficult to draw any firm conclusions about MCZ treatment from the small number of selected patients, nearly half of whom were moribund and virtually all of whom had received prior AMB therapy. The fact that five of eight nonmoribund patients[34] showed some clinical response is encouraging and is sufficient reason to continue investigation of the drug. At the present time MCZ is an acceptable drug for treating CM when AMB either fails or proves to be too toxic.

7.3. Adjunctive Neurosurgical Procedures

There are two complications of CM which can be treated with neurosurgical procedures. The complications are communicating hydrocephalus and coccidioidal infection of the lateral cerebral ventricles; and the procedures are ventricular shunt operations and ventriculostomy with an Ommaya reservoir.

Communicating hydrocephalus caused by obstruction to the flow of CSF is a well-known sequela of chronic basilar meningitis, including CM. This complication is responsible for both mortality and morbidity in CM. However, prompt and accurate diagnosis can lead to a neurosurgical shunt procedure (customarily a ventriculoperitoneal shunt) which results in decompression of the brain and, in some cases, improvement in clinical status. The occurrence of hydrocephalus in CM is probably related to duration of disease prior to diagnosis. The longer the delay in diagnosis the greater is the opportunity for the chronic inflammatory process to obstruct the flow of CSF. Winn[23] feels that early diagnosis and AMB treatment reduces the occurrence of hydrocephalus.

Communicating hydrocephalus is suspected if the CSF pressure is consistently elevated, if clinical signs of increased intracranial pressure develop, or if the patient does not respond to AMB treatment. The recent development of computerized axial tomography (CAT scans) provides a safe and accurate method for confirming the diagnosis. Serial CAT scans permit observation of ventricular size over a period of time and may increase the accuracy of early diagnosis.

When the presence of communicating hydrocephalus is established, neurosurgical consultation should be obtained and a shunt operation considered. A discussion of the various shunt procedures is beyond the scope of this chapter.

Decompression of the brain by an effective shunt can result in improved symptoms, and in some cases this is dramatic, but not all shunted patients will respond. Cheu and Waldmann[70] reported on five cases of CM managed with ventriculoatriostomy; three benefited and two did not. Zealer and Winn[35] reported on seven cases of CM requiring a shunt; six benefited and one did not.

All of the current shunt procedures can be complicated by bacterial infection, mechanical malfunction of the shunt, and/or migration (e.g., into brain tissue) of the ventricular catheter from its insertion site. These complications can be difficult to manage and may necessitate additional neurosurgery for revision or replacement of the shunt. In addition, Cheu and Waldmann[70] reported a unique complication of ventriculoatrial shunts in CM. Five patients who had V-A shunts and subsequently died were found to have fresh granulomas caused by *C. immitis* in their lungs and other viscera. These patients presumably redisseminated *C. immitis* from the cerebral ventricle via the shunt. Suppressive systemic chemotherapy might be contemplated in the presence of such shunts. The decision to use a shunt should be made on the basis of findings in each individual patient. The possible beneficial effects must be weighed against the potential hazards of the shunt.

Coccidioidal infection of the lateral cerebral ventricles is another complication of CM which requires neurosurgical intervention. Ventriculitis is difficult to treat with either lumbar or cisternal AMB because of downward flow of CSF. Intraventricular AMB, which can be administered safely via an Ommaya reservoir, provides intensive local treatment of ventriculitis.

Winn[23] states that coccidioidal ventriculitis should be suspected when the "patient . . . does not show very rapid improvement upon intravenous and cisternal injections of AMB." He[23] recommends ventricular fluid examination and culture to establish the diagnosis. If ventriculitis is present, an Ommaya device is placed and intraventricular AMB treatment is begun.

Ommaya reservoirs are mixed blessings. They provide convenient access to the lateral ventricles and greatly facilitate the administration of AMB. In a few instances reservoirs are used for ease of drug administration only and without evidence of ventriculitis. Unfortunately, the reservoirs and their attached catheters have a high incidence of infectious and mechanical complications which can be serious and even lethal.[59,60] In my opinion, Ommaya reservoirs should be used for proven or suspected ventriculitis and avoided in patients without ventriculitis.

The frequency of ventriculitis in CM is not known. Winn[23,35] reported four culture-proven cases among 31 cases of CM, but authors of other series did not specifically report ventriculitis.

Ventriculitis may or may not be associated with communicating hydrocephalus. Winn[23] suggested use of the indigo carmine dye test at the time of ventricular aspiration to determine the extent of CSF block. Similar information can now be obtained from the use of radioisotopes and flow study scans. If significant obstruction to the flow of CSF is present, then both an Ommaya device and a shunt operation may be necessary. The disadvantages of using both of these devices are the rapid clearance of AMB from the ventricles via the shunt (although some shunting devices allow temporary occlusion of flow), and the possible spread of *C. immitis* from an infected ventricle, leading to ineffective local treatment on one hand and to redissemination of coccidioidomycosis on the other.

REFERENCES

1. W. C. Buss, T. E. Gibson, and M. A. Gifford, Coccidioidomycosis of the meninges, *Calif. Med.* **72**:167–169 (1950).
2. R. W. Huntington, Jr., Morphology and racial distribution of fatal coccidioidomycosis, *J. Am. Med. Assoc.* **169**:115–118 (1959).
3. R. W. Huntington, W. J. Waldmann, J. A. Sargent, H. O'Connell, R. Wybel, and D. Croll, Pathologic and clinical observations of 142 cases of fatal coccidioidomycosis with necropsy, in: *Coccidioidomycosis* (L. Ajello, ed.), University of Arizona Press, Tucson (1967), pp. 143–167.
4. R. G. Caudill, C. E. Smith, J. A. Reinarz, Coccidioidal meningitis: A diagnostic challenge, *Am. J. Med.* **49**:360–365 (1970).
5. D. Pappagianis and R. Crane, Survival in coccidioidal meningitis since introduction of amphotericin B, in: *Coccidioidomycosis: Current Clinical and Diagnostic Status* (L. Ajello, ed.), Symposia Specialists, Miami (1977), pp. 223–237.
6. W. A. Winn, The use of amphotericin B in the treatment of coccidioidal disease, *Am. J. Med.* **27**:617–635 (1959).
7. E. C. Dickson and M. A. Gifford, Coccidioides infection (coccidioidomycosis). II. The primary type of infection, *Arch. Intern. Med.* **62**:853–871 (1938).
8. E. C. Dickson, Coccidioidomycosis, *J. Am. Med. Assoc.* **111**:1362–1365 (1938).
9. W. D. Forbus and A. M. Bestebreutje, Coccidioidomycosis: a study of 95 cases of the disseminated type with special reference to the pathogenesis of the disease, *Mil. Surg.* **99**:619–653 (1946).
10. K. H. Abbott and O. I. Cutler, Chronic coccidioidal meningitis, *Arch. Pathol.* **21**:320–330 (1936).
11. F. E. Jackson, D. Kent, and F. Clare, Quadriplegia caused by involvement of cervical spine with Coccidioides immitis, *J. Neurosurg.* **21**:512–515 (1964).
12. S. D. Ingham, Coccidioidal granuloma of the spine with compression of the spinal cord, *Bull. Los Angeles Neurol. Soc.* **1**:41–49 (1936).
13. C. W. Rand, Coccidioidal granuloma, *Arch. Neurol. Psychiatry* **23**:502–511 (1930).
14. M. L. Gottlieb, Coccidioidomycosis localized to the thoracic spinal cord and brain, with a plea for early diagnosis, *Ariz. Med.* **13**:131–139 (1956).
15. C. B. Courville and K. H. Abbott, Pathology of coccidioidal granuloma of the central nervous system and its envelopes, *Bull. Los Angeles Neurol. Soc.* **3**:27–41 (1938).
16. H. G. Schlumberger, A fatal case of cerebral coccidioidomycosis with cultural studies, *Am. J. Med. Sci.* **209**:483–496 (1945).
17. A. E. Rhoden, Coccidioidal brain abscess, *Bull. Los Angeles Neurol. Soc.* **11**:80–85 (1946).
18. D. M. Goldstein and J. B. McDonald, Primary pulmonary coccidioidomycosis, *J. Am. Med. Assoc.* **124**:557–561 (1944).
19. C. E. Smith, R. R. Beard, E. G. Whiting, and H. G. Rosenberger, Varieties of coccidioidal infection in relation to the epidemiology and control of the diseases, *Am. J. Public Health* **36**:1394–1402 (1946).
20. C. E. Smith, M. T. Saito, R. R. Beard, R. M. Kepp, R. W. Clark, and B. U. Eddie, Serological tests in the diagnosis and prognosis of coccidioidomycosis, *Am. J. Hyg.* **52**:1–21 (1950).
21. P. C. Kelly, M. L. Sievers, R. Thompson, and C. Echols, Coccidioidal meningitis: results of treatment in 22 patients, in: *Coccidioidomycosis, Current Clinical and Diagnostic Status* (L. Ajello, ed.), Symposia Specialists, Miami (1977), pp. 239–251.
22. E. Rosen and J. P. Belber, Coccidioidal meningitis of long duration, *Ann. Intern. Med.* **34**:796–809 (1951).

23. W. A. Winn, Coccidioidal meningitis: A follow-up report, in: *Coccidioidomycosis* (L. Ajello, ed.), University of Arizona Press, Tucson (1967), pp. 55–62.
24. D. L. Reeves and C. F. Baisinger, Primary chronic coccidioidal meningitis: A diagnostic neurosurgical problem, *J. Neurosurg.* 2:269–280 (1945).
25. S. C. Deresinski and D. A. Stevens, Coccidioidomycosis in compromised hosts, *Medicine* 54:377–395 (1974).
26. N. Smithline, D. A. Ogden, A. I. Cohn, and K. Johnson, Disseminated coccidioidomycosis in renal transplant patients, in: *Coccidioidomycosis: Current Clinical and Diagnostic Status* (L. Ajello, ed.), Symposia Specialists, Miami (1977), pp. 201–208.
27. V. S. Rowland, R. E. Westfall, and W. A. Hinchcliffe, Fatal coccidioidomycosis: analysis of host factors, in: *Coccidioidomycosis: Current Clinical and Diagnostic Status* (L. Ajello, ed.), Symposia Specialists, Miami (1977), pp. 91–106.
28. H. Einstein, C. W. Holeman, Jr., L. Sandidge, and D. H. Holden, Coccidioidal meningitis, the use of amphotericin B in treatment, *Calif. Med.* 94:339–343 (1961).
29. D. D. Norman and Z. R. Miller, Coccidioidomycosis of the central nervous system, a case of ten years' duration, *Neurology* 4:713–717 (1954).
30. C. F. Sweigert, H. W. Turner, and J. B. Gillespie, Clinical and roentgenologic aspects of coccidioidomycosis, *Am. J. Med. Sci.* 212:652–673 (1946).
31. V. E. Jenkins and J. C. Postlewaite, Coccidioidal meningitis: report of four cases with necropsy findings in 3 cases, *Ann. Intern. Med.* 35:1068–1084 (1951).
32. F. Unterharnscheidt, M. DeBeukelaer, and J. L. Simon, Chronic untreated coccidioidomycosis of the central nervous system: a case of 7 1/2 years duration, *Tex. Rep. Biol. Med.* 27:513–524 (1969).
33. W. A. Winn, The treatment of coccidioidal meningitis. The use of amphotericin B in a group of twenty-five patients, *Calif. Med.* 101:78–89 (1964).
34. S. C. Deresinski, J. N. Galgiani, and D. A. Stevens, Miconazole treatment of human coccidioidomycosis: status report, in: *Coccidioidomycosis: Current Clinical and Diagnostic Status* (L. Ajello, ed.), Symposia Specialists, Miami (1977), pp. 267–294.
35. D. S. Zealear and W. A. Winn, The neurosurgical approach in the treatment of coccidioidal meningitis. Report of 10 cases, in: *Coccidioidomycosis* (L. Ajello, ed.), University of Arizona Press, Tucson (1967), pp. 43–53.
36. D. Pappagianis, N. J. Lindsey, C. E. Smith, and M. T. Saito, Antibodies in human coccidioidomycosis: immunoelectrophoretic properties, *Proc. Soc. Exp. Biol. Med.* 118:118–122 (1965).
37. Y. Sawaki, M. Huppert, J. W. Bailey, and Y. Yagi, Patterns of human antibody reactions in coccidioidomycosis, *J. Bacteriol.* 91:422–427 (1966).
38. R. W. P. Cutler, G. V. Watters, J. P. Hammerstad, and E. Merler, Origin of cerebrospinal fluid gamma globulin in subacute sclerosing leukoencephalitis, *Arch. Neurol.* 17:620–628 (1967).
39. S. Cohen and R. Bannister, Immunoglobulin synthesis within the central nervous system in disseminated sclerosis, *Lancet* 1:366–367 (1967).
40. C. E. Smith, M. T. Saito, and S. A. Simons, Pattern of 39,500 serologic tests in coccidioidomycosis, *J. Am. Med. Assoc.* 160:546–552 (1956).
41. D. Pappagianis, M. Saito, and K. H. Van Hoosear, Antibody in cerebrospinal fluid in non-meningitic coccidioidomycosis, *Sabouraudia* 10:173–179 (1972).
42. E. A. Petersen, B. A. Friedman, E. D. Crowder, and D. Rifkind, Coccidioidouria: clinical significance, *Ann. Intern. Med.* 85:34–38 (1976).
43. M. J. Fiese, *Coccidioidomycosis*, p. 152, Charles C. Thomas, Springfield, Ill. (1958).
44. J. J. Ellner and J. E. Bennett, Chronic meningitis, *Medicine* 55:341–370 (1976).
45. W. A. Winn, Coccidioidomycosis, *Med. Clin. North Am.* 47:1131–1148 (1963).
46. M. S. Collins and D. Pappagianis, Uniform susceptibility of various strains of *Cocci-*

dioides immitis to amphotericin B, *Antimicrob. Agents Chemother.* **11**:1049–1055 (1977).

47. D. D. Bindschadler and J. E. Bennett, A pharmacologic guide to the clinical use of amphotericin B, *J. Infect. Dis.* **120**:427–436 (1969).

48. C. W. Holeman and P. Johnson, Long term follow-up of amphotericin treated coccidioidal meningitis patients, *Proceedings of the Twenty-First Annual Coccidioidomycosis Study Group,* Abstract 1 (1976).

49. H. E. Einstein, Coccidioidomycosis of the central nervous system, in: *Advances in Neurology,* Vol. 6 (R. A. Thompson and J. R. Green, eds.), Raven Press, New York (1974), pp. 101–106.

50. H. W. Buchsbaum, Clinical management of coccidioidal meningitis, in: *Coccidioidomycosis: Current Clinical and Diagnostic Status* (L. Ajello, ed.), Symposia Specialists, Miami (1977), pp. 191–200.

51. J. J. Castellot, F. W. Pitts, and F. H. Mowrey, A case of coccidioidal meningitis arrested by prolonged therapy with amphotericin B., *Antibiot. Med. Clin. Ther.* **6**:480–485 (1959).

52. N. P. Alazraki, J. Fierer, S. E. Halpern, and R. W. Becker, Use of a hyperbaric solution for administration of intrathecal amphotericin B, *N. Engl. J. Med.* **290**:641–646 (1974).

53. K. P. Glynn, N. P. Alazraki, and T. A. Waltz, Coccidioidal meningitis–intrathecal treatment with hyperbaric amphotericin B., *Calif. Med.* **119**:6–9 (1973).

54. M. LeClerc and S. T. Giammona, Coccidioidal meningitis, the use of amphotericin B intravenously and intrathecally by repeated lumbar punctures, *West. J. Med.* **122**:251–254 (1975).

55. J. P. Sung and J. G. Grendahl, Clinical experimental therapy with miconazole for human disseminated coccidioidomycosis, in: *Coccidioidomycosis: Current Clinical and Diagnostic Status* (L. Ajello, ed.), Symposia Specialists, Miami (1977), pp. 293–310.

56. J. R. Keane, Cisternal puncture complications—treatment of coccidioidal meningitis with amphotericin B, *Calif. Med.* **119**:10–15 (1973).

57. A. Underman, Private communication of a paper delivered at the Third International Coccidioidomycosis Symposium, Tucson (1976).

58. D. L. Kelly, Lateral cervical puncture for myelography, *J. Neurosurg.* **29**:106–110 (1968).

59. R. A. Ratcheson and A. K. Ommaya, Experience with subcutaneous cerebrospinal—fluid reservoir, preliminary report of 60 cases, *N. Engl. J. Med.* **279**:1025–1031 (1968).

60. R. D. Diamond and J. E. Bennett, A subcutaneous reservoir for intrathecal therapy of fungal meningitis, *N. Engl. J. Med.* **288**:186–188 (1973).

61. A. J. Atkinson, Jr., and D. D. Bindschadler, Parmacokinetics of intrathecally administered amphotericin B, *Am. Rev. Resp. Dis.* **99**:917–924 (1969).

62. E. Goldstein, M. J. Winship, and D. Pappagianis, Ventricular fluid and the management of coccidioidal meningitis, *Ann. Intern. Med.* **77**:243–246 (1972).

63. J. P. Utz, J. E. Bennett, M. W. Brandriss, W. T. Butler, and G.J. Hill II, Amphotericin B toxicity, *Ann. Intern. Med.* **61**:334–354 (1964).

64. N. T. Carnevale, J. N. Galgiani, J. W. Langston, and D. A. Stevens, Myelopathy due to intrathecal amphotericin B, in: *Coccidioidomycosis: Current Clinical and Diagnostic Status* (L. Ajello, ed.), Symposia Specialists, Miami (1977), pp. 259–260.

65. N. T. Carnevale, J. N. Galgiani, J. W. Langston, D. A. Stevens, and M. K. Herrick, Amphotericin—induced myelopathy, *Neurology* **27**:359 (1977).

66. H. B. Levine, D. A. Stevens, J. M. Cobb, and A. E. Gebhart, Miconazole in

coccidioidomycosis. I. Assay of activity in mice and *in vitro*, *J. Infect. Dis.* **132**:407–414 (1975).

67. D. A. Stevens, H. B. Levine, and S. C. Deresinski, Miconazole in coccidioidomycosis. II. Therapeutic and pharmacologic studies in man, *Am. J. Med.* **60**:191–202 (1976).

68. S. C. Deresinski, R. B. Lilly, H. B. Levine, J. N. Galgiani, and D. A. Stevens, Treatment of fungal meningitis with miconazole, *Arch. Intern. Med.* **137**:1180–1185 (1977).

69. D. A. Stevens, Miconazole in the treatment of systemic fungal infections, *Am. Rev. Resp. Dis.* **116**:801–806 (1977).

70. S. H. Cheu and W. J. Waldmann, Unusual complications of ventriculo-atriostomy for communicating hydrocephalus in coccidioidal meningitis, in: *Coccidioidomycosis* (L. Ajello, ed.), University of Arizona Press, Tucson (1967), pp. 25–30.

12

Coccidioidomycosis of Bone and Joints

Stanley C. Deresinski

1. INTRODUCTION

Infection of bone or joint is one of the most frequent manifestations of dissemination in coccidioidomycosis, occurring in approximately 20% of cases.[1] Joas Furtado-Silveira, the second reported patient with coccidioidomycosis, had osteomyelitis of the tibia and the head of a metacarpal, both with sinus formation. In addition, one of his metacarpal-phalangeal joints was "thoroughly disorganized." Several years after Furtado-Silveira's death, Ophüls, upon writing the first review of coccidioidal granuloma, noted that 5 of the first 12 patients reported, including Furtado-Silveira, had musculoskeletal involvement.[2] These cases were, however, almost certainly not the first instances of coccidioidal infection, osseous or otherwise. Recent roentgenographic examination of the 1800-year-old bones of an Indian of the San Joaquin Valley of California, where the climate has not changed significantly in 10,000 years, revealed a lytic lesion of the patella as well as a "moth-eaten" lesion of the distal femur, both very likely due to *Coccidioides immitis*.[3]

The age, sex, and racial frequencies of bone and joint infection in this disease appear to be those of disseminated coccidioidomycosis in general. Infection at these sites occurs almost invariably, if not exclusively, as the result of hematogenous spread rather than direct inoculation, although joints may be involved as the result of spread from adjacent bone.

2. OSTEOMYELITIS

2.1. Sites of Involvement

Osteomyelitis is polyostotic in approximately 40% of cases; 20% have involvement of two bones, 10% have involvement of three, while 1% have involvement of as many as eight bones.[4] Any and all osseous sites may be involved, with the vertebral column being most frequently affected in the series of Iger.[4] This site was followed, in descending order of frequency, by the tibia, skull, metatarsals, metacarpals, femur, and ribs. Seventeen additional sites were involved in the 112 patients reported. Strangely, when multiple lesions are present, involvement is not infrequently symmetrical. Dalinka et al.[5] reported such a finding in 4 of 9 cases with polyostotic disease, including 1 patient with symmetrical bone involvement at four separate locations.

Lesions most frequently occur in the middle of flat bones and the metaphysis of long bones, with special predilection for bony prominences such as the tibial tubercle, the malleoli, and the styloid processes.[6] In the bones of the hands and feet the diaphysis is frequently involved.[6] Adjacent soft tissue abscesses resulting from periosteal rupture are relatively frequent; these may produce sinus tracts and drain through the skin. Similarly, vertebral lesions may lead to paraspinal and psoas abscesses which may dissect widely and drain at sites distant from the bony lesion. Rib lesions, which are usually marginal (these are usually central in tuberculosis), may produce extrapleural mass lesions on chest X-ray and may dissect widely before penetrating the skin. Epiphyseal lesions may penetrate joint spaces. Vertebral and skull lesions may lead to epidural involvement and, on occasion, to meningitis.

2.2. Laboratory and Clinical Findings

Roentgenographically, the lesions are initially lytic and are well demarcated, having the appearance of uniloculated or multiloculated cysts (Fig. 1), except when they occur in the small bones of the hands and feet, wherein the margins are frequently indistinct. Soft-tissue swelling is frequent as is regional osteoporosis. Sequestration is infrequent, occurring in 1 of 14 patients (these 14 had a total of 66 lesions) in Dalinka's series.[6] Periosteal new bone formation is also uncommon, occurring in 4 of 14 patients in that same series but being an early finding in only 2 of the 4. Sclerosis, cortical thickening, and, occasionally, walled-off cystic areas are also late findings.

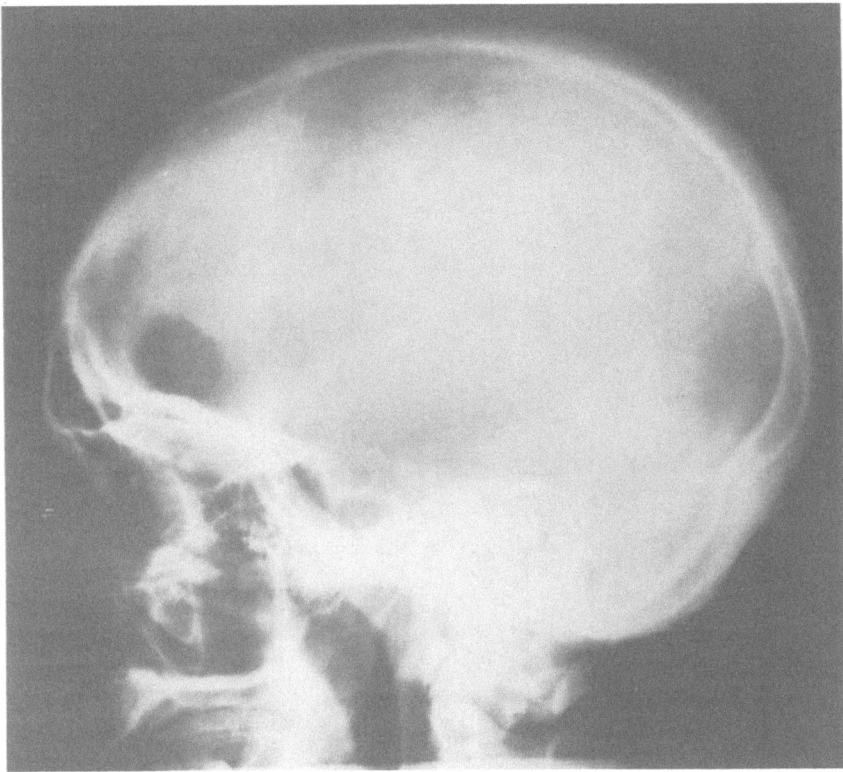

Figure 1. Typical lytic lesion of the skull with little or no reactive new bone formation.

Vertebral lesions occur most commonly in the dorsal and lumbar spines (Fig. 2). Multiple vertebral lesions are common (this is true in only 10% of tuberculous spinal disease). In one series of seven patients there were 17 discrete vertebral lesions. Three of the seven patients had solitary vertebral lesions, but even in these, contiguous vertebrae were involved. There is indiscriminate involvement of vertebral bodies and other vertebral elements. Of the 17 lesions mentioned above, 5 involved the pedicles, 3 the transverse processes, and 3 the spinous processes.[7] Thus, in contradistinction to tuberculous vertebral disease, these appendages may be involved as "primary" sites and not necessarily only as the result of extension from the vertebral body. When the thoracic vertebrae are involved with coccidioidal infection, contiguous rib involvement is not uncommon, a finding also not seen in tuberculosis. The intervertebral disk is relatively spared (and is usually involved early in tuberculous disease). Paraspinal masses are common as is sinus tract

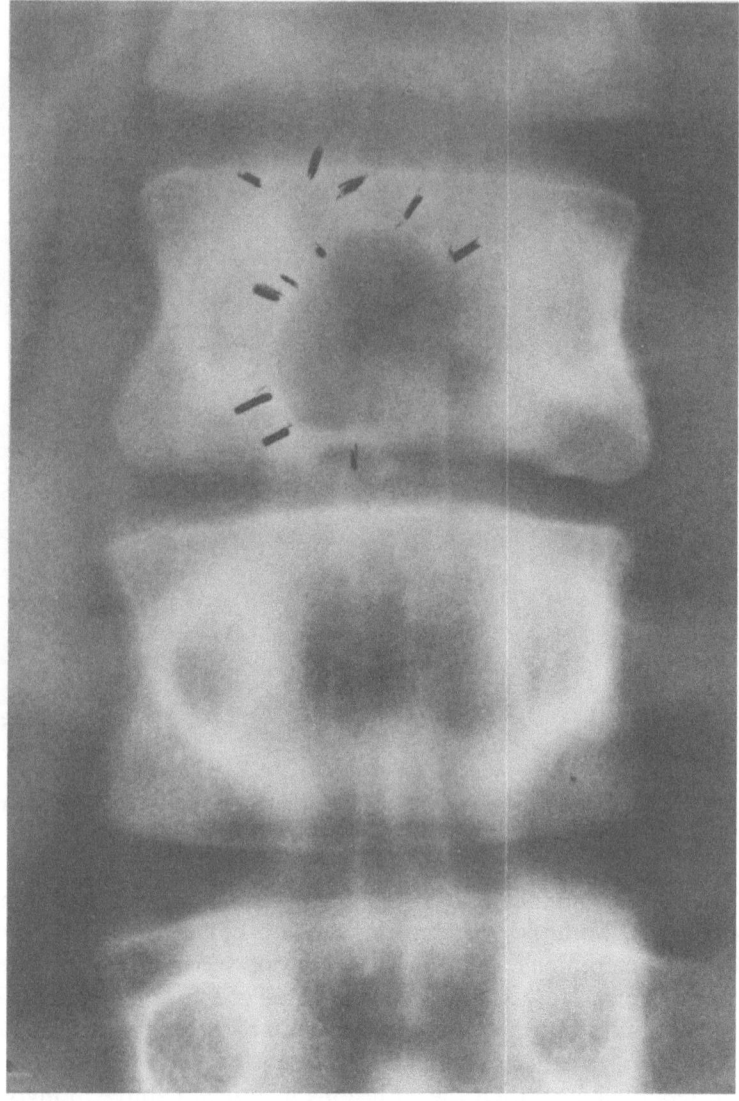

Figure 2. Multilocular vertebral osteomyelitic lesion.

formation. Vertebral collapse is unusual and, when it occurs, is a late manifestation.

As with other bony sites of infection, vertebral lesions are radiolucent with minimal or no early new bone formation. Sclerosis occurs as a late response to destructive lesions. However, uniform densely sclerotic vertebrae without associated destruction has been reported as a consequence of coccidioidomycosis. The affected vertebrae reverted to normal radiodensity after treatment with amphotericin B.[8] Another rarely reported roentgenographic manifestation is vertebra plana, which is characterized by a flat vertebra without narrowing of the adjacent disk spaces.[9] With healing, the commonly noted lesions, vertebral or nonvertebral, generally leave a sclerotic scar, although complete return to a normal roentgenographic appearance may occur, especially in children.[4]

The clinical features of coccidioidal osteomyelitis depend primarily upon the acuteness of the skeletal lesion as well as on the presence or absence of extraosseous foci of infection. The early infection may be characterized by all the signs and symptoms characteristic of the acute inflammatory process: swelling, local heat and systemic fever, erythema, pain and tenderness. With chronicity the lesion becomes "cold" with frequent abscess and sinus formation. Lesions may, however, be asymptomatic at either stage, and the stages are simply two ends of a continuous spectrum of the disease process.

The roentgenographic findings have been discussed above. Information concerning the usefulness of bone-scanning techniques in this disease is limited. Eller reported a positive strontium bone scan in a patient with radiographically apparent vertebral osteomyelitis.[8] Iger[4] reported a case with a transiently positive radioisotope study despite a normal X-ray of the site (L-4). More recently, Armbruster et al. have reported positive technetium pyrophosphate bone scans in five patients with disseminated coccidioidomycosis and osseous lesions.[10] The limited experience to date suggests that, as with other inflammatory conditions of bone, radioisotope scanning techniques are more sensitive than radiographic examination in coccidioidal osteomyelitis.

Anemia may be present. The peripheral leukocyte count may be normal or elevated, and eosinophilia may be seen. In a series of 11 patients in whom the erythrocyte sedimentation rate was reported, it was elevated in 5, and in 3 of these it was greater than 100 mm/hr. In the absence of acute widespread dissemination or secondary bacterial infection, fever is generally absent or low-grade.[11] The coccidioidin skin and serologic tests are useful to the same extent as that found in other forms of disseminated coccidioidomycosis. It should be noted, however, that vertebral involvement may lead to a positive complement-fixing antibody test for coccidioidomycosis in the cerebrospinal fluid in the absence of apparent meningitis. Hypercalcemia has been reported as a complication of disseminated coccidioidomycosis in three patients.[12] At least 1 of the patients, however, had no evidence of bony involvement (negative skeletal roentgenography and technetium bone scan), and the pathophysiology of the hypercalcemia in these patients was unknown.

2.3. Differential Diagnosis

While a variety of infectious and neoplastic lesions of bone and joint can mimic coccidioidomycosis, other fungal infections and tuberculosis constitute the primary differential diagnostic possibilities. Pyogenic infection is generally distinguished by the clinical findings and by early radiographic appearance of sclerosis. While histoplasmosis rarely affects bone, such involvement occurs in approximately 10% of patients with disseminated cryptococcosis.[13] Bone and joint infection in disseminated blastomycosis occurs with approximately the same frequency and sites of distribution as in disseminated coccidioidomycosis. The sites of distribution of the lesions in the two diseases are similar, as is the frequency of polyostotic involvement.[14] Unfortunately there appear to be no reliable means of roentgenographic differentiation between the various mycotic etiologies and specific diagnosis must therefore rely on serologic, histologic, and microbiologic techniques.

The basic lesion in skeletal tuberculosis is almost invariably a combination of osteomyelitis and arthritis. Fifty percent of such cases involve the vertebral column, followed by the hip and knee (15% each). Rib involvement occurs in approximately 5%; tuberculosis is said to be the most common infectious process of ribs. When rib involvement does occur, it does so as a result of dissemination directly to the site rather than by spread from adjacent thoracic vertebrae, as may occur with fungal disease. Also in contrast to fungal infection wherein lesions of the skull are not rare, such involvement occurs in fewer than 1% of cases of skeletal tuberculosis.[15] Roentgenographically, the initial finding in skeletal tuberculosis may be limited to soft-tissue swelling. In long bones this is followed by small localized areas of subchondral osteoporosis, often with a thin rim of sclerosis. Next is seen progressive cortical and cartilaginous destruction. The first finding in tuberculous spondylitis is generally slight narrowing of the intervertebral disk space. The adjacent vertebral bodies develop destructive lesions and eventually collapse. Paravertebral soft-tissue masses are common. While roentgenographic differentiation of tuberculous from fungal skeletal infection may frequently be impossible, possibly helpful points of contrast are listed in Table 1.

Coccidioidal lesions may also roentgenographically resemble those of multiple myeloma, sarcoidosis, histocytosis, and metastatic carcinoma.

2.4. Pathology

Drainage of a soft-tissue abscess may yield either caseous material or one that is serous but contains "lumps and shreds of fibrin and

TABLE 1
Differential Diagnosis of Skeletal Coccidioidomycosis and Tuberculosis

	C. immitis	M. tuberculosis
Nonvertebral		
Predilection for bony prominences	Yes	No
Associated joint involvement	Occasional	Usual
Draining sinuses	Common	Less common
Skull involvement	Third most frequent site	1% of skeletal tuberculosis
Rib Lesions:		
Location	Marginal	Central
Route by which involved	Hematogenous; may occur by contiguous spread from thoracic vertebrae	Hematogenous
Vertebral		
Disk space involvement	Late	Early
Vertebral collapse	Unusual, occurs late	Frequent, occurs early
Multiple lesions	Common ($\geq$ 50%)	10%
Vertebral appendages — route by which involved	Hematogenous or by contiguous spread	Contiguous spread

necrotic soft tissue.''[11] Areas of bone destruction show "replacement with soft tissue, [and a] xanthoma-like, yellow-appearing sac filled with gray-green, thin purulent fluid in which C. immitis sporangia may be demonstrated. . . . Greenish yellow granulation tissue may be found in sinus tracts and along the course of the neighboring tendons and muscles.'' Microscopically, the findings are similar to those seen elsewhere in the body.

2.5. Prognosis

The prognosis for survival depends primarily upon the extent of dissemination, i.e., the number of extrapulmonary foci of infection. Additional prognostic factors, as delineated by Conaty et al.[16] in 1959, include the general condition of the patient, the height of the complement-fixing-antibody titer, the duration of illness, the activity of the pulmonary lesions, and the histopathology (suppuration with the presence of many organisms bodes ill). With these factors in mind, the following data presented by Iger and Larson[17] in 1965 are of interest. Analysis of their cases during the time period 1949–1956 (prior to the use of amphotericin B) indicates that while the mortality of all cases of disseminated coccidioidomycosis was 47%, the mortality rate when bony involvement was present was 28%. This latter group constituted only 6% of all the deaths from disseminated coccidioidomycosis, while osteomyelitis occurred in 20% of cases of dissemination. This lesser mortality with osseous involvement undoubtedly represents the inclusion of a number of patients with single site involvement and chronic infection.

Coccidioidal spondylitis may lead to a fatal outcome in the absence of widespread dissemination because of the proximity of the infected site to the meninges. Iger and Larson reported a fatal result in 8 of 22 (36%) patients, all 8 dying with meningitis. However, only 4 of the 8 patients were treated with amphotericin B. A much improved prognosis was reported by Winter et al.,[18] all of whose patients received amphotericin B. An additional cause of mortality in these patients is spinal cord compression due to vertebral collapse or epidural abscess.

2.6. Treatment

The first therapeutic success in coccidioidal osteomyelitis (and in disseminated coccidioidomycosis in general) was reported in 1904[19] and included in Ophül's review of 1905.[2] An elderly railroad worker, otherwise "in perfect health," with chronic (4 years' duration) infection of the right fourth metatarsal underwent amputation of the foot with apparent cure.

The principles of management of coccidioidal osteomyelitis have been stated by Iger and Larson[4,17] and by Winter et al.[18] When infection is limited to a single site, surgical ablation, either by amputation, as in the case above, or by wide ostectomy, is effective and may in certain circumstances be indicated. Large abscesses may be drained, extensive bony lesions debrided, and sinus tracts excised. A further indication for surgical intervention is impending instability of the spinal column, in which grafting procedures may be useful. Immobilization is, of course, also indicated under such circumstances, but the role of immobilization in coccidioidal vertebral osteomyelitis in general is uncertain.

Littman's paper,[20] read to the First Coccidioidomycosis Symposium in 1957, probably represents the first report of the use of amphotericin B in coccidioidal osteomyelitis. While, as with other forms of coccidioidomycosis, there has been no controlled evaluation of the effectiveness of this polyene antimycotic in osseous coccidioidomycosis, retrospective analysis suggests that it has improved prognosis. In Iger and Larson's series,[17] the introduction of amphotericin B was associated with a 3.1-fold decrease in mortality (from 28% to 9%) in patients with osseous involvement. (The mortality in disseminated coccidioidomycosis decreased by a factor of 2.4 from 47% to 20% at the same institution after the introduction of amphotericin B.) Mortality in patients with osseous involvement during a subsequent period of time (1964–1976) at the same institution was 15%[4] for a combined mortality of 13% (8 of 63) since the introduction of amphotericin B. Death in these latter periods after the introduction of this polyene was either secondary to acute overwhelming widespread dissemination (4 of 8 deaths, 1 with meningitis) or to meningitis secondary to vertebral involvement (3 deaths), with 1 patient with an isolated tibial lesion dying of "old age and general debilitation." Forty-eight percent of survivors from the preamphotericin B cohort were symptom-free at follow up, while in those seen after 1957, 83% were similarly without apparent disease.

A further indication of improved prognosis since the introduction of amphotericin B is apparent from a comparison of the mortality rate of 36% (8 of 22) in Iger's series, in which only half the fatal cases received the drug, to 9% (1 of 11) in the series of Winter et al., in which all the patients received amphotericin B. In the latter series, after follow-up periods ranging from 2 to 30 years, 9 were disease-free and 1 had developed meningitis 2 years subsequent to treatment.

While it thus appears that parenterally administered amphotericin B has efficacy in at least some forms of osseous coccidioidomycosis, Winter et al. state that it is not indicated in "patients with isolated peripheral foci, relatively low complement fixation titers, no clinical or serologic evidence of progressive disease, or in patients who have successfully contained their foci already for years or decades."[18]

Amphotericin B is often locally administered directly into sites of osteomyelitis after surgical drainage and debridement.[4,21] Iger recommends this therapeutic modality in patients in whom the lesion is advancing during parenteral therapy. Specifically, he administers 50 mg of amphotericin B in 500 ml of distilled water once daily for approximately 1 week via a suction and drainage system. Local drug administration has also been used in the treatment of draining sinuses. The efficacy of topically administered amphotericin B in these settings is, however, unknown.

Of the new, potentially promising therapeutic modalites, coccidioidin-specific transfer factor or miconazole have been administered to patients with coccidioidal osteomyelitis.[22–24] Both improvement and failure have been noted with each mode of therapy. Additional clinical information is necessary in order to judge their efficacy and relative role compared to amphotericin.

3. ARTHRITIS

"Desert rheumatism," consisting of arthralgias and occasionally arthritis, occurs in 3–5% of patients with primary nondisseminated coccidioidomycosis. Such joint involvement is, however, probably an immunologic rather than a directly infectious phenomenon. It is usually accompanied by erythema nodosum and, like this skin manifestation of hypersensitivity, is transient.[6] Actual joint infection occurs as a result of hematogenous dissemination either directly to the synovium or by extension from an adjacent osteomyelitis. While early investigators felt that the latter pathogenetic mechanism was the most common, analysis of coccidioidal arthritis reported in the literature indicates that there was no roentgenographic evidence of adjacent bone involvement (other than erosion of articular surfaces) in the great majority of cases.

While the incidence of either bone or joint involvement in patients with acute extrapulmonary coccidioidomycosis appears to be approximately 20%,[1] the frequency of joint involvement alone in this setting is not entirely clear. Fiese states[6] that coccidioidal arthritis occurs in one-third of cases of chronic dissemination. Conversely, widespread dissemination at the time of presentation with joint disease was 25% in the series of Winter et al.[25]

3.1. Sites of Involvement

Review of 42 evaluable cases[23,25–36] reported in the literature indicates that only one joint was infected in greater than 90%. The knee was involved in 32 of 42 patients and in one of these, both knees were involved. Involvement of other joints occurred in 2 of these patients. Clear evidence of osteomyelitis adjacent to the knee joint (excluding simple erosion of the articular surface) was present in only 5 of these patients. Two of the patients with knee involvement clearly had Baker's cysts, and a third was described as having a "popliteal mass."

Four patients had involvement of the ankle joint and 2 had elbow involvement (1 each of these also had knee involvement). There were single cases of wrist, interphalangeal joint, and hip involvement. These numbers cannot be taken as reflecting the true frequency of involvement of various joints since they are obtained from series reported for disparate reasons. In a series of coccidioidal granuloma cases reported prior to the availability of amphotericin B, 79 of 254 patients had joint involvement. The sites of joint involvement, in decreasing order of frequency, were ankle, knee, foot, elbow, wrist, shoulder, finger, vertebral, hip, and sternoclavicular.[37]

3.2. Laboratory and Clinical Findings

In the 42 cases examined, the diagnosis was frequently delayed for extraordinary periods of time. In 80% the period of time from onset to diagnosis was >1 year, with diagnosis being delayed 5 or more years in 30%; the longest interval was 29 years.

Initially, affected joints may appear acutely inflamed. This stage may, however, be bypassed. In the "chronic" stage of the infection, the patient complains of pain and stiffness of the affected joint. Effusion, swelling, and thickened synovium with decreased range of motion are present on physical examination. The joint infection may drain spontaneously to the skin, producing indolent and persistent sinus tracts. As noted, Baker's cysts may occur as a result of a knee involvement.

Roentgenographic examination revealed joint narrowing in 60%, evidence of intraarticular "swelling" in 74% (of knees and ankles) and "periarticular periostitis" in 55%.[38] Erosion of articular cortex was totally absent in only 6 of 43 cases in this series, which was published in 1934. The erosion seen was present throughout the articular surface in 15, was localized to weight bearing regions in 2, and was localized to non-weight-bearing areas in 3. In 17 subjects the articular erosion was seen only adjacent to local areas of osteomyelitis. Adjacent osteoporosis was observed in all but a single case, which was seen early in its course. Sequestra were seen in two joints which were involved as a result of extension from a focus of osteomyelitis.

The most commonly seen associated sites of bony involvement include the tibial tubercle and patella, the malleoli and tarsal bones, the distal radius and ulna (especially the styloid processes), the metacarpal base and carpals, the humeral condyles, and the olecranon.

Synovial fluid from infected joints ranges from cloudy to transparent yellow in appearance. While there is a paucity of information concerning synovial fluid analysis, cell counts have ranged from 5800 to 50,000/mm³ with cell differentials ranging from 20% polymorphonuclear leukocytes and 80% mononuclear cells to the inverse. Protein is greater than 3.0 g/ 100 ml and glucose less than 50% of serum glucose, and the mucin clot is poor.[29,32,35,39] Culture of synovial fluid has yielded the organism in approximately half the cases in which this was attempted.[31,34] This finding is difficult to evaluate without knowledge of the amount of fluid that was studied as well as the mycological techniques used. Culture and histologic examination of synovial tissue has been more reliably productive. While such tissue has generally been obtained by open surgical procedures, needle biopsy of the synovium has provided diagnostic specimens in at least two cases.[31,40]

Serum complement-fixing antibody to coccidioidin was invariably present in the cases reported, with 3 having titers of 1 : 8 and the other 30 in whom this examination was reported having titers of 1 : 32 or greater, despite the fact that in most cases widespread dissemination was not apparent at the time of study. There is no evaluable data on the significance of complement-fixing antibody in synovial fluid.

3.3. Pathology

The affected synovium exhibits granulomatous villonodular inflammatory changes. The villous projections from this edematous hypertrophic tissue are numerous and are 5–30 mm in length and 3–15 mm thick. The entire synovium has been described as "yellow-red with pale gray tips."[30] While one author describes the pannus as well defined and noninvasive,[34] most have remarked on its ability to invade menisci, cruciates, and articular surfaces.[28,30]

3.4. Prognosis

The ultimate prognosis of the patient with coccidioidal arthritis depends upon the presence or absence of other sites of infection, e.g., widespread dissemination, progressive pulmonary disease, or meningitis. Later further dissemination from an articular or osseous focus of infection rarely, if ever occurs.

The prognosis for the untreated joint is poor, with resultant chronic disability which is generally progressive over the long term. The clinical activity may remit and relapse spontaneously, however, with relapses frequently occurring after trauma. One remarkable patient described by Pollock et al.[31] survived widespread dissemination, including involvement of the knee, prior to the availability of amphotericin. Within 2 years of onset, the knee became asymptomatic and continued so for 29 more years, when the infection finally relapsed!

3.5. Treatment

Thirteen of the 42 patients reported in detail were treated only surgically (1 of these received sulfas and radiotherapy, and 1 received cycloheximide). Five underwent amputation with assumed cure of the joint disease (2 of these died of disseminated infection, however). One patient underwent arthrodesis of the affected wrist joint and was without recurrence after 24 years of follow-up. One patient with involvement of the foot underwent synovectomy and debridement of the adjacent infected cuneiform but relapsed after 3 years. Six subjects with knee involvement underwent synovectomy, most often described as anterior synovectomy. Three continued with active infection; 1 became apparently inactive but recurred after 3 years; 1 persisted with culture positive effusion, but at 10 months this ceased and the patient became asymptomatic; 1 was felt to be inactive at 5 months but had markedly impaired joint function; and 1 remained asymptomatic after 18 months. Thus while amputation, and perhaps arthrodesis, alone can permanently eliminate active coccidioidal arthritis, synovectomy alone is largely unsuccessful. Winter et al.[25] have pointed out the impossibility of performing a total synovectomy in this disease. Consequently infected synovium invariably remains.

Twelve of the 42 subjects received amphotericin B intravenously (but not intraarticularly) as well as undergoing surgery. Three joints underwent arthrodesis: one, a hip, was felt to be inactive at 2 years, although pain was still present. Two patients with knee involvement (1 of which had remained active after synovectomy) appeared to have inactive joints after 15 months and after 11 years after arthrodesis. The remaining 9 patients underwent synovectomy of the knee. In one there was no follow-up. Four patients, who had received 948–1500 mg amphotericin B intravenously had active joint infection at last follow-up (1 died of coccidioidal meningitis). In 4 patients the joint infection was clinically inactive after follow-up periods of 1, 2, 3, and 5 years. Thus, in conjunction with intravenously administered amphotericin B, arthrodesis was successful in 3 of 3 and synovectomy was apparently successful in 4 of 8 patients.

Eight patients received amphotericin B intravenously but underwent no "definitive" surgical procedure (five underwent arthrotomy, one had excision of the distal ulna, and one underwent patellectomy). Two also received amphotericin B intraarticularly, and one of these appeared to be disease-free after 2 years of follow-up. One patient who received the drug only intravenously appeared cured after 11 years. The other six had active disease at follow-up.

Seven patients, all with knee involvement, both underwent surgery and received intraarticular amphotericin B. Three also received the drug intravenously; none of these had inactive disease after significant follow-up. The other four all had inactive disease after periods ranging from 1.5 to 5 years. The surgical procedures in this latter group included synovectomy in two and excision of Baker's cysts in two.

In the studies cited, it is frequently impossible to determine the functional state of the joints in which the infection has been designated by the author as inactive. Because of this, as well as frequently inadequate follow-up, it is impossible to determine the optimal mode of therapy from review of these cases. It does appear, however, that surgery alone, other than arthrodesis or amputation, is ineffective. While Winter et al.[25] have concluded that cure is rare if the mobility of the involved joint is allowed to persist, a significant proportion of joints can be maintained in a functionally satisfactory and clinically inactive state for reasonable periods of time by a combination of synovectomy and amphotericin B. The relative roles of intravenous and intraarticular drug administration in this combined approach is unclear, since responses have occurred when either or both routes were used. It has been reported, however, that amphotericin B administered intraarticularly in rabbits produces an intense synovial and superficial chondrocyte reaction.[41] Thus, it is possible that repeated administration by this route in humans may actually further compromise joint function.

Knowledge of the ability of amphotericin B to penetrate into synovial fluid after intravenous administration is based on limited data. Noyes et al.[42] found, in a single case of Candida arthritis, that the joint fluid concentration of amphotericin B after intravenous administration was similar to the serum concentration with values of 0.4–1.6 μg/ml 20 hr after a 4-hr intravenous infusion of 0.5 mg/kg. Miconazole, a newer antifungal agent which has been used in only a few patients with coccidioidal arthritis, with mixed results, achieves reasonable concentrations in infected joint effusions after intravenous administration.[23] The concentration of the drug in the synovial fluid of an infected ankle ranged from 0.5 to 0.9 μg/ml with intravenous doses of 600–2400 mg per day. The concentration in an infected knee effusion of a patient receiving 3.6 g per day was 1.35 μg/ml, which was 135% of the simultaneous serum concentration.

4. TENOSYNOVITIS

Coccidioidal tenosynovitis without joint or bone infection is a rare manifestation of dissemination. Tenosynovitis about the wrist has been reported in at least three patients. One, treated only surgically, had subsequent recurrence of disease.[43] A patient with Stage IV-B lymphocytic lymphoma underwent partial resection of infected tissue as well as receiving amphotericin B; functional result was good, but follow-up was only 6 weeks.[44]* A third patient, having failed with previous amphotericin B therapy, had a good clinical result after receiving 45.3 g of miconazole intravenously over 20 days.[23]

ACKNOWLEDGMENTS.   The author wishes to acknowledge the assistance of Mrs. Rosemarie Vila in the preparation of the chapter. Figure 2 is reprinted from reference 45, with permission.

REFERENCES

1. W. Forbus and A. M. Bestebreurtje, Coccidioidomycosis: A study of 95 cases of the disseminated type with special reference to the pathogenesis of the disease, *Mil. Surg.* **5**:653–719 (1946).
2. W. Ophüls, Coccidioidal granuloma, *J. Am. Med. Assoc.* **45**:1291–1296 (1905).
3. B. D. Poswall, Coccidioidomycosis and North American blastomycosis: Differential diagnosis of bone lesions in pre-Columbian American Indians, Presented at the Annual Meeting of the American Association of Anthropologists, April 14–18, 1976.
4. M. Iger, Coccidioidal osteomyelitis, in: *Proceedings of the Third International Coccidioidomycosis Symposium* (L. Ajello, ed.), Symposia Specialists, Miami (1977), pp. 177–190.
5. M. K. Dalinka, S. Dinnenberg, W. H. Greendyke, and R. Hopkins, Roentgenographic features of osseous coccidioidomycosis and differential diagnosis, *J. Bone J. Surg.* **53-A**:1157–1164 (1971).
6. M. J. Fiese, *Coccidioidomycosis,* Charles C. Thomas, Springfield, Ill. (1958).
7. M. K. Dalinka and W. H. Greendyke, The spinal manifestations of coccidioidomycosis, *J. Can. Assoc. Radio.* **22**:93–99 (1971).
8. J. L. Eller and P. E. Siebert, Sclerotic vertebral bodies: an unusual manifestation of disseminated coccidioidomycosis, *Radiology* **93**:1099–1100 (1969).
9. P. W. Nykamp, Vertebra plana: two cases due to disseminated coccidioidomycosis, *Ariz. Med.* **28**:165–167 (1971).
10. T. G. Armbruster, T. G. Goerzen, D. Resnick, and A. Catanzaro, Utility of bone scanning in disseminated coccidioidomycosis: case report, *J. Nucl. Med* **18**:450–454 (1977).

* This patient's cast was removed postoperatively on the hospital roof "in order to have adequate ventilation to prevent infection of other patients or physicians. . . . " This was perhaps inspired by the fact that the only known cases of human to human transmission (via fomite) of *C. immitis* occurred on an orthopedic service when a dressing, applied over a draining focus of osteomyelitis, was changed for the first time on the 22nd postoperative day. This delay apparently allowed arthrosporulation of the fungus on the dressing, and two interns, three nurses, and one resident, all of whom had cared for the patient, developed coccidioidomycosis [B. H. Eckmann, G. L. Schaefer, and M. H. Huppert, Bedside transmission of coccidioidomycosis via growth on fomites, *Am. Rev. Resp. Dis.* **89**:1175–1185 (1964)].

11. J. R. Schwartzmann, Coccidioidal bone infections, in: *Proceedings of the Symposium on Coccidioidomycosis, U.S. Public Health Serv. Publ.* No. 575, pp. 32–35 (1957).

12. J. C. Lee, A. Catanzaro, J. G. Parthemore, B. Roach, and L. J. Deftos, Hypercalcemia in disseminated coccidioidomycosis, *N. Engl. J. Med.* **297**:431–434 (1977).

13. V. P. Collins, Bone involvement in cryptococcosis (torulosis), *Am. J. Roentgenol.* **63**:102–112 (1950).

14. J. A. Gehweiler, M. P. Copp, and E. W. Chick, Observations on the roentgen patterns in blastomycosis of bone, *Am. J. Roentgenol. Radium Ther. Nucl. Med.* **108**:497–510 (1970).

15. P. T. Davidson and I. Horowitz, Skeletal tuberculosis: a review with patient presentations and discussion, *Am. J. Med.* **48**:77–84 (1970).

16. J. P. Conaty, M. Biddle, and F. M. McKeever, Osseous coccidioidal granuloma. An attempt to measure the prognosis, *J. Bone J. Surg.* **41-A**:1109–1122 (1959).

17. M. Iger and J. Larson, Coccidioidal osteomyelitis, in: *Coccidioidomycosis. Proceedings of the Second Coccidioidomycosis Symposium* (L. Ajello, ed.), University of Arizona Press, Tucson (1967), pp. 89–92.

18. W. G. Winter, Jr., D. Pappagianis, R. A. Huntington, and R. K. Larson, *Coccidioidal arthritis and spondylitis—1976*, in: *Proceedings of the Third International Coccidioidomycosis Symposium* (L. Ajello, ed.), Symposia Specialists, Miami (1977), pp. 169–176.

19. S. J. Gardner, An unusual infection in the bones of the foot, *Calif. J. Med.* **20**:386–388 (1904).

20. M. L. Littman, Preliminary observations on the intravenous use of amphotericin B, an antifungal antibiotic, in the therapy of acute and chronic coccidioidal osteomyelitis, in: *Proceedings of the Symposium on Coccidioidomycosis, U.S. Public Health Serv. Publ.* No. 575, pp. 86–94, (1957).

21. S. R. Stein, C. A. Leukens, and R. J. Bagg, Treatment of coccidioidomycosis infection of bone with local amphotericin B suction-irrigation, *Clin. Orthop.* **108**:161–164, (1975).

22. D. A. Stevens, H. B. Levine, S. C. Deresinski, Miconazole in coccidioidomycosis: II. Therapeutic and pharmacologic studies in man, *Am. J. Med.* **60**:191–202 (1976).

23. S. C. Deresinski, J. N. Galgiani, and D. A. Stevens, Miconazole treatment of human coccidioidomycosis: status report, in: *Proceedings of the Third International Coccidioidomycosis Symposium* (L. Ajello, ed.), Symposia Specialists, Miami (1977), pp. 267–292.

24. A. Catanzaro and L. Spitler (for the Coccidioidomycosis Cooperative Treatment Group), Clinical and immunologic results of transfer factor therapy in coccidioidomycosis, in: *Transfer Factor: Basic Properties and Clinical Applications* (M. S. Ascher, A. A. Gottlieb, and C. H. Kirkpatrick, eds.), Academic Press, New York (1976), pp. 477–494.

25. W. G. Winter, Jr., R. K. Larson, M. M. Honeggar, D.T. Jacobsen, D. Pappagianis, and R. W. Huntington, Coccidioidal arthritis and its treatment, *J. Bone Jt. Surg.* **57-A**:1152–1157 (1975).

26. E. F. Rosenberg, M. B. Dockerty, H. W. Meyerding, Coccidioidal arthritis, *Arch. Intern. Med.* **69**:238–248 (1942).

27. J. S. Thiemeyer, Monoarticular coccidioidal synovitis, *J. Bone Jt. Surg.* **36-A**:387–390 (1954).

28. F. Sotelo-Ortiz, Chronic coccidioidal synovitis of the knee joint, *J. Bone Jt. Surg.* **37-A**:49–56 (1955).

29. M. L. Littman, P. L. Horowitz, and J. G. Swadey, Coccidioidomycosis and its treatment with amphotericin B, *Am. J. Med.* **24**:568–592 (1958).

30. W. A. Haug and R. C. Merrifield, Coccidioidal villous synovitis, *Am. J. Clin. Pathol.* **31**:165–171 (1959).

31. S. F. Pollock, J. M. Morris, and W. R. Murray, Coccidioidal synovitis of the knee, *J. Bone Jt. Surg.* **49-A:**1397–1407 (1967).

32. H. P. Aidem, Intra-articular amphotericin B in the treatment of coccidioidal synovitis of the knee: Case report, *J. Bone Jt. Surg.* **50-A:**1663–1668 (1968).

33. A. M. Pankovich and M. M. Jevtic, Coccidioidal infection of the hip, *J. Bone Jt. Surg.* **55-A:**1525–1528 (1973).

34. R. Greenman, J. Becker, G. Campbell, and J. Remington, Coccidioidal synovitis of the knee, *Arch. Intern. Med.* **135:**526–530 (1975).

35. A. S. Bayer, T. T. Yoshikawa, J. E. Galpin, and L. B. Guze, Unusual syndromes of coccidioidomycosis, *Medicine* **55:**131–152 (1976).

36. R. S. Bisla and T. H. Taber, Coccidioidomycosis of bone and joints, *Clin. Orthop. Relat. Res.* **121:**196–204 (1976).

37. California Department of Public Health: Coccidioidal granuloma (Special Bulletin No. 57), Sacramento, California State Printing Office (1931).

38. R. A. Carter, Infectious granulomas of bones and joints with special reference to coccidioidal granuloma, *Radiology* **23:**1–16 (1934).

39. S. C. Deresinski and D. A. Stevens, Coccidioidomycosis in compromised hosts, *Medicine* **54:**377–395 (1974).

40. H. R. Schumacker and J. P. Kulka, Needle biopsy of the synovial membrane. Experience with Parker-Pearson technique, *N. Engl. J. Med.* **286:**416–419 (1972).

41. C. C. Edwards and R. H. Michael, The effects of intra-articular amphotericin B on articular cartilage, Presented at the Orthopedic Research Society, Las Vegas, Nev., February 1, 1976.

42. F. R. Noyes, J. D. McCabe, and F. R. Fekety, Jr., Acute candida arthritis. Report of a case and use of amphotericin B. *J. Bone Jt. Surg.* **55-A:**169–176 (1973).

43. O. R. Walker and R. H. Hall, Coccidioidal tenosynovitis. Report of a case, *J. Bone Jt. Surg.* **36-A:**391–392 (1954).

44. R. E. Iverson and L. M. Vistnes, Coccidioidal tenosynovitis in the hand, *J. Bone Jt. Surg.* **55-A:**413–417 (1973).

45. D. A. Stevens, *Coccidioides immitis,* in: *Principles and Practice of Infectious Diseases* (G. L. Mandell, R. G. Douglas, and J. E. Bennett, eds.), John Wiley (1979), Chapter 220.

13

Cutaneous Coccidioidomycosis

Paul H. Jacobs

In August of 1892, the first case of cutaneous coccidioidomycosis was reported by Alejandro Posada. The patient survived 11 years after the appearance of skin lesions.

Cutaneous coccidioidomycosis may be classified clinically, in order of prevalence, as follows: (1) hypersensitivity reaction coccidioidomycosis, including erythema multiforme and erythema nodosum; (2) toxic reaction coccidioidomycosis; (3) secondary (disseminated) cutaneous coccioidomycosis; and (4) primary chancriform cutaneous coccidioidomycosis. Manifestations (1) and (2) are also discussed in Chapter 9.

1. HYPERSENSITIVITY REACTION COCCIDIOIDOMYCOSIS

The hypersensitivity reactions of erythema multiforme and erythema nodosum are true allergic manifestations. They occur in approximately 10% of all coccidioidal infections[1] and in those patients with the least likely chance of contracting a disseminated form of the disease. These reactions are observed most often in white females, and infrequently in blacks and males. Although the development of these hypersensitivity reactions usually indicates a good prognosis, dissemination and death may occur in rare instances.

1.1. Clinical Features

Erythema multiforme presents with erythematous targetlike lesions that may have a bullous component (Fig. 1). Lesions usually appear in

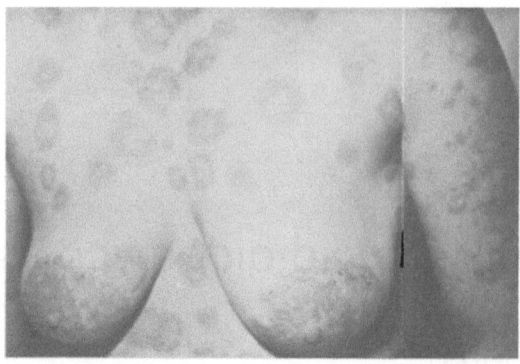

Figure 1. Erythema multiforme presents with erythematous targetlike lesions that occur most frequently on the upper body in adults or the lower body in children.

a single crop, but occasionally multiple, symmetrical crops of lesions may appear. They are often pruritic, and may desquamate. Lesions occur most frequently on the upper body in adults, or the lower body in children. In a study of 137 children with coccidioidomycosis, McKay[2] reported that more than 64% developed erythema multiforme. The inner thighs were a particular site of involvement.

Erythema nodosum presents in crops of red, tender, hot, pruritic, firm, elastic nodules that may reach several centimeters in diameter. Lesions occur most commonly on the anterior tibial region but may extend to the thighs and occasionally to the forearms. The distribution is symmetrical. The lesions gradually become violaceous and then regress within 1–2 weeks, leaving residual postinflammatory hyperpigmented macules ("desert bumps") that gradually fade over the next few weeks to months.

1.2. Diagnosis

Positive skin tests to coccidioidin will confirm the diagnosis of coccidioidomycosis hypersensitivity reaction. A coccidioidin dilution of 1 : 1000 or 1 : 10,000 must be used to prevent necrosis at the test site.[3]

2. TOXIC REACTION COCCIDIOIDOMYCOSIS

In approximately 10% of the cases of primary coccidioidomycosis, the patient develops a nonspecific toxic erythema.[4] The erythema commonly occurs in conjunction with an elevated temperature. In most cases, the eruption vanishes within 1 week and is only diagnosed retrospectively as coccidioidomycosis.

3. SECONDARY (DISSEMINATED) CUTANEOUS COCCIDIOIDOMYCOSIS

Cutaneous lesions of coccidioidomycosis almost always arise by dissemination from pulmonary foci rather than by primary cutaneous inoculation. The presence of skin lesions in an area in which trauma has previously occurred is common enough to indicate that the trauma creates a locus minoris resistentiae for secondary dissemination. Almost any system of the body may be infected through dissemination. However, the skin, because of its accessibility to clinical examination and diagnostic tests, is often the first organ in which the disease is noted.

3.1. Clinical Features

Lesions of secondary cutaneous coccidioidomycosis may present in numerous clinical forms (see Table 1).

The papule, the most common early lesion (Fig. 2), is usually ignored until it increases in size or until multiple lesions appear. The plaquelike lesion is a localized collection of papules. This lesion may appear as a solid plaque (Fig. 3) or it may develop a verrucous or warty appearance. Miliary lesions are generalized papules that appear scattered over the body surface.

The pustular lesion develops from the papule and may resemble a

TABLE 1
Lesions of Secondary (Disseminated) Cutaneous
Coccidioidomycosis

I. Papules	III. Granulomatous lesions
A. Solitary	A. Nodular
B. Multiple	B. Fungating
1. Grouped	C. Ulcerative
a. Plaquelike	D. Scarring
b. Verrucous	IV. Subcutaneous
2. Miliary	abscesses
II. Pustules	A. Ulcerating
A. Furuncular	B. Sinusal
B. Vegetating	

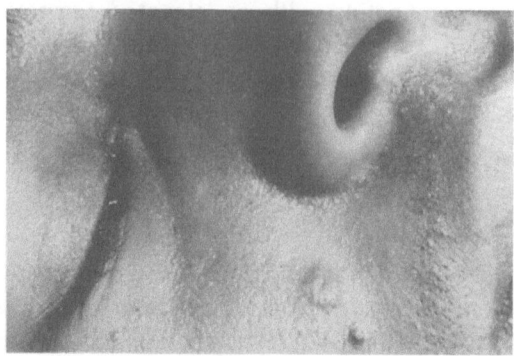

Figure 2. Secondary (disseminated) cutaneous coccidioidomycosis presents in numerous clinical forms. A single papule, as seen on the face of this patient, is usually the first type of lesion to appear.

bacterial furuncle or vegetating-type lesion with tumid nodules or plaques.

The granulomatous lesion (Fig. 4a) is usually seen as a direct extension of the papule and commonly appears in sites of trauma or scars. This lesion progresses through the nodular phase, develops central fungating changes, and eventually ulcerates (Fig. 4b); or, as in North American blastomycosis, the lesion may show central clearing with scar tissue.

The subcutaneous abscess begins as a nondescript erythematous nodule (Fig. 5) that gradually breaks down, leaving an ulcer or a sinus tract. Ophüls,[5] describing an abscess the size of a softball, reported large tubers that were similar to those found in mycosis fungoides and that later became suppurant. Scrofulodermalike lesions also have sinus tracts but initially arise in the lymph nodes and then extend to the skin. Sinus tracts also develop from underlying disease in other tissues, such as the joint spaces. Purulent drainage may be present from the sinus. Sinus tracts may dissect along or even across tissue planes for long distances.

3.2. Chronic Cutaneous Coccidioidomycosis

Smith and co-workers[6] reported that 18% of 409 patients with coccidioidomycosis had chronic forms of the disease. The chronic syndrome, characterized by a prolonged course sometimes lasting up to 30 years,[7] is more common in pigmented races than in whites. There is usually only one obvious extrapulmonary lesion involving the skin and not endangering life. The patient may have few or no systemic complaints. Skin lesions are occasionally very extensive and prominent and usually have a verrucous appearance. These lesions, like those of North American blastomycosis, may show central clearing with scarring.

If dissemination to the bone or joints occurs, the patient may develop a chronic draining sinus. Purulent material containing spherules may drain constantly to the skin surface. This form of the disease may persist for decades; however, dissemination throughout the body can eventually occur, sometimes resulting in death. Cox and Smith[8] produced arrested lesions of this type in white rats and guinea pigs by inoculating the animals intravenously with spherules of *Coccicioides immitis*.

3.3. Differential Diagnosis

Differential diagnosis of secondary cutaneous coccidioidomycosis includes tuberculosis, syphilis, leishmaniasis, glanders, tularemia, neoplasms, North American blastomycosis, South American blastomycosis, actinomycosis, cryptococcosis, nocardiosis, sporotrichosis, histoplasmosis, and mycetoma.

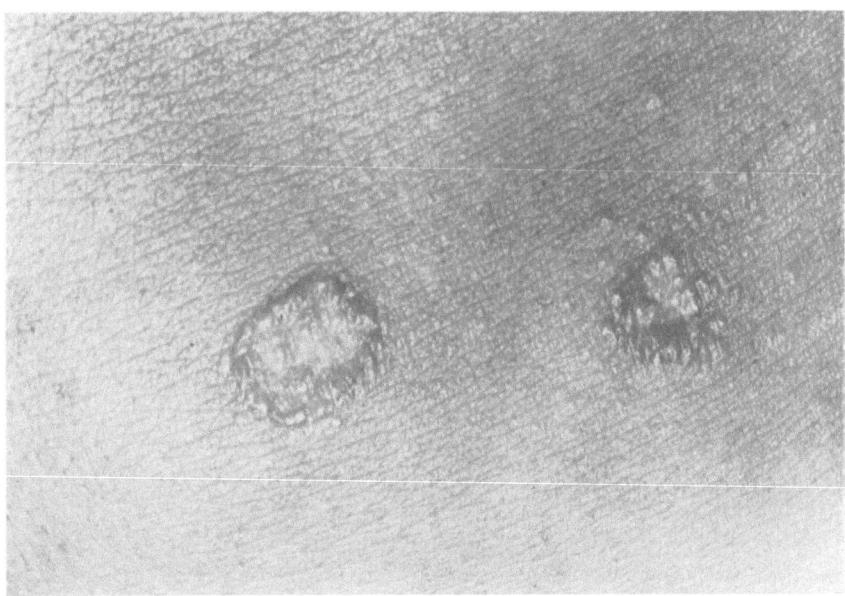

Figure 3. These solid plaque lesions of secondary (disseminated) cutaneous coccidioidomycosis show microabscesses that typically contain spherules.

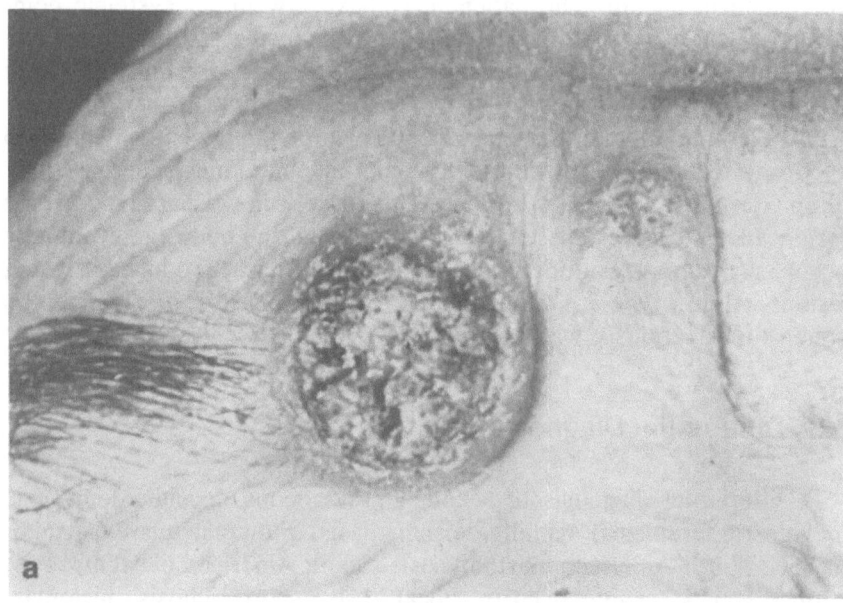

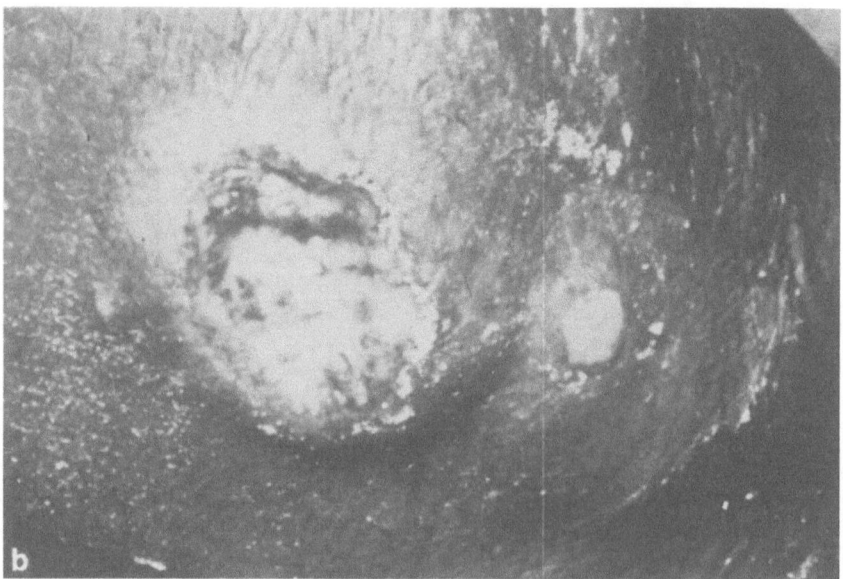

Figure 4. Granulomatous lesions of secondary (disseminated) cutaneous coccidioidomy-cosis progress through the nodular phase, develop central fungating changes (a), and eventually ulcerate and form scar tissue (b).

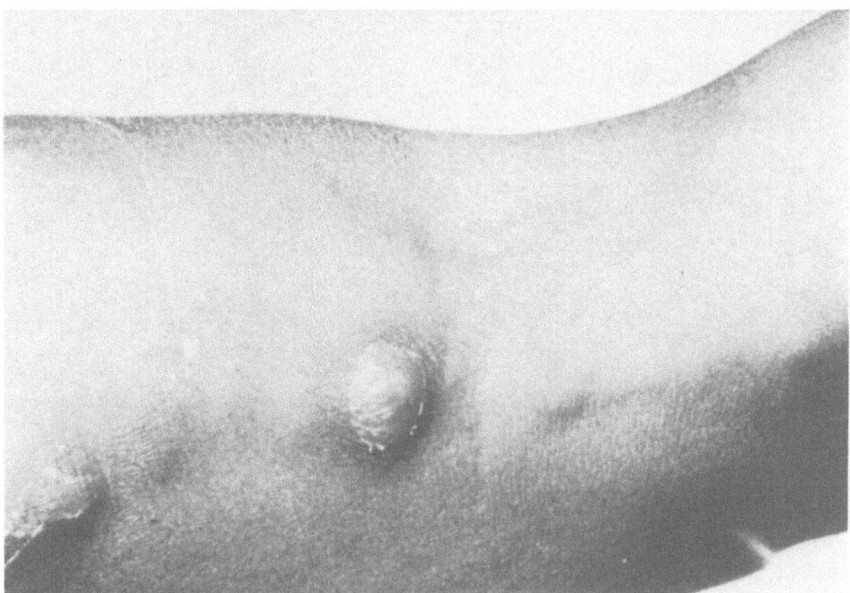

Figure 5. The subcutaneous abscess of secondary (disseminated) cutaneous coccidioido-mycosis begins as an erythematous nodule, as seen on the arm of this patient. The abscess gradually breaks down, leaving an ulcer or a sinus tract.

3.4. Diagnosis

Histologic findings of all types of secondary cutaneous coccidioi-domycosis lesions may show microabscesses that contain spherules.

Even in the very early papular stage of the disease, diagnosis of coccidioidomycosis may be confirmed by a direct saline preparation.[9] Purulent material may be obtained from the microabscesses or sinus drainage, or by gently scraping the sinus wall with a small curette. A droplet of purulent material is then diluted with a drop of saline on a glass slide. The edges of a coverslip are rimmed with petrolatum jelly. The coverslip is placed over the specimen and pressure is applied to seal the coverslip to the slide. Further details on processing these specimens are described in Chapter 3. An immediate microscopic search may demonstrate the characteristic spherules (Fig. 6a). Examination of the slide after it remains overnight (slide cultures) at room temperature may reveal germinating hyphae (see Fig. 6b). The simple punch biopsy or shave biopsy can also be diagnostic if spherules are found. Special stains,

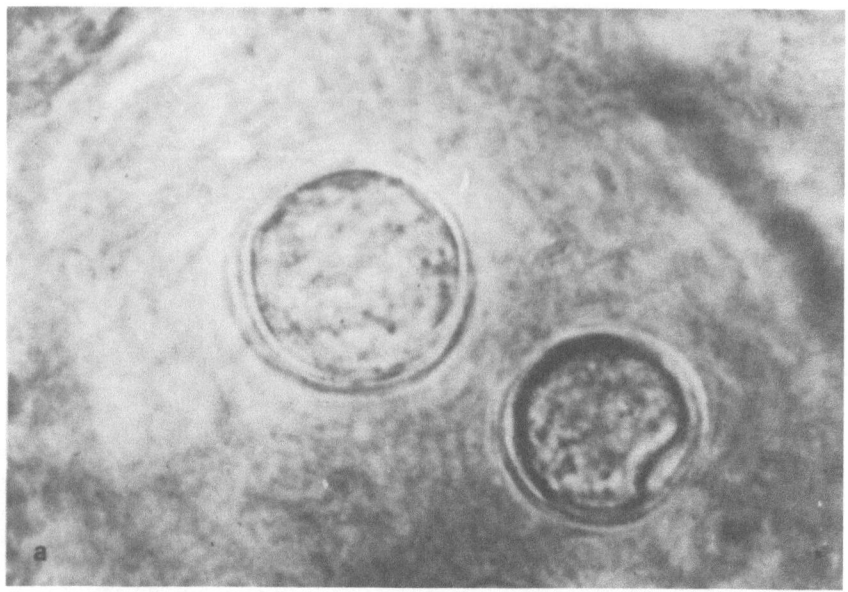

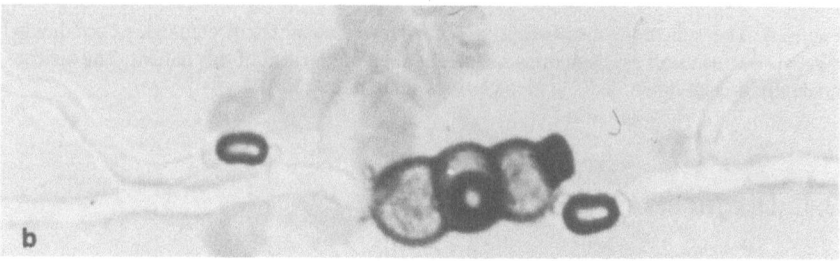

Figure 6. Diagnosis of coccidioidomycosis may be confirmed by a direct saline preparation. An immediate microscopic search may demonstrate the characteristic spherules (a). Examination of the slide after it remains overnight at room temperature may reveal germinating hyphae (b).

such as the periodic acid Schiff, Gridley, and Gomori, may be superior, but the simple hematoxylin and eosin will usually suffice.

Culture of the organism is also a useful diagnostic tool. Those who use a dermatophyte test medium (DTM) should be forewarned that *C. immitis* will turn it to a red color within 7 days. The change in color is similar to that of several of the dermatophytes.[10] The cautions in handling *C. immitis* in the laboratory, because of its infectious biohazard risk, and the variations in colonial morphology, have been discussed in Chapters 2 and 3.

4. PRIMARY CHANCRIFORM CUTANEOUS COCCIDIOIDOMYCOSIS

Of an estimated 10 million persons infected with coccidioidomycoses, the total number of primary cutaneous cases reported to date is less than 20.[11] Thus, primary coccidioidomycosis infection through the skin is extremely rare.

4.1. Criteria for Determining Primary Cutaneous Infection

According to Wilson and co-workers,[12] presence of the following factors in a case of coccidioidomycosis will establish that the skin is the portal of entry.

1. A negative history of pulmonary disease preceding the skin lesion.

2. A break in the skin and the presence of an inoculation at the site of the skin lesion. (Simple bumps or bruises may represent a site of locus minoris resistentiae for a disseminated lesion.)

3. A short incubation period of 1–3 weeks.

4. A chancre-type lesion (see Fig. 7) that is a relatively painless, indurated nodule or nodular plaque with ulceration.

5. A positive precipitin reaction that declines more slowly than it does in the case of a pulmonary lesion.

6. A positive coccidioidin skin test with increased sensitivity, i.e., sensitivity to a 1 : 1000 dilution. (This may be negative in cases in which the patient is immunosuppressed or dissemination of the disease has occurred.)

7. An early negative complement-fixation reaction which may become weakly positive.

8. Lymphangitis and lymphadenopathy only in the region of drainage and similar to that seen in sporotrichosis of the skin.

9. Spontaneous healing of the primary cutaneous chancre within a few weeks unless the patient is defective immunologically.

4.2. Differential Diagnosis

The primary cutaneous coccidioidomycosis lesion must be differentiated clinically from a primary inoculation of the skin with etiologic agents of the following disease processes: sporotrichosis, histoplasmosis,

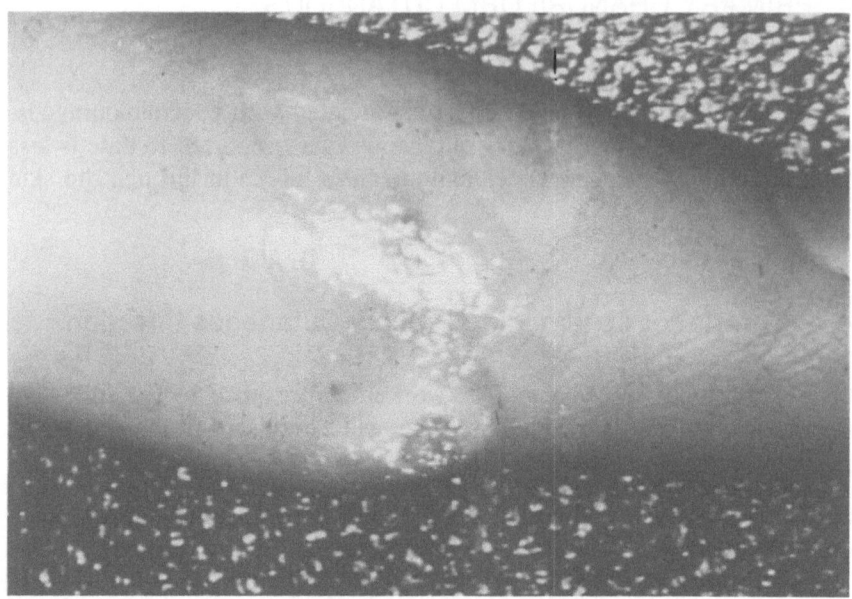

Figure 7. This chancriform lesion with surrounding induration is typical of primary cutaneous coccidioidomycosis.

North American blastomycosis, tuberculosis, other mycobacteriosis, syphilis, leishmaniasis, nocardiosis, actinomycosis, and botryomycosis.

4.3. Diagnosis

Early histologic findings of primary cutaneous coccidioidomycosis show polymorphonuclear leukocytes and the presence of spherules. The inflammation later becomes granulomatous with epithelial cells, giant cells, and lymphocytes. Fewer spherules are seen in the more mature lesions.

A direct saline preparation is often diagnostic, especially if performed early while the spherules are more prominent.

Patients should be skin tested. A patient with primary cutaneous coccidioidomycosis who fails to react to this skin test could be suffering from disseminated disease or be immunologically suppressed.

In addition to the skin test, the tests for IgM antibodies are useful in an early stage.[13] If the complement-fixing antibodies (IgG) become positive in the 8th to 10th week following inoculation, dissemination should be suspected, especially if the titers are high (see Chapter 6).

4.4. Dissemination and Reinfection

Many clinicians believe that primary cutaneous coccidioidomycosis is a benign, self-healing disease; however, the possibility of dissemination does exist. Winn[14] reported a case in which a patient later developed meningitis.

Judging from the serological response and the few available case reports, the patient usually develops resistance to further infection.

Sorensen and Cheu[15] reported the case of a laboratory worker who recovered from pulmonary coccidioidomycosis and developed a resistance to the disease. When this patient was accidentally reinoculated with *C. immitis*, he did not develop a typical chancriform lesion. This case differed from the typical chancriform syndrome in the following ways: the immune response was more rapid, with the complement-fixation titer rising within the first week; the coccidioidin skin test was positive before reinfection occurred; the lymphatic system was not involved; and the infection was localized and small, 2 mm in diameter. Smith and co-workers[16] documented a similar case presented by Triggert at a conference. In this case, a laboratory worker known to have a positive coccidioidin skin test accidentally inoculated his wrist with a suspension of *C. immitis* and developed coccidioidal osteomyelitis.

The rarity of primary cutaneous infections and cutaneous reinfections indicates that infection through the skin is difficult. This has been further demonstrated by Wright and Winer,[17] who were unable to produce infections in guinea pigs by abrading the skin and rubbing an inoculum of *C. immitis* into the abraded area. Primary infection of the skin or subcutaneous tissues in the majority of cases usually produces some immunity to reinfection via the skin and the pulmonary route as well. The latter was demonstrated by Pappagianis and co-workers[18] in their work on monkeys.

It may thus be concluded that multiple factors—such as development of host immunity, number of organisms inoculated, type of trauma, and factors of race and sex prevalence for the disease—are involved in the primary cutaneous coccidioidomycosis disease process.

REFERENCES

1. J. W. Rippon, *Medical Mycology: The Pathogenic Fungi and the Pathogenic Actinomycetes*, W. B. Saunders, Philadelphia (1974), p. 365.
2. International Medical News Service, Coccidioidomycosis possible if rash accompanies cold (article regarding study of B. M. McKay), *Skin & Allergy News* 2(1):9 (1971).

3. J. W. Wilson and W. R. Bartok, Immunoallergic aspects of coccidioidomycosis, *Int. J. Dermatol.* **9**:253–258 (1970).

4. C. W. Emmons, C. H. Binford, J. P. Utz, and K. J. Kwon-Chung, *Medical Mycology*, 3rd ed., Lea and Febiger, Philadelphia (1977), p. 233.

5. W. Ophüls, Further observations on a pathogenic mould formerly described as a protozoon *(Coccidioides immitis, Coccidioides pyogenes)*, *J. Exp. Med.* **6**:443–485 (1905).

6. C. E. Smith, M. T. Saito, R. R. Beard, R. M. Kepp, R. W. Clark, and B. U. Eddie, Serological tests in the diagnosis and prognosis of coccidioidomycosis, *Am. J. Hyg.* **52**:1–21 (1950).

7. M. J. Fiese, *Coccidioidomycosis*, Charles C. Thomas, Springfield, Ill. (1958), pp. 167–168.

8. A. J. Cox and C. E. Smith, Arrested pulmonary coccidioidal granuloma, *Arch. Pathol.* **27**:717–734 (1939).

9. J. W. Wilson, Primary inoculation coccidioidomycosis: discussion (Society Transactions), *Arch. Dermatol.* **79**:118–120 (1959).

10. P. H. Jacobs and B. Russell, Dermatophyte test medium for systemic fungi (Letter), *J. Am. Med. Assoc.* **224**:1649 (1973).

11. J. W. Wilson, The importance of the portal of entry in certain microbial infections: The primary cutaneous "chancriform" syndrome, *Dis. Chest* **54**(Suppl. 1):43–48 (1968).

12. J. W. Wilson, C. E. Smith, and O. A. Plunkett, Primary cutaneous coccidioidomycosis: The criteria for diagnosis and a report of a case, *Calif. Med.* **79**:233–239 (1953).

13. L. Kaufman, Serology: Its value in the diagnosis of coccidioidomycosis, cryptococcosis, and histoplasmosis, in: *Proceedings, International Synposium on Mycoses, Pan Am. Health Organ. Sci. Publ.* No. 205, Washington, D.C. (1970), pp. 96–100.

14. W. A. Winn, Primary cutaneous coccidioidomycosis: reevaluation of its potentiality based on study of three new cases, *Arch. Dermatol.* **92**:221–228 (1965).

15. R. H. Sorensen and S. H. Cheu, Accidental cutaneous coccidioidal infection in an immune person: A case of an exogenous reinfection, *Calif. Med.* **100**:44–47 (1964).

16. C. E. Smith, D. Pappagianis, H. B. Levine, and M. Saito, Human coccidioidomycosis, *Bacteriol. Rev.* **25**:310–320 (1961).

17. E. T. Wright and L. H. Winer, The natural history of experimental primary-inoculation *Coccidioides immitis* infection, *Int. J. Dermatol.* **10**:17–23 (1971).

18. D. Pappagianis, R. L. Miller, C. E. Smith, and G. S. Kobayashi, Response of monkeys to respiratory challenge following subcutaneous inoculation with *Coccidioides immitis*, *Am. Rev. Resp. Dis.* **82**:244–250 (1960).

14

Genitourinary Coccidioidomycosis

Eskild A. Petersen

1. INTRODUCTION

Coccidioidomycosis of the genitourinary tract occurs frequently in patients with disseminated disease. In two autopsy series, the kidneys were involved in 35 and 60% of patients with fatal dissemination.[1,2]

Contrasting with the findings at autopsy has been the clinical impression that involvement of the genitourinary tract producing evident disease occurs only rarely. The apparent discrepancy between clinical impression and pathological findings can be partially accounted for by considering the routine diagnostic armamentarium employed in the diagnosis of coccidioidomycosis.

The definitive procedures for diagnosing coccidioidomycosis include isolating the organism and demonstrating typical coccidioidal spherules in body fluids or in histologic examination. Sputum, spinal fluid, abscess drainage, and biopsy specimen are common clinical sources of the fungus.

In contrast, urine specimens have only rarely been examined for coccidioidouria. Consequently, the incidence of genitourinary coccidioidomycosis has been underestimated.

2. PATHOGENESIS AND PATHOLOGY

Genitourinary coccidioidomycosis usually follows pulmonary infection sustained after inhalation of *Coccidioides immitis* arthroconidia. Data regarding the relative frequency of blood stream invasion and the occurrence of secondary foci during the primary pulmonary infection is lacking. Genitourinary involvement, however, has been demonstrated in both fatal disseminated disease and in chronic cavitary pulmonary coccidioidomycosis.[3] In some instances, the prostatic gland or the epididymis has been the only anatomic site with evidence of active infection.[4-8] Coccidioidouria, during the primary pulmonary infection, has not yet been demonstrated. Other modalities for acquiring the infection are rare, but include the following possibilities:

1. Primary inoculation of *C. immitis* in the genital area has been described but is an exception.

2. Genital coccidioidomycosis acquired through sexual contact with a patient with genitourinary disease is an unproven theoretical possibility.

3. Transmission of renal coccidioidomycosis from donor kidney to a recipient transplant patient may have taken place.[3]

Genitourinary coccidioidomycosis occurs primarily in males; involvement of female genitalia is very rare[9-12] (see Section 4). The majority of patients are immunosuppressed secondary to primary underlying disease and/or iatrogenic intervention.

Renal transplant patients seem to be at special risk[13,14] (5% of renal transplant patients at University of Arizona have urinary coccidioidomycosis).

The pathology findings are no different from coccidioidomycosis of other organs except that involvement of kidneys tends to be microscopic, i.e., granulomas and abscesses. The anatomical sites involved are, in decreasing frequency, kidneys, epididymis, prostate, bladder, uterus, and salpinges.[15-22]

3. CLINICAL PRESENTATION

The clinical symptomatology of genitourinary coccidioidomycosis is determined by two factors: anatomical localization of coccidioidomycosis within the genitourinary tract, and degree of dissemination of *C. immitis* outside the genitourinary system. With upper urinary tract involvement, specific symptomatology referrable to the kidneys is virtually absent. Symptoms are predominantly those associated with disseminated disease, i.e., fever, chills, etc. In lower urinary tract disease, on the contrary, symptomatology primarily reflects the organ involved, e.g., chronic epididymitis and chronic prostatitis. Rectal examination may reveal asymptomatic cases of prostatitis. Often few other signs are present, indicating coccidioidomycosis activity elsewhere in the patient. Upper- and lower-tract disease may be present simultaneously.

Coccidioidomycosis of female genital organs is rare, as mentioned. The data available from the few case reports seem to indicate no characteristic pattern of presentation. Chronic pelvic inflammatory disease and cervicitis may be the only signs of infection.

4. DIAGNOSIS

The most readily available body fluid for culture in genitourinary coccidioidomycosis is urine.[23] The census of fungi in the urine is low, ranging in one study from 0.03 to 17 colonies/ml.[3] Consequently, if urine specimens are cultured without prior concentration, most instances of coccidioidouria will go undetected. The following procedure is recommended: Collect a first-voided morning urine specimen. Centrifuge the specimen and resuspend to 0.5% of the original volume. Plate 1-ml aliquots on media. Colony counts in prostatic secretions are higher (15–120 colonies/ml).[3]

Following the demonstration of coccidioidouria, the most practical procedure for identifying the site of infection within the urinary tract is culture of fractional urine specimens.[3] In addition, more-precise data can be obtained by such invasive procedures as ureteral catheterization and biopsy of the kidney and prostate.

Intravenous pyelography is of some help, but the findings usually are not specifically diagnostic. Routine urinalysis and measurements of the BUN and serum creatinine give little information on the presence, extent, or localization of urinary tract coccidioidomycosis.

If female genital coccidioidomycosis is suspected, use of curettage of the uterine cavity and laparoscopy with cul-de-sac or salpingeal culture are often necessary to make the diagnosis.[10]

The application and interpretation of skin tests and serological parameters has been covered elsewhere in this book (Chapters 4 and 6).

Urinalysis, in general, is not strikingly abnormal.[3] Small amounts of proteinuria are noted, and most have pyuria.

5. TREATMENT

The treatment modalities include antifungal chemotherapy with either amphotericin B or miconazole and surgical intervention. The indications, duration, and dosage of chemotherapeutic agents as well as indications for surgery in genitourinary coccidioidomycosis have not been developed in detail. Absolute indications for systemic chemotherapy include coccidioidouria in the patient with classical disseminated disease, as well as in the immunosuppressed patient, where coccidioidouria might well be the first indication of incipient disseminated disease.

The decision on how to treat localized disease is more difficult. Chronic coccidioidal prostatitis, epididymitis, and pelvic inflammatory disease (PID) appear to be cured only rarely by antifungal chemotherapeutic intervention, and in the immune-competent host no evidence is present to suggest that later dissemination from a genitourinary focus takes place. Surgical intervention is only occasionally called for. If chronic PID or epididymitis results in a high degree of discomfort to patients, surgery may be indicated.

REFERENCES

1. W. D. Forbus and A. M. Bestebreurtje, Coccidioidomycosis: A study of 95 cases of the disseminated type with special reference to the pathogenesis of the disease, *Mil. Surg.* **99**:653–719 (1946).
2. R. W. Huntington, Jr., W. J. Waldmann, J. A. Sargent, H. O'Connell, R. Wybel, and D. Croll, Pathologic and clinical observations on 142 cases of fatal coccidioidomycosis with necropsy, in: *Coccidioidomycosis* (L. Ajello, ed.), University of Arizona Press, Tucson (1967), pp. 143–167.
3. E. A. Petersen, B. A. Friedman, E. D. Crowder, and D. Rifkind, Coccidioidouria: Clinical significance, *Ann. Intern. Med.* **85**:34–38 (1976).
4. H. M. Weyrauch, F. W. Norman, and J. B. Bassett, Coccidioidomycosis of the genital tract, *Calif. Med.* **72**:465–468 (1950).
5. G. Amromin and C. M. Blumefeld, Coccidioidomycosis of the epididymis, *Calif. Med.* **78**:136–138 (1953).
6. J. M. Pace, Coccidioidomycosis of the epididymis, *South. Med. J.* **48**:259–260 (1955).
7. B.G. Steward, Epididymytis and prostatitis due to coccidioidomycosis: a case report with 5-year rollowup, *J. Urol.* **91**:280–281 (1964).
8. S. F. Cheng, Bilateral coccidioidal epididymitis, *Urology* 3:362–363 (1977).
9. E. C. Saw, L. E. Smale, H. Einstein, and R. W. Huntington, Female genital coccidioidomycosis, *Obstet. Gynecol.* **45**:199–202 (1975).
10. W. R. Hart, R. P. Prins, and J. C. Tsai, Isolated coccidioidomycosis of the uterus, *Hum. Pathol.* 7:235–239 (1976).
11. L. C. Wormley, L. Manoil, and M. Rosenthal, Coccidioidomycosis of female adnexa, *Am. J. Surg.* **80**:958–960 (1950).
12. E. W. Page and L. M. Boyers, Coccidioidal pelvic inflammatory disease, *Am. J. Obstet. Gynecol.* **50**:212–215 (1945).
13. G. P. J. Schroter, K. Bakshandeh, B. S. Husberg, and R. Weil, Coccidioidomycosis and renal transplantation, *Transplantation,* **23**:485–489 (1977).
14. N. Smithline, D. A. Ogden, A. I. Cohn, and K. Johnson, Disseminated coccidioidomycosis in renal transplant patients, in: *Coccidioidomycosis* (L. Ajello, ed), Symposia Specialists, Miami, Fla. (1977), pp. 201–206.
15. T. G. McDougall and A. H. Kleiman, Prostatitis due to *Coccidioides immitis*, *J. Urol.* **49**:472–477 (1943).
16. J. G. Rohn, J. C. Davila, and T. E. Gibson, Urogenital aspects of coccidioidomycosis: review of the literature and report of two cases, *J. Urol.* **65**:660–667 (1951).

17. H. Bodner, A. H. Howard, and J. H. Kaplan, Coccidioidomycosis of the spermatic cord: roentgen therapy, *J. Int. Coll. Surg.* **32**:530–533 (1958).
18. E. J. Gritti, F. E. Cook, Jr., and H. B. Spencer, Coccidioidomycosis granuloma of the prostate: a rare manifestation of the disseminated disease, *J. Urol.* **89**:249–252 (1963).
19. S. Weitzner, Coccidioidomycosis of prostate and epididymis—case report and review of literature, *Southwest Med.* **49**:67–69 (1968).
20. H. J. Bellin and B. S. Bhagavan, Coccidioidomycosis of the prostate gland, *Arch. Pathol.* **96**:114–117 (1973).
21. J. E. Gottsman, Coccidioidomycosis of prostate and epididymis, with urethrocutaneous fistula, *Urology* **4**:311–314 (1974).
22. W. T. Conner, G. W. Drach, and W. C. Bucher, Jr., Genitourinary aspects of disseminated coccidioidomycosis, *J. Urol.* **113**:82–88 (1975).
23. M. J. Goldman and E. Movitt, Disseminated coccidioidomycosis: isolation of causative organism from the urine, *Calif. Med.* **69**:456–458 (1948).

15

Ophthalmic Coccidioidomycosis

John N. Galgiani

1. INTRODUCTION

Coccidioidal infection of the eye is thought to be a rare complication of disseminated disease. It is, however, of historical interest that ocular involvement was described by Rixford and Gilchrist in their first patient.[1] Furthermore, eye findings have been reported as the only manifestation of dissemination in some patients.[2,3] Since previous reviews,[4–6] additional case reports have been published and are included in this report. Also discussed is new information concerning potentially beneficial antifungal agents that have become available.

2. NONSPECIFIC OCULAR FINDINGS

The most common form of eye involvement associated with coccidioidomycosis is phlyctenular conjunctivitis. This complication of a primary infection usually is associated with erythema nodosum or arthritis and is thought to be a manifestation of developing immunity to the fungus.[4] It occurs in at least 4–6% of persons with acute illness.[4,7] Symptoms improve over a period of days to weeks. Minor abnormalities, however, may persist for years.

Coccidioidal meningitis, when it causes increased intracranial pressure, may produce the typical ocular signs such as retinal hemorrhages and papilledema. In addition, such infection can involve the optic nerve[8,9] and extend into the orbit.[10]

3. PERIORBITAL INVOLVEMENT

The lid[11,12] and conjunctiva[13] can both be involved as part of cutaneous dissemination. In a report by Wood,[3] a granuloma of the lid, demonstrating *Coccidioides immitis* by culture and biopsy, was the only evidence of dissemination in a child with a primary illness. Resolution in this patient occurred without specific therapy. Thus, the natural course of periorbital infection is as variable and difficult to predict as for dissemination to most other sites. Since contiguous extension to the globe is rare (see Section 4), decisions concerning therapy should be made in a manner similar to those for extrapulmonary disease in other parts of the body.

4. INTRAOCULAR INFECTIONS

Infection of the globe can involve either the anterior or posterior uvea, but usually not both together. A patient reported by Brown *et al.*[14] demonstrated anterior uveitis with subsequent development of juxtapapillary chorioretinitis. Postmortem findings included spherules within granulomas of the ciliary processes and iris. Similar anterior ocular pathology has also been reported in another person[15] and in dogs.[16,17] In a patient described by Pettit,[2] an aqueous tap yielded *C. immitis* in culture. Of particular interest in this patient was the absence of any other evidence of coccidioidomycosis except for serum complement-fixing antibodies to the fungus. In addition, the early stages of his uveitis did not appear granulomatous. This underscores the need to consider *C. immitis* as the cause of perhaps any inflammation of the anterior chamber in persons traveling to or residing in the areas endemic for this organism.

Focal chorioretinal lesions have been observed by funduscopic examination in one[14,18,19] or both[9,20-25] eyes. In most of these earlier reports, eye complaints led to the discovery of the eye lesions. In a recent study, 54 persons who had previously had either serologic or culture evidence of a coccidioidal infection were examined prospectively. Chorioretinal scars were found in five persons (9.3%), four of whom had had neither eye complaints nor antifungal therapy.[25a] In another prospective study of ten patients who had more severe infections, four had evidence of intraocular involvement at some point in their clinical course.[26] Figure 1 shows the lesions in one of these patients. These recent studies indicate that chorioretinal lesions may be more frequently present than previous reports would suggest.

In some cases pathologic material has demonstrated spherules, residing within choroidal granulomas microscopically[9,23,25] as well as

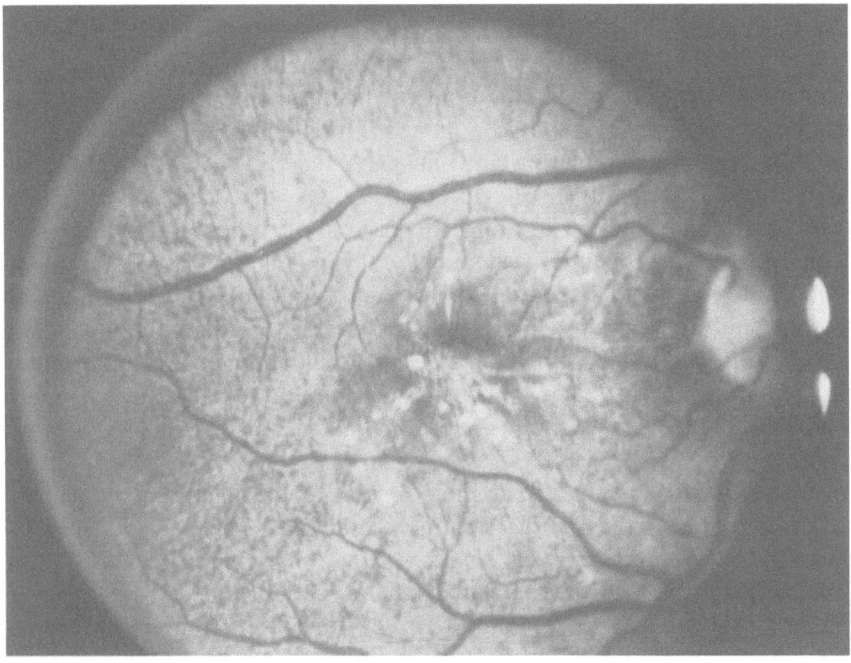

Figure 1. Chorioretinal lesions seen in a patient with *C. immitis* infection.

yielding positive cultures.[24] Serous detachment of the macula and retinal lipid deposition and hemorrhage has also been described, presumably secondary to foci of choroidal involvement.

Either anterior or posterior uveal infection indicates hematogenous dissemination to the globe in almost all cases. A possible exception might be the periorbital lesions which led to destruction of the eyes in Rixford's first patient.[1] Even in this case, however, contiguous spread of the fungus may not actually have taken place. Chorioretinal lesions in association with meningitis have been demonstrated histologically[24] in autopsy material and observed funduscopically in another patient who responded to therapy.[27] There was no evidence of direct extension in either case.

Although anterior chamber or vitreous taps may lead to cultural confirmation of intraocular dissemination, treatment is often recommended on the presumption that the funduscopic findings indicate active infection. Pathologic corroboration, when sought, has not always been demonstrable. For example, Brown[14] could not find spherules with careful microscopic examination of his patient's chorioretinal lesions.

Furthermore, Levitt[20] observed resolution of the vitreous lesions over 1 month in a patient with a pulmonary infiltrate and *C. immitis* cultured from the sputum. Again, it would seem that ocular lesions are no more predictable than other complications of this fungal infection, and claims of therapeutic efficacy should be judged in this context.

Until recently, amphotericin B has been the only available antifungal agent against *C. immitis*. Chorioretinal lesions have been observed to resolve in some patients[19,27] and to progress in others[9,25,28] where the drug has been administered systemically. It is not clear whether treatment failures are related to inadequate drug penetration, although experimental work would suggest that this is not the case.[29,30] Subconjunctival and intraocular injection have been used for other oculomycoses.* In treating coccidioidal infections, however, only one report of anterior chamber administration has been published.[31] In this instance, enucleation was eventually required.

Miconazole is a new broad-spectrum antifungal agent which has had extensive clinical trials in the treatment of various types of *C. immitis* infections.[32] Preliminary work indicates that therapeutic levels of this drug may be achieved in the human eye.[33] Miconazole may become a less toxic alternative to amphotericin B. Its role in the treatment of intraocular coccidioidomycosis deserves further study, but preliminary results suggest it may be inferior to amphotericin.[34]

ACKNOWLEDGMENTS. This manuscript has been reviewed by M. S. Blumenkranz, R. L. Stamper, J. C. Cavender, and W. H. Spencer, and their helpful comments are gratefully acknowledged. Figure 1 is reproduced from reference 34 with permission of the publisher.

REFERENCES

1. E. Rixford and T. C. Gilchrist, Two cases of protozoan (coccidioidal) infection of the skin and other organs, *Johns Hopkins Hosp. Rep.* 1:209–268 (1896).
2. T. H. Pettit, R. N. Learn, and R. Y. Foos, Intraocular coccidioidomycosis, *Arch. Ophthalmol.* 77:655–661 (1967).
3. T. R. Wood, Ocular coccidioidomycosis, *Am. J. Ophthalmol.* 64:587–590 (1967).
4. D. H. Trowbridge, Ocular manifestations of coccidioidomycosis, *Trans. Pac. Coast Oto-Ophthalmol. Soc.* 33:229–244 (1952).
5. M. J. Fiese, *Coccidioidomycosis,* Charles C. Thomas, Springfield, Ill. (1958).
6. J. Francois and M. Rysselaere, *Oculomycoses,* Charles C. Thomas, Springfield, Ill. (1972).

---

* This topic has been reviewed by Francois and Rysselaere.[6]

7. F. M. Willett and A. Weiss, Coccidioidomycosis in Southern California: report of a new endemic area with a review of 100 cases, *Ann. Intern. Med.* **23**:349–375 (1945).

8. W. D. Forbus and A. M. Bestebreurtje, Coccidioidomycosis. A study of 95 cases of the disseminated type with special references to the pathogenesis of the disease, *Mil. Surg.* **99**:653–719 (1946).

9. E. A. Rainin and H. L. Little, Ocular coccidioidomycosis. A clinico-pathologic case report, *Trans. Am. Acad. Ophthalmol. Otolaryngol.* **76**:645–651 (1972).

10. J. W. Wilson and O. A. Plunkett, *The Fungus Diseases of Man,* University of California Press, Berkeley and Los Angeles (1965).

11. D. M. Perry and W. M. M. Kirby, Acute disseminated coccidioidomycosis: two cases treated with amphotericin B, *Arch. Intern. Med.* **105**:929–934 (1960).

12. A. R. Irvine, Jr., Coccidioidal granuloma of lid, *Trans. Am. Acad. Ophthalmol. Otolaryngol.* **72**:751–754 (1968).

13. R. F. Faulkner, Ocular coccidioidomycosis. Report of a case of coccidioidal granuloma of the conjunctiva associated with cutaneous coccidioidomycosis, *Am. J. Ophthalmol.* **45**:822–827 (1958).

14. W. C. Brown, R. E. Kellenberger, and K. E. Hudson, Granulomatous uveitis associated with disseminated coccidioidomycosis, *Am. J. Ophthalmol.* **45**:102–104 (1958).

15. R. Bell and R. L. Font, Granulomatous anterior uveitis caused by *Coccidioides immitis, Am. J. Ophthalmol.* **74**:93–98 (1972).

16. R. M. Cello, Ocular manifestations of coccidioidomycosis in a dog, *Arch. Ophthalmol.* **64**:897–903 (1960).

17. J. N. Shively and C. E. Whiteman, Ocular lesions in disseminated coccidioidomycosis in two dogs, *Pathol. Vet.* **7**:1–6 (1970).

18. W. C. Brown, K. E. Hudson, and A. A. Nisbet, Pulmonary coccidioidomycosis associated with Jensen's disease, *Am. J. Ophthalmol.* **43**:965–967 (1957).

19. P. B. Alexander and E. L. Coodley, Disseminated coccidioidomycosis with intraocular involvement, *Am. J. Ophthalmol.* **64**:283–298 (1967).

20. J. M. Levitt, Ocular manifestations in coccidioidomycosis, *Am. J. Ophthalmol.* **31**:1626–1628 (1948).

21. N. J. Conan and G. A. Hyman, Disseminated coccidioidomycosis. Treatment with protoanemonin, *Am. J. Med.* **9**:408–413 (1950).

22. L. G. Lovekin, Coccidioidomycosis. Report of a case with intraocular involvement, *Am. J. Ophthalmol.* **34**:621–623 (1951).

23. R. Olavarria and L. F. Fajardo, Ophthalmic coccidioidomycosis. Case report and review, *Arch. Pathol.* **92**:191–195 (1971).

24. B. S. Boyden and D. S. Yee, Bilateral coccidioidal choroiditis. A clinicopathologic case report, *Trans. Am. Acad. Ophthalmol. Otolaryngol.* **75**:1006–1010 (1971).

25. K. A. Zakka, R. Y. Foos, and W. J. Brown, Intraocular coccidioidomycosis, *Surv. Ophthalmol.* **22**:313–321 (1978).

25a. H. T. Rodenbeker, J. P. Ganley, J. N. Galgiani, and S. G. Axline, Prevalence of chorioretinal scars associated with coccidioidomycosis, *Arch. Ophthalmol.* (in press).

26. M. S. Blumenkranz and D. A. Stevens, Endogenous coccidioidal endophthalmitis, *Ophthalmology* (in press).

27. W. R. Green and J. E. Bennett, Coccidioidomycosis. Report of a case with clinical evidence of ocular involvement, *Arch. Ophthalmol.* **77**:337–340 (1967).

28. A. J. Hagele, D. J. Evans, and T. R. Larwood, Primary endophthalmic coccidioido-mycosis: Report of a case of exogenous primary coccidioidomycosis of the eye diagnosed prior to enucleation, in: *Coccidioidomycosis* (L. Ajello, ed.), University of Arizona Press, Tucson (1967), pp. 37–39.

29. W. R. Green, J. E. Bennett, and R. O. Goos, Ocular penetration of amphotericin B.

A report of laboratory studies and a case report of postsurgical cephalosporium endophthalmitis, *Arch. Ophthalmol.* **73**:769–775 (1965).

30. K. K. Sethi and J. Schwarz, Amphotericin B in ocular histoplasmosis of rabbits, *Arch. Ophthalmol.* **75**:818–825 (1966).

31. J. E. Cutler, P. S. Binder, T. O. Paul, and J. Beamis, Metastatic coccidioidal endophthalmitis, *Arch. Ophthalmol.* **96**:689–691 (1978).

32. D. A. Stevens, Miconazole in the treatment of systemic fungal infections, *Am. Rev. Resp. Dis.* **116**:801–806 (1978).

33. L. I. Lutwick, J. N. Galgiani, R. H. Johnson, and D. A. Stevens, Visceral fungal infections due to *Petriellidium boydii (Allescheria boydii). In vitro* drug sensitivity studies, *Am. J. Med.* **61**:632–640 (1976).

34. M. S. Blumenkranz and D. A. Stevens, Therapy of endogenous fungal endophthalmitis: miconazole or amphotericin for coccidioidal and candidal infection, *Arch. Ophthalmol.* (in press).

16

Other Coccidioidal Syndromes

David A. Stevens

The major sites involved in human coccidioidal infection have been detailed in the preceding chapters (Chapters 10 through 15) under the heading of each organ system. Uncommonly, other sites in the body may be involved in disseminated disease.

1. *Miliary.* That disseminated coccidioidomycosis may involve any organ system in the body is best exemplified in miliary coccidioidomycosis. This entity has been discussed, with particular reference to its presentation in the lungs, in Chapter 10.

2. *Peritonitis.* Coccidioidal peritonitis may be seen as part of generalized coccidioidomycosis or as an independent process.[1,2] Concomitant pleuritis and/or pericarditis has been noted. The symptoms are generalized (fever, anorexia) and/or referable to the abdomen (pain, distension, ascites) and not pathognomonic. Cases are often diagnosed at exploratory laparotomy for these symptoms, although asymptomatic cases have been diagnosed incidentally at the time of abdominal surgery. The appearance at surgery or postmortem examination with numerous miliary nodules suggests that laparoscopy would be diagnostic, in most cases, of a diffuse granulomatous peritonitis (in addition to suggesting the need for coccidioidal serology as part of the further workup); and biopsies at that time could yield the specific etiologic agent in many instances. Protein content of ascitic fluid has varied from 4 to 8 g/100 ml. Many cases have resolved without surgery.

3. *Otomycosis.* Involvement of the middle ear has been reported, as apparent reactivations of hematogenously disseminated foci.[3] Coccidioidal otomycosis appears to behave as other invasive fungi (e.g., mucor species and mycetoma organisms) in this regard, and not as the locally restricted disease generally seen with others (e.g., *Aspergillus* and

Candida species). Serologic titers may not be high (see Chapter 6) if the ear is the only focus affected.[3] A combined chemotherapeutic-surgical approach seems warranted.[3]

4. *Upper respiratory infection.* The nasopharynx, epiglottis, larynx, and trachea have all been reported to be involved in various cases.[4-6] Paraspinal cervical abscesses may present in the retropharynx (Chapter 12).

5. *Pleuritis.* Pleuritis may occur, with or without effusion. This has been discussed in Chapter 9.

6. *Myocarditis.* The association of this entity with coccidioidomycosis has been discussed in Chapter 7.

7. *Endocarditis.* The endocardium is extremely rarely involved in coccidioidomycosis.[7,8] Occasionally endocardial involvement may occur secondary to the distal end of a ventriculoatrial or ventriculovenous shunt for central nervous system involvement (Chapter 11).

8. *Pericarditis.* Pericarditis may occur acutely, usually as a concomitant of pleuritis at the time of primary infection with pleuritis (Chapter 9), or as part of generalized dissemination.[9] Tamponade may occur.[10] Electrocardiographic changes involving T waves or low voltage, as seen with other etiologies of acute pericarditis, have been noted.[11] Chronic constrictive pericarditis may occur secondary to acute pericardial involvement, with the insidious onset of the former entity as seen, due to several etiologies, in the modern era.[12]

9. *Liver.* Miliary dissemination may be diagnosed as a result of liver biopsy.[13] Liver involvement may be present in half the cases of disseminated disease that come to autopsy.[9]

10. *Lymphoid.* Lymph node involvement has been discussed in connection with primary and/or pulmonary infection (Chapters 9 and 10).

11. *Spleen.* Splenic involvement in disseminated coccidioidomycosis may be documented in the majority of cases at autopsy. A mass or miliary granulomas may be present.[14]

12. *Adrenal.* Granulomatous involvement of the adrenal glands has been noted at postmortem examination,[9] and Addison's disease consequent to involvement has been noted during life in several instances.[15,16] The latter appears to be less common than seen in tuberculosis.

13. *Thyroid.* We have seen thyroid abscess due to *Coccidioides immitis* in two patients. A mass was present, which led to the diagnosis of involvement at surgery (in one case it was the most prominent manifestation of disseminated coccidioidal disease and led to the diagnosis of the disease). Endocrine dysfunction of the thyroid was not apparent clinically prior to surgery.

14. *Gastrointestinal.* Involvement of the gastrointestinal tract, aside from the pharynx or serosal involvement in peritonitis, is extremely rare.[17]

REFERENCES

1. P. R. Meis, T. R. Larwood, and W. A. Winn, Coccidioidal peritonitis, in: *Coccidioidomycosis* (L. Ajello, ed.), University of Arizona, Tucson (1967), pp. 85–88.
2. E. C. Saw, S. J. Shields, T. P. Comer, and R. W. Huntington, Granulomatous peritonitis due to *Coccidioides immits*. *Arch. Surg.* **108**:369–371 (1974).
3. R. P. Harvey, D. Pappagianis, J. Cochran, and D. A. Stevens, Otomycosis due to coccidioidomycosis, *Arch. Intern. Med.* **138**:1434–1435 (1978).
4. J. H. Childrey and P. A. Gray, Coccidioidal granuloma primary in the nasopharynx, *Calif. West. Med.* **37**:250–252 (1932).
5. L. S. Mumma, Coccidioidomycosis of the epiglottis, *Arch. Otolaryngol.* **58**:306–309 (1953).
6. H. Singh, C. J. Yast, and J. H. Gladney, Coccidioidomycosis with endolaryngeal involvement, *Arch. Otolaryngol.* **63**:244–247 (1956).
7. E. Epstein, Prognostic significance of cutaneous lesions in coccidioidal granuloma, *Arch. Dermatol. Syphilol.* **38**:752–755 (1938).
8. T. E. Townsend and R. W. McKey, Coccidioidomycosis in infants, *Am. J. Dis. Child.* **86**:51–53 (1953).
9. W. D. Forbus and A. M. Bestebreurtje, Coccidioidomycosis: a study of 95 cases of the disseminated type with special reference to the pathogenesis of the disease, *Mil. Surg.* **99**:653–719 (1946).
10. A. S. Bayer, T. T. Yoshikawa, J. E. Galpin, and L. B. Guze, Unusual syndromes of coccidioidomycosis: diagnostic and therapeutic considerations, *Medicine* **55**:131–152 (1977).
11. P. B. Tudbury, The electrocardiogram in primary coccidioidomycosis, *Calif. Med.* **83**:89–90 (1955).
12. R. Larson and R. E. Scherb, Coccidioidal pericarditis, *Circulation* **7**:211–217 (1953).
13. J. R. Ward and R. C. Hunter, Disseminated coccidioidomycosis demonstrated by needle biopsy of the liver, *Ann. Intern. Med.* **48**:157–163 (1958).
14. M. J. Fiese, *Coccidioidomycosis,* Charles C. Thomas, Springfield, Ill. (1958), p. 111.
15. E. M. Butt and A. Hoffman, A study of latent lesions of coccidioidomycosis correlated with coccidioidin skin tests, *Am. J. Pathol.* **17**:579–580 (1941).
16. P. J. Maloney, Addison's disease due to chronic disseminated coccidioidomycosis, *Arch. Intern. Med.* **90**:869–878 (1952).
17. F. C. Greaves, Coccidioidal granuloma with lesions in the small intestine, *U.S. Nav. Med. Bull.* **32**:201–204 (1934).

17

Coccidioidomycosis in Pregnancy

Robert P. Harvey

Coccidioidomycosis is a serious infection in pregnancy. In endemic regions it has been reported to be the leading cause of maternal mortality.[1] The first reported case was by Mendenhall in 1948.[2] Since that time 69 cases have appeared in the world literature.[2-11] Fifty-nine cases have had sufficient clinical details provided to preclude duplication in analysis. This chapter is based on an assessment of these 59 cases.

The generally stated statistics on rates of dissemination and fatality of disease in coccidioidomycosis are inaccurate when applied to the gravid female. In endemic regions it has been estimated that 1 in 1000 pregnancies is complicated by coccidioidomycosis.[5] Twenty percent of these disseminate—a rate 40–100 times the general population. Furthermore, overall mortality in treated and untreated cases is 88%. This is compared with an estimated 50% mortality in untreated disseminated disease in the general population.[12] Although the appearance of cases in nonendemic regions is considerably less frequent, the disease is equally as serious and recognition extremely important.[6,7,11]

Calculated age-specific attack rates for coccidioidomycosis in pregnancy reflect the childbearing years, with most cases occurring in females 20–29 years old. The frequency of dissemination by age is the same for all childbearing years, except for a slightly increased dissemination rate in gravid females more than 30 years of age.

Ethnic origin is an important determinant of disease in both the pregnant and nonpregnant patient.[13] Most cases of coccidioidomycosis in pregnancy in the medical literature have been reported from Kern County, California. The population of this county is about 8% blacks, but 29% of the reported cases in pregnant women are in blacks. The overall percentage of cases of pregnant women with dissemination in the literature is 59%. In whites the percentage of dissemination is 35%, in all dark-skinned races combined 96%, and in blacks 100%. These figures are probably high and may reflect the bias of increased reporting of disseminated infections.

Gestational stage at the onset of infection appears also to be prognostically important. A history of antecedent coccidioides infection prior to pregnancy as manifested by a positive skin test does not predispose to relapse, dissemination, or any recognized gestational complication.[5] However, active nondisseminated infections acquired weeks to a few months before the onset of pregnancy disseminate at a higher frequency than in the general population.[8] Infections occurring during pregnancy produce dissemination rates and mortalities that correlate with the trimester of onset of infection. In the first trimester the dissemination rate is 31%, in the second trimester 70%, and in the third trimester 80%. (See also Table 6 in Chapter 4.)

The central nervous system is involved in approximately one-third of the patients with disseminated disease. All patients with central nervous system infection for whom adequate follow-up was described died. In the reported literature, dissemination to the meninges is more common in whites than in blacks. In whites with disseminated disease, 45% have meningitis, while in blacks, only 23% have meningitis. Central nervous system involvement occurs more often in late gestational onset coccidioidomycosis than in early gestational disease.

Coccidioidomycosis occurring in the pregnant female has serious adverse effects on the developing fetus. Only 60% of the pregnancies produce offspring that survive beyond the neonatal period, and one-third of these are delivered prematurely. Twenty percent of patients with early gestational onset infection have spontaneous first trimester abortions. Ten percent of patients die with their offspring undelivered. A documented case of maternal–fetal transmission of *Coccidiodes immitis* has been reported.[14] The absence of well-documented congenital infections is remarkable in view of the fact that placental infection is common and is recognized in 23% of the disseminated cases in the literature.[4] Examination of the placenta is useful in diagnosis and should be done if the diagnosis is considered and early spontaneous abortion occurs.

Because of the severity of disease, special caution should be exercised in prenatal care in endemic regions or when a patient has recently traveled to an endemic area. A serological study should be performed at the time of the first antenatal visit. If it is negative, patients should be seen promptly for febrile illnesses which occur during the pregnancy, and this diagnosis considered. An elevated or rising titer suggests that disseminated infection is present and an intensive diagnostic workup should ensue. Abortion or early delivery should be considered depending on the stage of pregnancy in patients with active infection, and they should be treated with amphotericin as if pregnancy were not present. The existing literature on infection in pregnant females suggests that amphotericin B used early may reduce mortality from 88% to 57%.[8-10] The effect of miconazole, combination therapy of other drugs with amphotericin, or immunotherapy on mortality has not been assessed, nor has the effect of these therapies on the fetus. If mortality is to be reduced, early recognition and treatment are essential.

The reasons for increased dissemination and severity of disease in pregnancy are not understood. It has been reasoned that the maternal host is immunocompromised in order to accept the fetal graft.[1] Indeed, maternal lymphocytes have decreased responsiveness to mitogens and in mixed lymphocyte cultures during the gestational period.[15] One may speculate that hormonal alterations in pregnancy play a role in these phenomena. Human chorionic gonadotropin produced by the placenta is immunosuppressive *in vitro* but only in supraphysiologic concentration.[15] The observation that diethylstilbestrol, a synthetic female estrogenic hormone, has *in vitro* coccidioidostatic properties is of interest.[16,17] However, *in vivo* tests with diethylstilbestrol have failed to show any therapeutic benefit.[18] The effect of diethylstilbestrol is probably related more to its structural similarity with stilbamidine than to its estrogenic properties.

In summary, coccidioidomycosis occurring in pregnancy is a serious infection with high morbidity and mortality. The mortality and dissemination rates are influenced by ethnic origin and the stage of gestation at the onset of infection. Infection in pregnancy is associated with high rates of fetal wastage and prematurity. These occur without evidence of maternal–fetal transmission of disease. Therapeutic intervention with amphotericin B improves survival statistics.

REFERENCES

1. S. C. Deresinski and D. A. Stevens, Coccidioidomycosis in compromised hosts, *Medicine* **54**:377–395 (1974).
2. J. C. Mendenhall, W. C. Black, and G. E. Pottz, Progressive (disseminated) coccidioidomycosis during pregnancy, *Rocky Mount. Med. J.* **45**:472–476 (1948).
3. L. E. Smale and J. W. Birsner, Maternal deaths from coccidioidomycosis, *J. Am. Med. Assn.* **140**:1152–1154 (1949).
4. R. Cohen, Placental coccidioides, *Arch. Pediat.* **68**:59–66 (1951).
5. J. E. Vaughan and H. Ramirez, Coccidioidomycosis as a complication of pregnancy, *Calif. Med.* **74**:121–123 (1951).
6. R. L. Baker, Pregnancy complicated by coccidioides: Report of two cases, *Am. J. Obstet. Gynecol.* **70**:1033–1038 (1955).

7. H. N. Harrison, Fatal maternal coccidioidomycosis. A case report and review of sixteen cases from the literature, *Am. J. Obstet. Gynecol.* **75**:813–820 (1958).

8. R. E. Harris, Coccidioidomycosis complicating pregnancy. Report of three cases and review of the literature, *Obstet. Gynecol.* **28**:401–405 (1966).

9. L. E. Smale and K. G. Walchter, Dissemination of coccidioidomycosis in pregnancy, *Am. J. Obstet. Gynecol.* **107**:356–359 (1970).

10. F. J. Hadsall and M. J. Acquarelli, Disseminated coccidioidomycosis presenting as facial granuloma in pregnancy: A report of two Cases and a review of the literature, *Laryngoscope* **83**:51–58 (1973).

11. W. S. Van Bergen, F. J. Fleury, and E. L. Cheattle, Fatal maternal disseminated coccidioidomycosis in a nonendemic area, *Am. J. Obstet. Gynecol.* **124**:661–663 (1976).

12. C. E. Smith, R. R. Beard, E. G. Whiting, and H. G. Rosenberger, Varieties of coccidioidal infection in relation to the epidemiology and control of the disease, *Am. J. Public Health* **36**:1394–1402 (1946).

13. M. A. Gifford, W. C. Bass, and R. J. Douds, Data on coccidioides fungal infection, Kern County, Calif. 1900–1936, in: Kern County Health Dept. Annual Report (1936–1937), p. 39.

14. T. R. Larwood, Maternal-fetal transmission of coccidioidomycosis. Transactions of the VII Annual Meeting of the VA-Armed Forces Coccidioidomycosis Study Group (1962), pp. 28–29.

15. M. J. Hobart and I. McConnell, *The Immune System,* Blackwell Scientific Publishers, Oxford (1975).

16. R. Cohen, Diethylstilbestrol—A coccidioidal fungicide, *Arch. Pediatr.* **71**: 291–292 (1954).

17. R. Cohen and J. Bos, Two new fungicides for *Coccidioides immitis, Arch. Pediat.* **69**:33–35 (1952).

18. W. N. Piper and R. W. Goldblum, Two treatment failures using diethylstilbestrol in treatment of coccidioidomycosis, *Arch. Dermatol. Syphilol.* **70**:805–812 (1954).

18

Coccidioidomycosis in Pediatrics

Allan Lavetter

While coccidioidomycosis is an uncommon infection in children in most of the United States, it is widely endemic in the arid regions of southern California, central and southern Arizona and New Mexico, and northwestern Texas.[1] In those areas the frequency of positive coccidioidin skin tests is higher among children living in rural areas than among those living in urban areas. Positive coccidioidin skin tests are more common among darker-skinned children (e.g., in one area, Indian 60%, Spanish-American 42%, black 32%, white children 30%).[2] Positive coccidioidin reactions are especially prevalent among Indian children living on reservations in central and southern Arizona, where 70% to 80% of all such children have been reported to have positive coccidioidin skin tests by the age of 14 years.[3,4]

Less than half of naturally acquired infections are clinically manifest.[5] Only a small proportion of coccidioidal infections progress to the disseminated form of the disease (approximately 1 in every 500 infections in whites).[6] This appears not to be different in children. Though dissemination is more common in adult males than adult females, there appears to be no sex difference prior to puberty.[5,7] Studies among Indians in Arizona suggest that survival with disseminated coccidioidomycosis is less likely for those under 5 years or over 50 years of age.[7] (See also Chapter 4, Section 4.4.)

There are three clinical presentations of coccidioidomycosis in children:

1. *Primary pulmonary coccidioidomycosis*—a benign pneumonia difficult, if not impossible, to differentiate from a pneumonia of viral or bacterial etiology.

2. *Primary coccidioidal granuloma*—a benign localized granuloma resulting from direct inoculation or trauma.

3. *Disseminated coccidioidomycosis*—most often a malignant, chronic, systemic disease.

Several authors have commented that coccidioidomycosis tends to be milder in children than in adults, but in those infected children requiring medical attention, dissemination, especially to bones and meninges, is relatively common. The mortality rate in infants with coccidioidomycosis is high.[1,8,9]

The clinical features of primary pulmonary coccidioidomycosis are variable. After an incubation period of 1–3 weeks, symptoms of a mild lower respiratory tract disease may develop, though most infected children remain asymptomatic. Characteristically, a dry, nonproductive cough develops, often accompanied by fever (generally low grade), anorexia, malaise, chest pain, and occasionally respiratory distress. The acute illness may be of variable duration, but symptoms generally wane after 1–2 weeks.[1,10]

When dissemination occurs, signs and symptoms may develop indicating the area(s) involved. Dissemination to the central nervous system may be missed because of the initially vague and nonspecific signs. Nuchal rigidity is infrequent early in this form of coccidioidomycosis. As the infection progresses, confusion, obtundation, coma, and seizures may occur.[1,8,9]

From 1–3 weeks after the onset of the infection, 5–20% of children with clinical disease may develop some cutaneous manifestation. These appear to represent allergic responses and are frequently accompanied by eosinophilia and exacerbation of constitutional symptoms. The rashes described include (1) a *"toxic"* erythema which may occur at the onset of symptoms,[10,11,12] (2) *erythema nodosum* not unlike that seen accompanying other infections such as tuberculosis,[13,14] and (3) *erythema multiforme,* including a vesicular type which has been mistaken for varicella.[15] An erythematous maculopapular rash prominent over the inner thighs appears to be unique to childhood infection. The literature suggests that there is a difference in the skin manifestations of children with coccidioidomycosis in different geographic areas, though no difference in the etiologic agent has been noted.

There is one well-described case of congenital coccidioidal infection, but infection has been observed during the early infancy period.[16–20] There is even one reported instance of apparent transmission of coccidioidomycosis to an infant rhesus monkey from its infected mother at some time during the infant's first 2 months of life.[21] There is no record of any such occurrence in humans. Placental involvement with coccidioidomycosis has been observed, but the placenta apparently remains an effective barrier against infection of the fetus.[22-24] Two explanations offered for the placenta's barrier effect are (1) that the average size of the endospores (40–70 μm) prevents them from passing through the placenta unless a tear exists, and (2) that the characteristic thrombotic segregation of organisms coupled with the acute neutrophilic response may eliminate the viable capillaries in the region of the organism and thus prevent their transmission to the fetus.

Establishing a diagnosis of coccidioidomycosis may be difficult, and in a young infant it may be very difficult. The coccidioidin skin test, the complement fixation antibody test, and the precipitin antibody test are all used diagnostically, but all are apt to remain negative in the young infant. Radiographic evidence of a nonresolving pulmonary infiltrate may be the earliest clue to the diagnosis in an infant in an endemic area. Early confirmation of the diagnosis may depend on microscopic examination of gastric washings and sputum and demonstration of *Coccidioides* spherules.

Amphotericin B is the most commonly used agent for the treatment of systemic fungal infections and the treatment of choice for disseminated coccidioidomycosis. There are almost no data regarding its use in newborns or older infants, and very little data from studies in older children. Consequently the guidelines for amphotericin B usage and toxicity in children are almost completely based on experience in adults. Its effectiveness and toxicity in children do seem to be similar to that in adults.[19,25] Intrathecal and intraarticular administration of amphotericin B has been described in one infant.[26] There are few data yet on the effectiveness of miconazole in children with this disease, and little on its toxicity for this age group.[27]

REFERENCES

1. C. E. Smith, Coccidioidomycosis, *Pediat. Clin. North Am.* **2**:109–117 (1955).
2. I. L. Doto, F. E. Tosh, S. F. Farnsworth, and M. L. Furcolow, Coccidioidin, histoplasmin, and tuberculin sensitivity among school children in Maricopa County, Arizona, *Am. J. Epidemiol.* **95**:464–474 (1972).
3. R. D. Geller, J. E. Maynard, and V. Jones, Coccidioidin sensitivity among Southwestern American Indians, *Am. Rev. Resp. Dis.* **107**:301–302 (1973).
4. M. L. Sievers, Coccidioidomycosis among Southwestern American Indians, *Am. Rev. Resp. Dis.* **90**:920–926 (1964).
5. C. E. Smith, R. R. Beard, E. G. Whiting, and H. G. Rosenberger, Varieties of coccidioidal infection in relation to the epidemiology and control of the disease, *Am. J. Public Health* **36**:1394–1402 (1946).

6. J. L. Dennis and A. E. Hansen, Coccidioidomycosis in children, *Pediatrics* **14**:481–493 (1954).

7. M. L. Sievers, Disseminated coccidioidomycosis among Southwestern American Indians, *Am. Rev. Resp. Dis.* **109**:602–612 (1974).

8. J. Dykes, J. K. Segesman, and J. W. Birsner, Coccidioidomycosis of bone in children, *Am. J. Dis. Child.* **85**:34–42 (1953).

9. R. G. Caudill, C. E. Smith, and J. A. Reinarz, Coccidioidal meningitis. A diagnostic dilemma, *Am. J. Med.* **49**:360–365 (1970).

10. H. B. Richardson, J. A. Anderson, and B. M. McKay, Acute pulmonary coccidioidomycosis in children, *J. Pediatr.* **70**:376–382 (1967).

11. M. J. Fiese, Coccidioidomycosis, Charles C. Thomas, Springfield, Ill. (1958), p. 133.

12. R. Cohen, Coccidioidomycosis. Case studies in children, *Arch. Pediatr.* **66**:241–265 (1949).

13. H. K. Faber, C. E. Smith, and E. C. Dickson, Acute coccidioidomycosis with erythema nodosum in children, *J. Pediatr.* **15**:163–171 (1939).

14. J. E. Thorner, Erythema nodosum in childhood associated with infection by the oidium coccidioides, *Arch. Pediatr.* **56**:628–638 (1939).

15. C. E. Smith, Diagnosis of pulmonary coccidioidal infections, *Calif. Med.* **75**:385–391 (1951).

16. T. E. Townsend, and R. W. McKey, Coccidioidomycosis in infants, *Am. J. Dis. Child.* **86**:51–53 (1953).

17. J. R. Christian, S. G. Sarre, J. H. Peers, E. Salazar, and J. de Rosario, Pulmonary coccidioidomycosis in a twenty-one-day-old infant, *Am. J. Dis. Child.* **92**:66–74 (1956).

18. H. W. Hyatt, Coccidioidomycosis in a three-week-old infant, *Am. J. Dis. Child.* **105**:93–98 (1963).

19. W. H. Ziering, and H. R. Rockas, Coccidioidomycosis: Long-term treatment with amphotericin B in a three-month-old baby, *Am. J. Dis. Child.* **108**:454–459 (1964).

20. C. R. Westley, and W. Haak, Neonatal coccidioidomycosis in a Southwestern Pima Indian, *South. Med. J.* **67**:855–857 (1974).

21. M. W. Castleberry, J. L. Converse, and J. E. Del Favero, Coccidioidomycosis transmission to infant monkey from its mother, *Arch. Pathol.* **75**:459–461 (1963).

22. R. Cohen, Placental *Coccidioides*, *Arch. Pediatr.* **68**:59–66 (1951).

23. R. E. Harris, Coccidioidomycosis complicating pregnancy, *Obstet. Gynecol.* **28**:401–405 (1966).

24. L. E. Smale, and K. G. Waechter, Dissemination of coccidioidomycosis in pregnancy, *Am. J. Obstet. Gynecol.* **107**:356–361 (1970).

25. J. D. Cherry, C. A. Lloyd, J. F. Quilty, and F. Laskowski, Amphotericin B therapy in children. *J. Pediatr.* **75**:1063–1069 (1969).

26. J. O. Klein, T. Yamauchi, and S. P. Horlick, Neonatal candidiasis, meningitis and arthritis, *J. Pediatr.* **81**:31–34 (1972).

27. T. J. Fischer, R. B. Klein, H. E. Kershnar, T. C. Borut, and E. R. Stiehm, Miconazole in the treatment of chronic mucocutaneous candidiasis: a preliminary report, *J. Pediatr.* **91**:815–819 (1977).

19

Coccidioidomycosis in Immunocompromised Hosts

David A. Stevens

In Chapter 5, the apparent centrality of the host immune response in determining the outcome of coccidioidal infection has been detailed—in particular, cell-mediated immunity. This suggests that instances of deficiencies of such responses would lead to severe and progressive disease. In fact, observations made in patients with immunodeficiencies have provided strong evidence for our current understanding of the role of immunity in the normal host–pathogen interaction.

Fungal infections are a significant cause of morbidity and mortality in immunocompromised hosts,[1-5] and in some series with some malignancies are the most common infections at death. The fungi most commonly implicated in such infections are *Candida* or *Aspergillus* species, *Cryptococcus neoformans,* and infections due to zygomycetes. Such opportunistic invaders are present in normal host flora or are organisms which may be encountered commonly in the environment in a variety of geographic areas, and are prevented from causing infection in most circumstances by the defense mechanisms of the unimpaired host, unless anatomic barriers are breached. However, coccidioidal infection can also be a severe problem in such patients if they have or have had the opportunity of exposure to the organism.

Review of the literature indicates that coccidioidomycosis has been reported in association with a variety of malignancies and with immunosuppression for transplantation and for other conditions. Many cases have been reported in association with corticosteroid or cytotoxic chemotherapy or both. The special case of coccidioidal infection in pregnancy is discussed in detail in Chapter 17. The association of insulin-dependent diabetes mellitus with chronic and/or progressive pulmonary disease, particularly with cavitation,[6] has been referred to in Chapter 10.

In a referral center adjacent to the endemic zone, a series of patients with immune impairment and coccidioidomycosis was analyzed in reference to the host populations with both conditions.[7] Some features of this association emerge in this analysis. Disseminated disease was noted to be 100 times more common (50%) than expected in the normal population. This was particularly clear if the infection occurred after the immune impairment, although infection which resolved and became quiescent prior to development of an immune-impairing condition sometimes can reactivate and disseminate after impairment. The increased risk of dissemination in males and in dark-skinned races each appeared to be accentuated with the presence of the risk associated with immune impairment. Coccidioidomycosis could be an early or late complication of underlying malignancies, unlike the opportunistic invaders which commonly are seen late in the course of the patient's illness.[2] Recent chemotherapy was a more important correlate of dissemination than was radiotherapy or the specific underlying diagnosis. Lymphocytopenia correlated closely with dissemination. Among the Hodgkin's disease patients, dissemination was associated with advanced stages of disease (III and IV).

Dissemination was highly lethal in these patients, whereas pulmonary coccidioidomycosis which remained localized to the lung appeared not necessarily worse than in normal hosts. (In another series,[8] subclinical relapses were also noted in renal transplant recipients. Urine cultures became positive before frank illness.) An unusual feature of disseminated infection was concomitant rapidly progressive pulmonary involvement, with bilateral infiltrates, with patients dying rapidly from the time of their first abnormal X-ray. Miliary coccidioidal disease has also been noted in other immunocompromised patients, and patients with immune impairment comprise a large segment of series of patients with that form of coccidioidal disease (see Chapter 10). Fungemia may also be seen in such patients.

Although the skin test reaction appears blunted in these patients, the serological response was at least qualitatively intact (positive test although titers are reduced). Whereas others have also noted the latter,[6] this is apparently not always the case,[8] particularly with specimens taken at the start of the illness.

An unfortunate number of these patients were diagnosed as having coccidioidal infection only just antemortem or at postmortem examination. The major problem in diagnosis of these patients was lack of suspicion of the diagnosis of coccidioidomycosis, although difficulties in laboratory identification of *Coccidioides immitis* isolates caused problems in some (see Chapter 3). This experience makes it clear that individuals with a positive coccidioidal skin test or a history of a positive test, a history of coccidioidal infection, or a history of residence or even travel in an endemic area who become immunocompromised need be considered at risk of reactivation of a latent focus of coccidioidal infection. Routine serological testing of such patients might give advance warning of early or reactivating infection and avert delays in diagnosis of their rapidly fatal infections, and may avoid dangerous diagnostic procedures. Such testing should certainly be used promptly in immuno-suppressed patients with febrile illnesses or abnormal chest X-rays who are at risk as just defined. The possible utility of routine culturing of urine, sputum, etc., remains conjectural at this time.

The problems of this association are likely to be more important in the future for several reasons: the endemic areas have high population growth, the population is more mobile (and individuals with residual coccidioidal foci will migrate to areas unfamiliar with the disease and not used to considering it in differential diagnosis), interest in transplantation for dysfunction of various organs is increasing, and some groups of cancer patients are living longer as a result of successful therapy (albeit often in the immunosuppressed state).

ACKNOWLEDGMENT. Appreciation is expressed to Stanley C. Deresinski, M.D., who collaborated in the analysis of the Stanford experience.[7]

REFERENCES

1. G. P. Bodey, Fungal infections complicating acute leukemia, *J. Chronic Dis.* **19**:667–687 (1966).
2. A. R. Cassaza, C. P. Duvall, and P. P. Carbone, Infection in lymphoma, *J. Am. Med. Assoc.* **197**:710–716 (1966).
3. D. Rifkind, T. I. Marchioro, S. A. Schneck, and R. B. Hill, Systemic fungal infections complicating renal transplantation and immunosuppressive therapy, *Am. J. Med.* **43**:28–38 (1967).
4. P. D. Hart, E. Russell, and J. S. Remington, The compromised host and infection. II. Deep fungal infection, *J. Infect. Dis.* **120**:169–191 (1969).
5. J. P. Utz, Pulmonary infections due to opportunistic fungi, *Adv. Intern. Med.* **16**:427–445 (1970).
6. D. Pappagianis, Opportunism in coccidioidomycosis, in: *Opportunistic Fungal Infections, Proceedings of the Second International Conference* (E. W. Chick, A. Balows, and M. L. Furcolow, eds.), Charles C. Thomas, Springfield, Ill. (1975), p. 221.

7. S. C. Deresinski, and D. A. Stevens, Coccidioidomycosis in compromised hosts. Experience at Stanford University Hospital, *Medicine* **54**:377–395 (1975).
8. N. Smithline, D. A. Ogden, A. I. Cohn, and K. Johnson, Disseminated coccidioido-mycosis in renal transplant patients, in: *Coccidioidomycosis: Current Clinical and Diagnostic Status* (L. Ajello, ed.), Symposia Specialists, Miami, Fla. (1977), pp. 201–207.

20

Chemotherapy of Coccidioidomycosis

David A. Stevens

Therapy of the various manifestations of coccidioidal disease has been discussed in the pertinent chapters. In this chapter the few drugs available for therapy of the disease are discussed, along with some general therapeutic guidelines.

1. AMPHOTERICIN B

The drug "standard" for therapy is amphotericin B, by virtue of over 20 years of experience with it in coccidioidomycosis.[1] Its structure resembles erythromycin; it differs in that erythromycin lacks the conjugated double bonds seen with amphotericin. This likely accounts for the biological differences between these two compounds. Erythromycin acts at 50 S ribosomal RNA inside the bacterial cell. Amphotericin B, like the other polyenes, acts at the cell membrane. The ability to do so probably depends on the fact that there are both hydrophilic and hydrophobic parts of the molecule. The hydroxylated portion of the molecule is hydrophilic, whereas double bonds represent the lipophilic part of the molecule. The probable mechanism of action is that amphotericin binds to the sterol in the cell membrane, thus changing the permeability of the membrane. The high affinity of this drug for the membrane has been shown in experiments using labeled compound. Cellular constituents are lost after exposure to the drug for brief periods of time, and the size of the constituents leaking from the cell increases as the dose of amphotericin increases. Further evidence of this specificity comes from the observation that this drug is inhibitory to fungi, most algae, protozoa, and mammalian cells, but not to bacteria or to blue-green algae. These latter organisms lack sterols in their cell membrane. Experiments with mycoplasma have shown that mycoplasma grown with cholesterol, which incorporate cholesterol in their cell membrane, are susceptible to the drug, whereas the same mycoplasma species grown in the absence of the cholesterol were resistant to the drug. Ergosterol is the principal sterol in the fungus cell membrane; cholesterol is the principal sterol in the human cell. Further evidence for this mechanism of action is that in the few instances when there was resistance development on therapy, these fungal mutants were ergosterol-poor.

In practice, it appears that although amphotericin has a fungicidal activity *in vitro,* in concentrations that are attainable in body fluids clinically the drug has only fungistatic action. *In vitro,* all isolates of *Coccidioides immitis* appear susceptible.[2]

The drug has an unusual and perhaps unique pharmacology. Peak serum levels up to 1–2 μg/ml are attained immediately after infusion of the usual doses used clinically. Immediately after the infusion, less than 10% of the administered drug is found in the serum. It is felt that the drug must bind to some membranes of the host rapidly. The drug has a large volume of distribution, which is greater than body weight. This suggests the affinity of this drug for membranes is greater than its distribution in blood and binding to blood constituents. One is unable to account for all the administered drug, even if one adds the totals in the extracellular fluid and the amount excreted in the urine.

Biliary excretion, recently suggested to be a major metabolic pathway, now appears not to be a significant excretory route. The serum half-life is 24 hr, an unusually long period. The elimination half-life, that is, the tail of the elimination curve, is 15 days. Active drug can be detected in the serum up to 7 weeks after the last administered dose. These peculiar pharmacokinetics are consistent with uptake into a reservoir from which the drug is later slowly released. It has also been observed that the dose–response curve flattens at doses greater than 50 mg. This is consistent with saturation of a releasing reservoir and filling of a "one way" storage reservoir. A model which best explains these pharmacological observations is as follows: Intravenously administered drug enters the central compartment. This compartment equilibrates with two other compartments, one a rapidly equilibrating compartment and the other a slowly equilibrating compartment. The drug leaves the central compartment by some nonrenal pathways of elimination. These are not entirely clear at the present time. Two to 5% of the drug is excreted in the urine.

Renal insufficiency has no apparent effect on serum levels. The reason for the standard practice of reducing the dose in the face of amphotericin-induced nephrotoxicity is not because the pharmacokinetics of the drug is changed, but due to fear of exacerbating nephrotoxicity already present.

Amphotericin is unique among the currently available drugs for systemic fungal infections in that its onset of action is rapid and apparently unrelated to the metabolic state of the fungus. This, plus the unusual pharmacokinetics described above, provide the rationale for every-other-day therapy with amphotericin. It has been shown that with high doses of intravenous drug, therapeutic levels will be maintained in the serum even 48 hr after the dose. This has significant advantages in the treatment of chronic disease: it means patients can be treated as outpatients, they will retain their appetite at least on the day that they are not receiving the drug, and they will not be tied to their intravenous line and be up and about on that day; in addition, every-other-day therapy is sparing of veins.

The penetration of this drug into body fluid is limited, perhaps because of its size. It penetrates well into inflamed pleural cavities and into joints, but poorly into the parotid gland, bronchial secretions, cerebrospinal fluid (where levels are less than 10% of serum levels), aqueous humor of the eye, brain, pancreas, muscle, and bone. The poor penetration into the cerebrospinal fluid means that for coccidioidal meningitis amphotericin therapy must be given by the intrathecal route.

It has been shown that mannitol or bicarbonate is capable of reducing the nephrotoxicity of amphotericin in dogs. However, trials in man have not confirmed the reduction of nephrotoxicity by these agents. A final pharmacological point worthy of mention is that the drug precipitates in solutions other than 5% dextrose in water, and should not be mixed with other intravenous fluids such as normal saline.

The other common toxic side effects of amphotericin are phlebitis, fever, chills, nausea, vomiting, azotemia, renal tubular acidosis, hypokalemia, hypomagnesemia, shock, and anemia. There is disagreement in the literature about the relationship between total dose administered and nephrotoxicity. What is clear is that creatinine clearance is an indicator of early nephrotoxicity. Other side effects reported include anaphylactic reactions, arrhythmias, coagulopathy, hemorrhagic enteritis, tinnitus, vertigo, pruritis, neuropathy, seizures, leukopenia, and thrombocytopenia. Clinicians experienced with this drug will commonly add modifiers to the therapy of patients receiving the intravenous drug, with the desired effect of reducing the subjective side effects of amphotericin such as the chills, nausea, and fever. These modifiers include salicylates, antihistamines, antiemetics, and low doses of steroids (e.g., 20 mg of hydrocortisone succinate).

New information about amphotericin that has been discovered in recent years concerns its effects on the immune system. It has been shown that in some circumstances this drug can be an immunosuppresant and in others an immunostimulator, and this will depend on the animal species, the antigen, the dose, the timing of the drug in relation to the antigen, and the assay of the immune response. Since immune function appears to be very important in how the host deals with fungal infections, the relationship of this effect to outcome in antifungal therapy will need further study.

The usual method of administering the drug is to give a test dose of 1 mg, and then on succeeding days to build up gradually in 5- to 10-mg increments to a total dose of 0.5–1.5 mg/kg every day or every other day. However, since with the gradual method of increasing the dose therapeutic levels in the blood are not reached for several days, in urgent situations it is wiser to follow the 1-mg test dose with a dose of 25 mg the same day, and on the following day move to the full desired therapeutic dose as tolerated.

A new development in amphotericin chemotherapy is a molecular modification resulting in the development of the amphotericin B methyl ester.[3] This drug is markedly more soluble than amphotericin B, and animal studies indicate that it is less toxic than amphotericin B. However, it also appears to be less effective on a milligram-for-milligram basis, so it is not clear that the decreased toxicity allowing administration of higher doses is not counterbalanced by the decreased efficacy. Moreover, its distribution in the body may not have a pattern as desirable as that of the parent compound. Initial clinical trials have not resolved whether this will represent a therapeutic advance, the incidence of ototoxicity has been disturbing, and presently further investigation with this compound has been halted because of possible neurotoxicity.

2. MICONAZOLE

The newest addition to the group of antifungal drugs is miconazole, a synthetic imidazole.[4] It is in the side chains that this drug differs from an earlier imidazole antifungal drug, clotrimazole, which has serious drawbacks in its ability to induce in the liver the enzymes which degrade it, side effects of marked gastrointestinal and neurologic toxicity, and lack of convincing efficacy *in vivo*. Miconazole has a broad spectrum of activity against pathogenic fungi; the only to date found to be relatively resistant are agents of the zygomycoses (mucor and rhizopus genera). Development of fungal resistance *in vitro* or *in vivo* has not been shown.

The postulated mechanism of action is inhibition of ergosterol synthesis by blocking demethylation at the 14 position in the intermediaries between lanosterol and ergosterol. This drug has been shown efficacious in topical use in cutaneous, oral, and vaginal infections in humans. Published series have indicated efficacy in systemic use in some patients with coccidioidomycosis, paracoccidioidomycosis, esophageal candidiasis, chronic mucocutaneous candidiasis, and petriellidiosis. We have studied this drug in chronic and disseminated coccidioidomycosis in patients who have failed to respond to amphotericin therapy, in patients who have relapsed after apparently successful amphotericin therapy, and in patients who either refused amphotericin therapy because of the subjective side effects or in whom it was deemed unwise to proceed with amphotericin because of other toxic side effects (mostly nephrotoxicity). No concurrent chemotherapy or immunotherapy directed at the fungal disease was given to these patients, who also had a high incidence of serious underlying diseases. The isolates from these patients were universally susceptible to miconazole *in vitro;* the range of minimal inhibitory concentrations was 0.1–1.7 μg/ml. Responses occurred in 67, 50, 41, and 35% of evaluable treatment courses in patients with chronic pulmonary, skin or soft-tissue, musculoskeletal, and meningitis disease due to coccidioidomycosis, respectively. Intrathecal therapy was given to several patients, with minimal toxicity. However, treatment courses were relatively brief (mean, 5 weeks' duration). With courses of this duration, the relapse rate has been disturbing, amounting to one-third to two-thirds of patients with objective clinical responses. With longer treatment courses, it is expected that the relapse rate may be lower; in fact, more recent experience with musculoskeletal disease indicates that this is indeed the case.

After administration of a 600- to 1000-mg intravenous dose, peak blood levels of approximately 10 μg/ml are achieved. The drug has a rapid initial disappearance phase ($t_{\frac{1}{2}}$ = 20–30 min, with a true half-life of 20–24 hr). Infusion doses greater than 350 mg/m^2 body surface area consistently produced peak blood levels greater than 1 μg/ml. The rapid decline of initial levels of biological activity necessitate giving the drug several times a day. The $t_{\frac{1}{2}}$ is minimally affected by renal insufficiency or hemodialysis, and only 10% of the drug is excreted in the urine, almost all of that as inactive metabolites. Over 90% of the drug is bound to serum protein. In the presence of meningitis, peak cerebrospinal fluid concentrations on intravenous therapy range from less than 3% to 48% of the serum concentrations. This is remarkable in view of the responses seen with intravenous therapy alone in some patients with coccidioidal meningitis, but there is a parallel with intravenous amphotericin therapy of cryptococcal meningitis. Intrathecal doses of 20 mg produce cerebro-spinal fluid concentrations greater than 1 μg/ml for 24 hr. The drug penetrates well into inflamed joints, the vitreous body of the eye, and the peritoneal cavity and poorly into the sputum and saliva. Absorption after oral administration is poor.

The most significant side effect is hyponatremia, which occurred in 50% of our cases. Simultaneous studies of serum and urine sodium osmolality suggest inappropriate antidiuretic hormone secretion as the mechanism in at least some patients. We recommend assay of the serum sodium three times weekly, and if hyponatremia begins, appropriate fluid and electrolyte management needs to be instituted. Phlebitis occurs in approximately 40% of patients with the current intravenous formulation. A significant decline in hematocrit due to normoblastic hypoplasia occurs in approximately 40% of patients. The platelet count is elevated in approximately 30% of patients on therapy, although this appears to be of no clinical significance. There appears to be an interaction with coumarin drugs, resulting in enhancement of anticoagulant affect. Elevation of serum lipids is noted in some patients on therapy; this appears to be due to the cremophor carrier which is used to solubilize the drug for its intravenous form. Nausea occurs in about 40% of patients, almost always transient or easily controlled, and pruritis occurs in 25%, occasionally severe and persistent. Other side effects are rare, the most notable being toxic acute psychosis. The intravenous infusion should be given for no less than 15 min, because of cardiac arrhythmias that have been noted with more rapid infusion rates. All toxicities that have been noted have reversed after discontinuing the drug. Irrigation of joints, bone, urinary bladder, infected wounds, the renal pelvis, pulmonary cavities, and the ear and intrapleural therapy were well tolerated by the few patients in whom it was tried. Nebulized drug is moderately irritating. The place of this new agent in our therapy of fungal diseases is at present uncertain, and awaits randomized comparisons. Its relative lack of toxicity vis-à-vis amphotericin B is encouraging.

3. OTHER DRUGS

Further molecular modifications of the imidazole ring are in progress to attempt to produce a drug with less toxicity and one which can be given by the oral route. Preliminary experience with one such compound, ketoconazole, appears promising.[5]

Several other drugs have been shown to be effective in therapy of this infection in animal models, such as ambruticin and R34,000,[6,7] as well as the combination of amphotericin B and polymyxin or tetracyc-line,[8,9] but clinical experience is absent or minimal.

4. GENERAL GUIDELINES

Data from comparative trials are lacking, and recommendations are based on empirical observations. Fortunately, as noted, most sympto-matic primary infections recover without therapy. It is generally agreed that severe primary infections, however, should receive chemotherapy. Because of the possibility of incipient dissemination, patients with complement-fixing antibody (CFA) titers >1 : 16–1 : 32 (see Chapter 6) should be considered for treatment. Other criteria utilized to determine the need for treatment are: persistent fever (>6 weeks); prostration; extensive, enlarging, or persisting pulmonary involvement; persisting precipitins; negative skin test; infancy; debilitation; pregnancy; concur-rent diseases (such as diabetes, asthma, and emphysema) likely to be adversely affected by coccidioidal infection or those associated with compromised immunity, e.g., malignancy, congenital immunodeficiencies or immunosuppressive therapy, e.g., steroids; or racial group predisposed to handle the infection poorly. Amphotericin B has been given intrave-nously to such patients, 1 mg/kg daily tapering to 1–1.5 mg/kg thrice weekly to a total dose of 0.1–1.5 g if a clinical response is obtained, and more if a response hasn't been obtained (CFA and skin test may be utilized to follow the disease as well as objective clinical parameters such as X-ray).

Once the disease has disseminated outside the lungs, chemotherapy is always indicated. With amphotericin B, courses of 1–2.5 g intrave-nously are usually employed, and more prolonged courses if remission isn't achieved. The same parameters as indicated in the preceding paragraph are followed. As is true for therapy of primary infection, duration of therapy may be as important or more important than total dose. Treatment until the complement-fixing-antibody titers fall to zero or to very low levels, and until X-rays (for example) become normal, is not a feasible goal in most patients, and may not be necessary. Tipping the balance in favor of the host defense may allow continued resolution after therapy is stopped.

In addition, local irrigation of sinuses and fistulae with antifungal drugs, tattooing into skin lesions, and instillation into abscesses and into body cavities have been tried. Because of the likelihood of relapse in this disease, and the toxicities of chemotherapy, incision and even excision when feasible should be considered as part of therapy for a variety of manifestations of coccidioidal disease. The role of surgery in pulmonary disease has been discussed in Chapter 10. An exception to the indication to treat all disseminated disease is the culture-positive but clinically inactive focus in a nonthreatening site which is stable for many years, and this is occasionally seen (e.g., a solitary skin lesion in a cosmetically insignificant area).

REFERENCES

1. J. M. T. Hamilton-Miller, Chemistry and biology of the polyene macrolide antibiotics, *Bacteriol. Rev.* **37**:166–196 (1973).
2. M. S. Collins and D. Pappagianis, Uniform susceptibility of various strains of *Coccidioides immitis* to amphotericin B, *Antimicrob. Agents Chermother.* **11**:1049–1055 (1977).
3. R. M. Lawrence and P. D. Hoeprich, Comparison of amphotericin B and amphotericin B methyl ester: efficacy in murine coccidioidomycosis and toxicity, *J. Infect. Dis.* **133**:168–174 (1976).
4. D. A. Stevens, Miconazole in the treatment of systemic fungal infections, *Am. Rev. Resp. Dis.* **116**:801–806 (1977).
5. D. Borelli, J. L. Bran, J. Fuentes, R. Legendre, E. Leiderman, H. B. Levine, A. Restrepo-M., and D. A. Stevens, Ketoconazole, an oral antifungal: laboratory and clinical assessment of imidazole drugs, *Postgrad. Med. J.* **55**:657–661 (1979).
6. H. B. Levine, S. M. Ringel, and J. M. Cobb, Therapeutic properties of oral ambruticin (W7783) in experimental pulmonary coccidioidomycosis of mice, *Chest* **73**:202–206 (1978).
7. H. B. Levine, R34,000, a dioxolane imidazole in the therapy of experimental coccidioidomycosis, *Chest* **70**:755–759 (1976).
8. M. S. Collins and D. Pappagianis, Treatment of murine coccidioidomycosis with polymyxin B, *Antimicrob. Agents Chemother.* **10**:318–321 (1976).
9. M. Huppert, S. H. Sun, and K. R. Vukovich, Combined amphotericin B—tetracycline therapy for experimental coccidioidomycosis, *Antimicrob. Agents Chemother.* **5**:473–478 (1974).

21

Immunotherapy-Transfer Factor in Coccidioidomycosis

David A. Stevens

Since, as indicated in Chapter 5, defective immunity, notably cell-mediated immunity, is closely associated with progressive coccidioidomycosis, attempts to treat the disease by altering the host response are eminently logical. In coccidioidomycosis, almost all the clinical experience with this approach has been by the use of transfer factor. Conversely, probably no disease has provided more rationale for further clinical study of transfer factor.

1. TRANSFER FACTOR

The literature is encumbered by reports of several preparations which have been given this term. The general term is used here to refer to leukocyte extracts capable, on injection, of transferring the cell-mediated immune response from the leukocyte donor to a recipient. The recipient may then react as if he is already sensitized, possessing donor reactivities even though he was not primed with such antigens. Some of these preparations reported are not dialyzable without loss of activity. Others have been characterized as RNA species. The present discussion principally focuses on a dialyzable extract of <10,000 molecular weight, originally described by Lawrence and co-workers, hereafter designated TF.[1,2] (Alternative nomenclatures have used this term to apply to only some components of such extracts.) The following summarizes material reviewed in greater detail elsewhere,[1-4] and these sources should be consulted for more extensive discussion and bibliographic citation not possible here because of space and the focus on data relevant to the use of TF in coccidioidomycosis.

Studies suggest this substance(s) is present in T lymphocytes, and can be released into the supernatant *in vitro* after exposure for 30–60 min to an antigen to which the donor is immune. Such studies suggest this results in depletion of activity relating to this antigen from the cell pellet, though activity relevant to other antigens is retained.

In vivo, the effect of transfer can be demonstrated in 4 hr after injection of the extract. The reactivity conferred persists at least a year, even in the absence of exposure to antigen, as was originally demonstrated with coccidioidin.[5] The amount of donor cells needed to produce TF to transfer dermal delayed hypersensitivity to normal subjects is only the number of leukocytes present in 10 ml of blood. TF has essentially no adverse reactions, with the exception of occasional local tenderness at the injection site. Serial transfer has been shown from a recipient, originally immunologically naive, to another recipient, etc., by preparation of TF from the leukocytes of each recipient in the chain after successful transfer. Transfer of some biological activities via TF can also be demonstrated *in vitro* by mixing TF, antigen to which the TF donor is immune, and naive lymphocytes.

TF has several potentially desirable features relevant to use as therapy: it doesn't affect antibody production (as would be harmful in the case of "blocking antibodies," which interfere with cell-mediated immune reactions), nor sensitize the donor to leukocyte antigens, nor transfer hepatitis B virus, nor cause graft-vs.-host reactions.

The precise biochemical definition of TF awaits resolution of questions from purification studies performed in numerous laboratories. A prevailing view is that TF is a polypeptide, possibly linked to a polynucleotide. Several lines of evidence indicate it is not a form of antigen— e.g., its dialyzability (implying a smaller size than some defined antigens that have been used in TF studies), and the serial transfer experiments. Some skin graft rejection studies, focusing on transplantation antigens, indicated that if skin from subject A was grafted to B, and TF prepared from B then given to C, C would show an accelerated rejection of A skin but not B skin. Attempts to remove activity from TF preparations with antigen-specific immunoadsorbents have failed. Lymphocytes of a highly reactive recipient will not react *in vitro* to the TF from the donor unless antigen is added.

TF is resistant to deoxyribonuclease, trypsin, and pancreatic ribonuclease, which acts on single stranded RNA. Some studies have described TF as susceptible to the action of ribonuclease III, which acts on double-stranded RNA, and to pronase. Some have reported TF susceptible to destruction of activity by 56°C for 30 min; others found it resistant to 80°C for 1 hr. Once lyophilized, TF is stable at 4°C for 5 years.

Initial skepticism was abetted by the difficulties in demonstrating similar activity in animal models, but more recently successes have been reported in guinea pigs, rabbits, rats, and monkeys. Much speculation has occurred concerning the mechanism of TF action, attempting to explain how such a small molecule(s) can transfer reactivity to multiple complex antigens. Postulated mechanisms include action as antigen receptor on T lymphocytes, promoter of differentiation of T cell precursors, nonspecific adjuvant, recruiter of T effector cells, amplifier of inflammatory response, peripheralization of T cells from more central compartments and/or derepressor of DNA sequences (either programming for the initiation of a reaction to an antigen, which would be a specific action, or for facilitating the response to an antigen—e.g., antigen processing, cell cooperation—which would be nonspecific).

It is of historical interest that it was in studies of transfer of coccidioidin reactivity that it was shown that transfer could occur even where there was a high probability of excluding boosting of latent reactivity in the recipient. This was done by performing transfers with recipients who had never visited the endemic areas and who remained outside them.[5] But the question arose in this, which has continued to plague the field, whether the recipients were complete strangers to the antigen or related antigens (e.g., other fungi). Evidence for the specificity of TF includes skin-grafting experiments where the recipient acquires accelerated rejection only to that individual(s) whom the donor similarly rejects, experiments showing transfer of the precise donor profile with a battery of antigen testing, transfer of reactivity from donors sensitized to keyhole limpet hemocyanin (latent reactivity to this or related antigens felt extremely remote in unselected subjects), studies with chemically produced new antigens (which don't require skin tests prior to transfer, to exclude reactors) demonstrating transfer even without exposure to antigen as occurs in pretransfer skin testing, and desensitization of a donor resulting in his TF losing the capability to transfer reactivity only to that antigen.

On theoretical grounds, it has been suggested that such a small molecule(s) could convey only limited information, and that therefore the recipient must already possess the genetic information for the responses studied. There is concrete evidence for nonspecific effects of TF. These include enhancement of recipient response to phytohemagglutinin (a nonspecific mitogen), increase (*in vivo*) in recipient erythrocyte-rosetting lymphocytes (a T-cell subset), conversions in recipients of reactivities not possessed by the donor (though in some of these instances

recipient exposure to antigen could not be excluded), increase in monocyte GMP, inability to transfer reactivity to artificial copolymers (suggesting the recipients must be primed somehow, such as by exposure to
related antigens), and experiments showing TF increased recipient lymphocyte blastogenesis more where the baseline levels were highest. This
latter finding was shown by Cohen *et al.*[6] in some elegant experiments
on the *in vitro* effect of TF. That finding is the opposite of what one
would expect if TF were engaging uncommitted cells. Moreover, response to antigen was augmented equally by TF prepared from donors
reactive to it and those nonreactive to it. By means of a radioactive pulse
in vitro ("suicide technique"), cells reactive to a specific antigen were
removed from a recipient population. TF was unable to restore reactivity
to the remaining population but could still augment reactivity to unrelated
antigens. This is excellent evidence for a nonspecific adjuvant effect—
that the response is a function of the recipient's underlying reactivity.
This, however, contrasts with the experiments of others with different
techniques for assaying cell-mediated immunity *in vitro*, such as leukocyte migration inhibition, which provided evidence for the specificity of
TF *in vitro*. Further experiments on purification of TF have led to reports
of fractions which increase lymphocyte blastogenesis only where the
donor is reactive to the antigen. Others have found[7-9] RNA preparations
extracted from leukocytes, which can transfer sensitivity to coccidioidal
and other antigens in similar fashion to classical TF and can be further
separated by dialysis into two RNA–peptide components, one of which
has a nonspecific immune-enhancing effect and the other an antigen-
specific effect. The RNA component of the latter carries the specific
information, whereas the peptide component appears responsible for
transport from the injection site and protection of the RNA from
ribonuclease.

2. CLINICAL EXPERIENCE WITH TF

TF has been reported to improve the clinical status of patients with
a variety of malignancies, as well as patients with a variety of congenital
immunodeficiencies, particularly the Wiskott–Aldrich syndrome. Delayed hypersensitivity has been restored not only in this condition but
also in immunodeficiencies such as X-linked and autosomal recessive
combined immunodeficiency (but not thymic aplasia), conditions thought
due to a stem cell defect and with absent T precursors. Also relevant to
the partial defects noted in the chapter on immunology of coccidioidomycosis is that whereas TF normally confers the full range of *in vivo* and
in vitro manifestations of cellular immunity including skin test reactivity,

lymphocyte blastogenesis *in vitro,* and lymphokine production in healthy recipients, in immunodeficiencies conversions of some of these functions but not others have been noted. Studies have demonstrated that separate lymphocyte populations are responsible for blastogenesis and lymphokine production, and with these populations experiments suggest TF preferentially acts more on the subset involved in lymphokine production.

TF has also been employed in a variety of infectious diseases, such as tuberculosis, leishmaniasis, and progressive vaccinia, which are frequently associated with defective cellular immunity. Beneficial results have been claimed there, as well as in lepromatous leprosy, a disease similar to coccidioidomycosis in presence of large antigenic load, cutaneous unreactivity, and high antibody titers. Chronic mucocutaneous candidiasis is another fungus disease with these same features. Some of these patients have congenital immunodeficiencies, endocrinopathies, ectodermal defects, or thymomas; others are apparently otherwise normal but have selective defects in cell-mediated immunity, involving all or only some *in vivo* and *in vitro* assays, similar to those described in coccidioidomycosis. In such patients reactivity has been restored by TF, and in a minority clinical responses have been noted (in some, without concomitant chemotherapy).[10,11]

3. CLINICAL COCCIDIOIDOMYCOSIS AND TF FACTOR

In progressive coccidioidomycosis, several groups of investigators have attempted transfer factor (made from healthy coccidioidin-positive donors) therapy independently of or in conjunction with specific antifungal chemotherapy.[12-15] Various groups reported clinical responses in association with such attempts. It was important to pool and compare these results, which was mutually recognized and done by forming the Coccidioidomycosis Cooperative Treatment Group (CCTG) by workers at the University of California at Davis, San Diego, and San Francisco, the University of Texas at San Antonio, and Stanford University, and by private practitioners from endemic areas.[16-18] The pooled data revealed the immunologic potency of TF in progressive coccidioidomycosis. Table 1 indicates that TF therapy was associated with conversion of defective cell-mediated immune responses to coccidioidal antigen; in two-thirds if lymphokine production (specifically, migration inhibition factor or MIF) was assessed, in greater than one-half if lymphocyte blastogenesis was the criterion used, and less than one-half if delayed dermal hypersensitivity was the parameter studied.

Although the fact that almost all of these were patients followed for a long time, thus decreasing the likelihood that these conversions were

TABLE 1
Changes in Immune Response to Coccidioidal Antigens

	Total number of patients	Number with positive pretransfer factor	Number converting posttransfer factor
Skin test	44	8	24
Blastogenesis	32	9	18
MIF production	28	3	21

spontaneous, inspection of the timing of the paired studies before and after therapy (Table 2) also helps indicate the conversion was due to TF—the conversions were documented shortly after TF.

These studies strongly emphasize TF as a powerful biological phenomenon. Three-fifths of these patients were also judged to clinically improve in relation to TF therapy (Table 3). This suggests TF might be a therapeutically useful reagent as well. Patients considered cured or improved in relation to TF therapy included patients with pulmonary and/or disseminated disease or with meningeal disease.[17] Multiple doses appeared to be more effective than a single dose. There was no correlation between the "cured or improved" group and whether amphotericin was given concomitantly, or the dose used if it was given.[17] Nor was the "good outcome" group apparently a phenomenon of short followup–analysis by duration of follow-up showed no such facile correlation.[17] The "probable cure" group included four patients who had been followed more than 2 years.[17]

The CCTG realized that to confirm whether TF was therapeutically useful would require a multicenter cooperative trial, a double-blind format, approaches to the question of whether the TF needed to be prepared from people immune to coccidioidomycosis, one set of standardized reagents pretested in healthy subjects never exposed to *Coccidioides immitis,* stratification of patients by a variety of criteria, use of

TABLE 2
Time of *in Vitro* or *in Vivo* Conversion of Immune Response[a] to Coccidioidal Antigens

Neg → Pos	Duration between pre-/poststudies			
	<4 Days	4–10 Days	>10 Days	Total
Converted one or more tests	7	5	20	22
No conversions	3	3	8	14
TOTAL:	10	8	18	36

[a] See Table 1.

TABLE 3
Clinical Improvement[a] Following
Transfer Factor in 49 Patients

None	Modest/gradual	Dramatic
19	18	12

[a] See reference 17.

multiple doses, serial immunological observations, defined and standard-ized criteria of improvement, and probably a crossover design. Such a large undertaking could only be done with extensive financial research support. Such support was sought but not obtained. Unfortunately, this important chapter in the immunology of coccidioidomycosis in the 1970s must end at present on this uncertain note—it is still unanswered whether this potent immunologic reagent is a useful therapeutic agent, or thera-peutic adjunct, in this disease.

ACKNOWLEDGMENTS. I thank Elmer Brummer, Ph.D., for helpful re-view of the manuscript.

REFERENCES

1. H. S. Lawrence and F. T. Valentine, Transfer factor and other mediators of cellular immunity, *Am. J. Pathol.* **60**:437–450 (1970).
2. H. S. Lawrence, Transfer factor, *Adv. Immunol.* **11**:195–266 (1969).
3. F. M. Burnet, Transfer factor—a theoretical discussion, *J. Allergy Clin. Immunol.* **54**:1–13 (1974).
4. C. H. Kirkpatrick, Properties and activities of transfer factor, *J. Allergy Clin. Immunol.* **55**:411–421 (1975).
5. F. T. Rapaport, H. S. Lawrence, J. W. Millar, D. Pappagianis, and C. E. Smith, Transfer of delayed hypersensitivity to coccidioidin in man, *J. Immunol.* **84**:358–367 (1960).
6. L. Cohen, R. S. Holzman, F. T. Valentine, and H. S. Lawrence, Requirement of precommitted cells as targets for the augmentation of lymphocyte proliferation by leukocyte dialysates, *J. Exp. Med.* **143**:791–804 (1976).
7. E. A. Peterson, J. A. Frey, M. Dinowitz, and D. Rifkind, Transfer of delayed hypersensitivity to mice with human immune cell extracts, in: *Transfer Factor—Basic Properties and Clinical Applications* (M. S. Ascher, A. A. Gottlieb, and C. H. Kirkpatrick, eds.), Academic Press, New York (1976), pp. 387–398.
8. D. Rifkind, J. A. Frey, E. A. Peterson, and M. Dinowitz, Transfer of delayed-type hypersensitivity in mice to microbial antigens with dialyzable transfer factor, *Infect. Immun.* **16**:258–262 (1977).
9. D. Rifkind, J. A. Frey, and M. Dinowitz, Susceptibility of murine transfer factor to dimerized ribonuclease A, *Infect. Immun.* **16**:920–922 (1977).

10. R. E. Rocklin, R. A. Chilgren, R. Hong, and J. R. David, Transfer of cellular hypersensitivity in chronic mucocutaneous candidiasis monitored *in vivo* and *in vitro*, *Cell. Immunol.* **1**:290–299 (1970).

11. C. H. Kirkpatrick, J. W. Chandler, and R. N. Schimke, Chronic mucocutaneous moniliasis with impaired delayed hypersensitivity, *Clin. Exp. Immunol.* **6**:375–385 (1970).

12. J. R. Graybill, J. Silva, R. H. Alford, and D. E. Thor, Immunologic and clinical improvement of progressive coccidioidomycosis following administration of transfer factor, *Cell Immunol.* **8**:120–135 (1973).

13. D. A. Stevens, D. Pappagianis, V. A. Marinkovich, and T. F. Waddell, Immunotherapy in recurrent coccidioidomycosis, *Cell Immunol.* **12**:37–48 (1974).

14. A. Catanzaro, L. Spitler, and K. M. Moser, Immunotherapy of coccidioidomycosis, *J. Clin. Invest.* **54**:690–701 (1974).

15. P. Cloninger, L. D. Thrupp, G. A. Granger, and H. S. Novey, Immunotherapy with transfer factor in disseminated coccidioidal osteomyelitis and arthritis, *West. J. Med.* **120**:322–325 (1974).

16. A. Catanzaro, L. Spitler *et al.* (Coccidioidomycosis Cooperative Treatment Group), Clinical and immunologic results of transfer factor therapy in coccidioidomycosis, in: *Transfer Factor—Basic Properties and Clinical Applications* (M. S. Ascher, A. A. Gottlieb, and C. H. Kirkpatrick, eds.), Academic Press, New York (1976), pp. 477–494.

17. J. R. Graybill *et al.* (Coccidioidomycosis Cooperative Treatment Group), The clinical couse of coccidioidomycosis following transfer factor therapy, in: *Coccidioidomycosis: Current Clinical and Diagnostic Status* (L. Ajello, ed.), Symposia Specialists, Miami, Fla. (1977), pp. 335–345.

18. D. A. Stevens *et al.* (Coccidioidomycosis Cooperative Treatment Group), Transfer factor therapy of infectious diseases, in: *Recent Advances in Dermatopharmacology* (P. Frost, E. C. Gomez, and N. Zaias, eds.), Spectrum, Holliswood, N.Y. (1977), pp. 67–74.

22

Vaccination-Immunoprophylaxis in Coccidioidomycosis

David A. Stevens

1. HISTORY

Rixford and Gilchrist, in their original studies at the turn of the century, showed that experimentally infected animals were more resistant to superinfection.[1] A half century then elapsed before serious experimentation was conducted on the subject of the effect of vaccination. Negroni reported such studies with nonviable organisms,[2] and Smith with attenuated live organisms.[3] Levine, Kong, Savage and other workers at the Naval Biosciences Laboratory, and others, in the decade of the 1960s performed extensive studies which defined our present directions and concepts regarding vaccination. Much of the history of the immunoprophylactic approach to coccidioidomycosis is outlined in Chapter 1.

2. ANIMAL STUDIES

These animal studies showed that the spherule phase, grown *in vitro,* was superior to the mycelial phase as a vaccine immunogen.[4] Most of the studies to be detailed involved challenge of the vaccine recipients by the pulmonary route. Growth and development of the spherule is associated with increased immunogenicity,[4] the principal immunogens appearing to reside in the spherule wall.[5,6] Soluble extracts were not protective; the insoluble wall material appears necessary.[4] The components associated with protection and cell-mediated immunity after vaccination are mostly heat labile.[7] The concurrent use of Freund's adjuvant decreased the immunogenicity.[6]

The route of vaccination was very important; intramuscular or subcutaneous vaccination appears superior to the intravenous, intranasal, and footpad routes.[4,7,8,9] Amputation of the animal's intramuscularly vaccinated limb before a critical interval weakened the resultant immunity.[4] Intravenously administered vaccine ends up in the lungs, and stimulates humoral immunity well but cellular immunity poorly by comparison with the intramuscular route.[7,10] In fact, intravenous vaccination could interfere with the immunity associated with an intramuscular immunization which preceded it.[9] Intramuscularly administered vaccine is ultimately distributed better to all other internal organs, and after respiratory infection mimicking the natural route or intraperitoneal challenge, replication of the challenge inoculum is retarded more in the lung and other organs compared with the intravenous vaccine route.[7,8,10]

The effect of vaccination is not to prevent infection but to increase the early inflammatory response to a subsequent live challenge; to decrease the multiplication *in vivo* of that challenge, an effect detectable soon after challenge; to prevent extrapulmonary dissemination, and to prevent death.[4,11-13] The route studies referred to suggest the primacy of cellular immunity in the stimulation of protection, and transfer experiments conferring protection from vaccinated donors via cells but not serum make this case convincingly.[14] Protection, however, occurs even though dermal delayed hypersensitivity following vaccination is not consistent.[5,8,9,15]

Several important observations were also made with regard to dose and timing of vaccination. Vaccine-induced resistance developed rather slowly, becoming optimal in the mouse at 35 days.[5] As time elapsed between vaccination and this optimal time, progressively greater live challenges could be resisted.[4] Dividing a dose into two or more sites at a single vaccination was superior to a single site, and dividing the dose into three fractions given at weekly periods markedly enhanced the effect.[4] A booster dose 2 months later provided further marked enhancement.[14]

Vaccination has been shown protective in the experimental situation in several species, including mice, guinea pigs, dogs, and monkeys.[2,4,5,12,13] The resistance engendered by vaccine prepared from a single strain of *Coccidioides immitis* protects against challenge with a wide variety of *C. immitis* strains of diverse morphological characteristics.[16]

3. HUMAN VACCINATION

It is an expectation that vaccination will be as effective in man as in other species, and a hope that it will be an efficacious means of reducing the morbidity and mortality associated with this disease. To date, 78 human volunteers have received the spherule vaccine.[17] Side effects appear to be minimal. In the skin-test-negative population, which is the eventual candidate for the vaccine, these consisted of local induration, swelling, and axillary adenopathy in some cases. A few skin-test-positive volunteers who received the vaccine developed fever. The maximal tolerable dose appears to be 5 mg. Few conversions of skin tests (or lymphocyte transformation) or development of antibody occurred in recipients, although, as noted above in animal studies, this may not be significant in terms of protection.

REFERENCES

1. E. Rixford and T. C. Gilchrist, Two cases of protozoan (coccidioidal) infection of the skin and other organs, *Johns Hopkins Hosp. Rep.* **1**:209–268 (1896).
2. P. Negroni, D. Viroli, and H. Bonfiglioli, Estudios sobre el *Coccidioides immitis* Rixford and Gilchrist. VII. Reacciones immunoalergicas en la infección experimental del cobayo, *Rev. Inst. Bacteriol. Dep. Nac. Hig. (Argent.)* **14**:273–286 (1949).
3. C. E. Smith, Annual Progress Report, Commission on Acute Respiratory Diseases, Armed Forces Epidemiological Board, Washington, D.C. (1951).
4. H. B. Levine, Y. M. Kong, and C. E. Smith, Immunization of mice to *Coccidioides immitis:* dose, regimen and spherulation stage of killed spherule vaccines, *J. Immunol.* **94**:132–142 (1965).
5. H. B. Levine, D. Pappagianis, and J. M. Cobb, Development of vaccines for coccidioidomycosis, *Mycopathol. Mycol. Appl.* **41**:177–185 (1970).
6. Y. M. Kong and H. B. Levine, Experimentally induced immunity in the mycoses, *Bacteriol. Rev.* **31**:35–53, 1967.
7. H. B. Levine and G. M. Scalarone, Deficient resistance to *Coccidioides immitis* following intravenous vaccination. III. Humoral and cellular responses to intravenous and intramuscular doses, *Sabouraudia* **9**:97–108 (1971).
8. G. M. Scalarone and H. B. Levine, Attributes of deficient immunity in mice receiving *Coccidioides immitis* spherule vaccine by the intravenous route, *Sabouraudia* **7**:169–177 (1969).
9. H. B. Levine, G. M. Scalarone, and J. W. Fresh, Some immune responses to *Coccidioides immitis,* in: Proceedings of the International Symposium on the Mycoses, *Pan Am. Health Organ. Sci. Publ.* **205**:142–148 (1970).
10. G. M. Scalarone and H. B. Levine, Deficient resistance to *Coccidioides immitis* following intravenous vaccination. I. Distribution of spherules after intravenous and intramuscular doses, *Sabouraudia* **9**:81–89 (1971).
11. M. W. Castleberry, J. L. Converse, J. T. Sinski, E. P. Lowe, S. P. Pakes, and J. E. Del Favero, Coccidioidomycosis: studies of canine vaccination and therapy, *J. Infect. Dis.* **115**:41–48 (1965).

12. H. B. Levine, R. L. Miller, and C. E. Smith, Influence of vaccination on respiratory coccidioidal disease in cynomolgous monkeys, *J. Immunol.* **89**:242–251 (1962).
13. D. C. Savage and S. H. Madin, Cellular responses in lungs of immunized mice to intranasal infection with *Coccidioides immitis, Sabouraudia* **6**:94–102 (1968).
14. Y. M. Kong, D. C. Savage, and H. B. Levine, Enhancement of immune responses in mice by a booster injection of *Coccidioides immitis, J. Immunol.* **95**:1048–1056 (1966).
15. Y. M. Kong, D. C. Savage, and L. N. L. Kong, Delayed dermal hypersensitivity in mice to spherule and mycelial extracts of *Coccidioides immitis, J. Bacteriol.* **91**:876–883 (1966).
16. M. Huppert, H. B. Levine, S. H. Sun, and E. T. Peterson, Resistance of vaccinated mice to typical and atypical strains of *Coccidioides immitis, J. Bacteriol.* **94**:924–927 (1967).
17. D. Pappagianis and H. B. Levine, The present status of vaccination against coccidioidomycosis in man, *Am. J. Epidemiol.* **102**:30–41 (1975).

23

Bibliography of Coccidioidomycosis

David A. Stevens

The following describes the essential reference library for the coccidioidomycologist, as well as serving as a guide for the reader seeking to pursue a particular point.

The praises of the monograph by Fiese[1] have already been sung in the Preface. It was appropriately referred to as a "classic,"[2] and a distant student of the disease expressed our gratitude as "the help obtained from the compendium of knowledge of this disease that was presented in such scholarly fashion."[3] Unfortunately, the book is out of print now, and it is impossible to buy a copy even from bookhunters (I've tried).

Three times since World War II, approximately decades apart, there has been an International Symposium on Coccidioidomycosis, at which the interested parties have gathered to share the latest information. The proceedings of the last two of these symposia[4,5] are still generally available and contain a wealth of material of current interest on all aspects of study.

Two bibliographers have attempted to compile comprehensive lists of references on all published articles on coccidioidomycosis. Dr. Stephen H. Cheu of the Veterans Administration Hospital, Fresno, now retired, revised and updated periodically such a compendium for many years. The last of these, the 1972 edition, was reportedly complete from 1892 to 1972 and included 1844 citations.[6] It is organized by year in alphabetical order by the first author's name, and there is an alphabetical index of all first authors. Two authors assembled a similar but not complete bibliography covering the literature from 1892 to 1970,[7] arranged in alphabetical order by first author's name. Neither of these sources has a subject index, limiting its utility as a reference work.

Many review articles on coccidioidomycosis have been published over the years, and many of these were very helpful summaries, but they have been overshadowed by one recent work by Drutz and Catanzaro.[2] This two-part article is concise, thoughtful, easily digested, and thorough (322 references). As part of the "State of the Art" series in the *American Review of Respiratory Diseases,* it also appeared in a book published by the American Lung Association in 1979.

The Coccidioidomycosis Study Group began meeting in 1956 under the umbrella of a Veterans Administration–Armed Forces cooperative study and under the chairmanship of Dr. Salkin. The group has been meeting approximately annually since then (in 1980 it held its 25th meeting). In the intervening years the sponsorship of the group has passed from the VA–Armed Forces to the California Thoracic Society (all but 2 of the 25 meetings were held in California), Dr. Salkin has passed the chairman's gavel to Dr. Pappagianis, and I have the honor of being the secretary, succeeding Dr. Huppert after approximately 20 years. The meetings are open to all, confined presently to one day, are a mix of formal papers and informal (sometimes rowdy) discussion, cover basic science aspects of the fungus to purely clinical case reports and all mixes in between, and are felt to be informative interchanges, a valuable forum, and thoroughly enjoyable by those who regularly participate in them. Over the years, as a by-product of the meetings, the Group has published memoranda, minutes, transactions, progress reports, reviews (of the meetings), and currently, proceedings in the form of abstracts of presented papers (current issue available on request, c/o this author, who is the current editor). Complete sets are on file in the Library of Congress, National Library of Medicine in Bethesda (request #S038948), New York State Department of Health (Albany), and VA Hospital, Long Beach, California. The group, its continuity, and its ongoing "literature" of recent advances is unique, and reflects ongoing fascination of the students of the disease with its mysteries.

REFERENCES

1. M. J. Fiese, *Coccidioidomycosis,* Charles C. Thomas, Springfield, Ill. (1958).
2. D. J. Drutz and A. Catanzaro, Coccidioidomycosis, *Am. Rev. Resp. Dis.* 117:559–585, 727–771 (1978).
3. W. St. C. Symmers, Cases of coccidioidomycosis seen in Britain, in: *Coccidioidomycosis* (L. Ajello, ed.), University of Arizona, Tucson (1967), p. 301.
4. L. Ajello, ed., *Coccidioidomycosis,* University of Arizona, Tucson (1967).

5. L. Ajello (ed.), *Coccidioidomycosis: Current Clinical and Diagnostic Status*, Symposia Specialists, Miami (1977).
6. S. H. Cheu (ed.), *Coccidioidomycosis Bibliography Research Service Publication*, 1972 ed., Veterans Administration Hospital, Fresno, Calif. (1972).
7. Y. Al-Doory and R. Pairon, A bibliography of coccidioidomycosis, *Mycopathol. Mycol. Appl.* **46:**113–188 (1972).

Index